Safety in
Everyday Living

Joseph H. Mroz

Memphis State University

Safety in Everyday Living

WM. C. BROWN COMPANY PUBLISHERS
Dubuque, Iowa

Copyright © 1978 by Wm. C. Brown Company Publishers

Library of Congress Catalog Card Number: 77-91276

ISBN 0–697–07371–8

Printed in the United States of America

For my parents
who provided the opportunity . . .

Contents

Chapter 5. Pedestrian Accidents

Chapter 6. Bicycle Accidents

Chapter 7. Falls

Chapter 8. Fires

Foreword

There is a time worn cliché about the weather: Everyone talks about it, but no one does a thing about it. Paraphrased, the saying easily could apply to safety in our everyday living. Fortunately, however, some thoughtful educators like Joseph Mroz are making a concerted effort to expose and reduce the dangers which attend even the most common of our activities, such as automobile driving, swimming, and boating. Sharp focus is also drawn to fire hazards and other timely subjects which should be of major concern to everyone. Easily the most exciting and timely is Mroz's treatment of "poisonings," a topic which will excite the student as well as the instructor.

The feeling that "it won't happen to me" only increases the hazards of common place accidents, for we never seem to prepare for that moment when quick thinking can avoid a catastrophe. Worse, we are not prepared to take the next step when accidents occur, because we have not learned proper treatment. This book, carefully and thoughtfully studied, will provide an ounce of prevention as well as a pound of cure.

Joseph H. Mroz has made a very worthwhile contribution to an important subject.

Billy M. Jones, President
Memphis State University

Preface

Throughout history, man viewed accidents as chance occurrences caused by mysterious, unseen forces. Shrouded in ignorance and superstition, he saw himself as weak and utterly helpless in the presence of these mighty forces. Such was the situation until recent times, when a more sophisticated modern man first dared to suggest that he could prevent or at least mitigate many accidents. Today, man is probably more conscious of accidents and their causes than at any other time in history, and it is indeed fortunate that he is. In this country accidents are the fourth leading cause of death for persons of all ages, and the leading cause of death for persons between the ages of one and thirty-eight years.

In the face of the accident problem in this country, a need arises for a book which provides basic safe-living information for persons of all ages. This textbook is designed to meet this need. Although the book was written primarily for use in college safety and safety education courses, industrial supervisors, fleet supervisors, community safety officials, school administrators, and high school health, physical education, and driver education teachers will find the textbook to be a useful reference addition to their libraries. Unlike many other textbooks, *Safety in Everyday Living* does not "hide" resource addresses, learning activities, and review materials within a special "Instructor's Manual."

In general, this textbook deals with positive action which can be taken to prevent, or to reduce the severity of accidents while in traffic, in the home, in the school, at work, and in leisure pursuits. Appropriate safe actions are suggested and discussed; inappropriate, unsafe actions are discouraged through a discussion of their possible undesirable consequences. Nowhere is there a list of "DO's" or "DON'T's," for the individual reader must ultimately decide upon his own actions and accept responsibility for them. The book does, however, attempt to provide a sound basis for decision making.

While numerous individuals have assisted in the preparation of this textbook, a few deserve special recognition. More than any other persons, Dr. Milton Medeiros and Erci Medeiros were responsible for the "spark" which initiated the writing of this book. To them, special thanks is offered. In continuation of a professional, as well as a personal, relationship, Don Carter, Charles R. Schroeder, Geddes Self Jr., and Elijah V. Turman were instrumental in providing the encouragement that the author needed to complete this book. As they already know, their support was greatly appreciated. Art Grider, Mike Maple, Gil Michael, Phyliss Smith, and Tom Wofford, all associated with Photo Services of Memphis State University, Fred Griffith Jr., an independent photographer in Memphis, and Mark Raeber, Editor of *The Waterloo Times* in Waterloo, Illinois, went well beyond professional duty in producing many of the photographs in this book. Sincere gratitude is extended to them. As a personal favor, Stephanie Seals and Mary Ann Garey drew several of the diagrams and illustrations in this book, and Kathleen Hand and Marcy Kinkennon read many of the proofs. To them, special appreciation is given. Finally, the author's wife, Patricia, was indispensable in typing the manuscript and reading the proofs. Deepest appreciation is offered to her for this "service beyond the call of duty."

Joseph H. Mroz

The Accident Problem

1

As the space age dawned, astronaut John Glenn Jr. became an overnight legend. Being the first American to orbit the earth, Glenn was asked upon his return about his thoughts during the lift-off of his Friendship 7 spacecraft from Cape Canaveral. According to the astronaut, one thought filled his mind: "Just think, this was all built by the lowest bidder."[1] Ironically, while the spacecraft proved to be reliable, just two years later, John Glenn, the man who had traveled out of this world and back again without even being scratched, slipped on a throw rug in the bathroom and cracked his head against the bathtub. This "reentry," as Glenn referred to his fall, left him with periodic dizzy spells for several months.

As Glenn's mishap clearly shows, no one is immune to accidents. According to recent figures, in this country accidents are the leading cause of death among persons between the ages of one and thirty-eight. For persons of all ages, accidents are the fourth leading cause of death. Altogether, accidents account for over 100,000 deaths and approximately 10.3 million disabling injuries every year. (See Figure 1.1.) Obviously, the consequences are staggering: an untold amount of grief is suffered over the loss of loved ones, children are left without the guidance of one or both parents, and families are forced to bear the burden of hospital bills and lost wages.

Definition of an Accident

What is an accident? Unfortunately, even experts in the safety field disagree on the definition. However, all of them concur on one point: An accident is a multifaceted concept.

As defined by Strasser and his collaborators, "An accident may be thought of as an unplanned act or event resulting in injury or death to persons or damage to property."[2] According to this definition, an event must

---

1. "Pioneer in Orbit," *Newsweek,* February 7, 1972, p. 8.
2. Marland K. Strasser and others, *Fundamentals of Safety Education* (2d ed.; New York: The Macmillan Company, 1973), p. 4.

Leading causes of all deaths

	No. of Deaths	Death Rate*
All Ages	1,892,879	889
Heart disease	716,215	336
Cancer	365,693	172
Stroke**	194,038	91
Accidents	**103,030**	**48**
Motor-vehicle	45,853	21
Falls	14,896	7
Drowning	8,000	4
Fires, burns	6,071	3
Other	28,210	13
Under 1 Year	50,525	1,641
Anoxia	12,577	408
Congenital anomalies	8,582	279
Complications of pregnancy and childbirth	6,344	206
Immaturity	4,398	143
Pneumonia	2,171	71
Accidents	**1,337**	**43**
Ingestion of food, object	360	12
Mech. suffocation	268	9
Motor-vehicle	255	8
Fires, burns	135	4
Falls	68	2
Other	251	8
1 to 4 Years	9,060	71
Accidents	**3,611**	**28**
Motor-vehicle	1,321	10
Drowning	760†	6
Fires, burns	617	5
Ingestion of food, object	144	1
Falls	129	1
Other	640	5
Congenital anomalies	1,141	9
Cancer	711	6
5 to 14 Years	13,479	36
Accidents	**6,818**	**18**
Motor-vehicle	3,286	9
Drowning	1,300†	3
Fires, burns	580	2
Other	1,652	4
Cancer	1,807	5
Congenital anomalies	742	2
15 to 24 Years	47,545	119
Accidents	**24,121**	**60**
Motor-vehicle	15,672	39
Drowning	2,520†	6
Poison (solid, liquid)	1,332	3
Firearms	758	2
Other	3,839	10
Homicide	5,493	14
Suicide	4,736	12

	No. of Deaths	Death Rate*
25 to 44 Years	104,732	196
Accidents	**22,877**	**43**
Motor-vehicle	11,969	22
Poison (solid, liquid)	1,853	4
Drowning	1,740†	3
Fires, burns	961	2
Other	6,354	12
Cancer	16,645	31
Heart disease	14,922	28
45 to 64 Years	450,066	1,034
Heart disease	160,384	368
Cancer	128,371	295
Stroke**	25,789	59
Accidents	**19,643**	**45**
Motor-vehicle	7,663	18
Falls	2,449	6
Fires, burns	1,602	4
Drowning	1,120†	2
Other	6,809	15
Cirrhosis of liver	18,235	42
Diabetes mellitus	8,238	19
65 to 74 Years	442,496	3,189
Heart disease	183,667	1,324
Cancer	107,604	776
Stroke**	42,056	303
Diabetes mellitus	10,432	75
Accidents	**9,220**	**66**
Motor-vehicle	3,047	22
Falls	2,148	15
Fires, burns	795	6
Surg. complications	785	6
Other	2,445	17
Pneumonia	8,915	64
Emphysema	7,127	51
75 Years and Over	774,976	9,087
Heart disease	355,004	4,163
Stroke**	121,435	1,424
Cancer	107,725	1,263
Pneumonia	29,517	346
Arteriosclerosis	23,872	280
Accidents	**15,403**	**181**
Falls	8,510	100
Motor-vehicle	2,640	31
Surg. complications	976	12
Fires, burns	879	10
Ingestion of food, object	594	7
Other	1,804	21
Diabetes mellitus	14,865	174
Emphysema	6,722	79

Source: Deaths are for 1975, latest official figures from National Center for Health Statistics, Health Services and Mental Health Administration, U.S. Department of Health, Education and Welfare.
*Deaths per 100,000 population in each age group. Rates are averages for age groups, not individual ages.
**Cerebrovascular disease.   †Partly estimated.

Figure 1.1   Deaths in the United States. (Reproduced from *Accident Facts—1977 Edition,* p. 8, courtesy of the National Safety Council)

result in injury or property damage before it can be properly classified as an accident. Consequently, if a driver loses control of his car on an icy road and the vehicle skids completely in a circle without causing damage to itself or injury to the driver, an accident did not occur.

Another definition of an accident is given by Licht. According to this definition, "An accident is a sudden, unplanned event which has the potential for producing injury or damage."[3] Thus, applying this definition to the previously mentioned example of the icy road and the skidding car, an accident did occur, since the event certainly had the potential for producing injury or property damage.

As specified by the National Safety Council, "An accident is that occurrence in a sequence of events which usually produces unintended injury, death or property damage."[4] While this definition is similar to Licht's, one additional important concept is included in the Council's definition. This concept is "that occurrence in a sequence of events." In comparison to Licht's meaning, the National Safety Council's definition suggests that all accidents are caused by multiple factors.

For use in this book, the following definition of an accident is suggested: **An accident is a sequence of sudden, unplanned events which has the potential for producing personal injury or property damage.** According to this definition, an accident has at least four different components. *First,* several different events, rather than a single event, are involved in the production of an accident. This statement recognizes that all accidents are caused by multiple factors, each interacting in a sequence with the others. *Second*, all accidents are sudden occurrences. While safety experts can accurately foretell the occurrence of certain accidents, they cannot predict exactly when a particular accident will occur. *Third,* accidents are unplanned. Thus, an injury sustained by the victim of a robbery would not be considered an accident, since the robbery was deliberately planned. *Fourth,* all accidents have the potential for producing personal injury or property damage. For example, a bolt of lightning striking an unoccupied body of water would not be an accident. However, the same occurrence in a crowded swimming pool would certainly be considered an accident.

As the accident is defined in this book, personal injury and property damage are possible only after the passage of a particular sequence of events. Consequently, any alteration or interruption of this sequence has the potential for preventing an accident. If this were not true, then safety education would be a worthless pursuit.

---

3. Kenneth F. Licht, "Safety and Accidents—A Brief Conceptual Analysis, and A Point of View," *The Journal of School Health,* November, 1975, p. 532.
4. National Safety Council, *Accidents Facts—1977 Edition* (Chicago: NSC, 1977), p. 97.

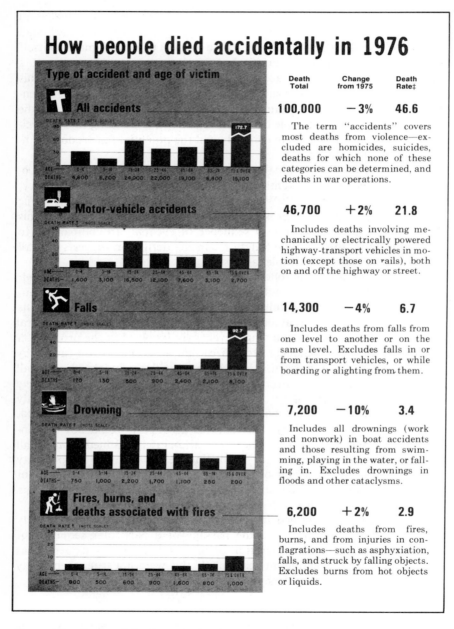

Figure 1.2   Types of death-producing accidents in the United States. (Reproduced from *Accident Facts—1977 Edition,* pp. 6-7, courtesy of the National Safety Council)

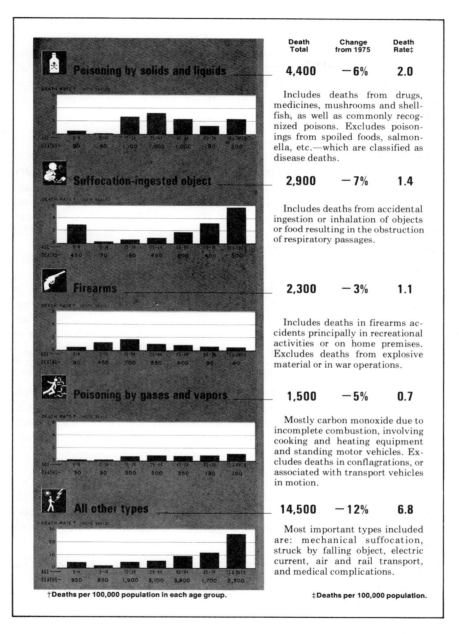

	Death Total	Change from 1975	Death Rate‡

Poisoning by solids and liquids — 4,400   −6%   2.0

Includes deaths from drugs, medicines, mushrooms and shellfish, as well as commonly recognized poisons. Excludes poisonings from spoiled foods, salmonella, etc.—which are classified as disease deaths.

Suffocation-ingested object — 2,900   −7%   1.4

Includes deaths from accidental ingestion or inhalation of objects or food resulting in the obstruction of respiratory passages.

Firearms — 2,300   −3%   1.1

Includes deaths in firearms accidents principally in recreational activities or on home premises. Excludes deaths from explosive material or in war operations.

Poisoning by gases and vapors — 1,500   −5%   0.7

Mostly carbon monoxide due to incomplete combustion, involving cooking and heating equipment and standing motor vehicles. Excludes deaths in conflagrations, or associated with transport vehicles in motion.

All other types — 14,500   −12%   6.8

Most important types included are: mechanical suffocation, struck by falling object, electric current, air and rail transport, and medical complications.

†Deaths per 100,000 population in each age group.   ‡Deaths per 100,000 population.

Figure 1.2.   Cont'd.

Classes of Accidents

According to the location where the accident occurred or the activity in which the person was participating, accidents may be classified into five major groups. These groups include (1) traffic accidents, (2) home accidents, (3) school accidents, (4) work accidents, and (5) public accidents.

Traffic Accidents

Every year nearly forty-seven thousand persons are killed in motor-vehicle accidents in this country. This means that almost one out of every two accidental deaths are caused by traffic accidents. In addition, approximately 1.8 million automobile drivers, motorcyclists, pedestrians, and bicyclists are disabled. According to the National Safety Council, improper driving and drinking of alcoholic beverages are implicated in most traffic accidents, both fatal and nonfatal.

Home Accidents

Annually, approximately twenty-four thousand persons are killed in home accidents in the United States, and another 3.7 million persons are disabled. Almost one out of every three deaths is attributable to falls, particularly by persons over the age of sixty-five years. Ranked behind falls in seriousness are fires, poisonings, suffocations, and firearm accidents.

School Accidents

More than six thousand school-age children are killed in accidents every year in this country. However, probably less than one-tenth of the deaths are the result of school-related activities. Apparently, most of the school-related deaths are caused by accidents while the children move to and from school, whether on foot or by bicycle, automobile, or school bus.

Work Accidents

Each year in the United States almost thirteen thousand persons are fatally injured in work accidents. In addition, approximately 2.2 million persons are disabled. Of the many different types of jobs, construction work and agricultural work produce the most deaths.

Public Accidents

Annually, accidents in public places or places used in a public way account for almost twenty-two thousand deaths in this country and almost 2.7 million disabling injuries. In nearly two-thirds of the fatal public accidents, the victims are engaged in recreational activities. Water-related sports, such as boating, swimming, and scuba diving, account for most of the recreational deaths.

A Philosophy of Safety

"When your number's up, it's up, and there's nothing you can do about it." "I'll watch out for myself, don't worry about me." "Accidents are the price you have to pay for progress." "When God wants me, he'll take me, and until he does, there's no sense in worrying." Undoubtedly, most people have heard these or similar comments by relatives, friends, and neighbors. While the comments are all stated differently, each expresses the same underlying belief: risk taking is an inevitable part of living.

Obviously, no one can deny that risks are an inherent part of life. Even getting out of bed in the morning involves risk. However, not all risks are equal. Different activities may present different levels of risk. For example, exploring an old shipwreck on the ocean bottom is a riskier pursuit than playing golf. Furthermore, a particular activity may involve more risk for one person than for another. Driving a motorcycle, for instance, is a greater risk for a beginner than for an experienced motorcyclist. Finally, during an activity, a person may experience more risk on one occasion than on another. For example, driving a car while fatigued is a riskier activity than driving while relaxed and rested. Thus, while risks are unavoidable, most of them can be chosen or at least lessened by an individual.

Apparently, good risk taking is one of the most important personal precautions against accidents. In good risk taking, a person must decide before performing any activity whether or not the risk is worthwhile. He must recognize any undesirable consequences of the activity, assess the probability of these consequences occurring, and determine any reward or other desirable outcomes of the activity. When this appraisal is realistically applied to the problem, an activity may then be viewed as a calculated risk rather than a haphazardous risk based on inadequate knowledge or foolish judgment. Naturally, people with such beliefs or attitudes as "when your number's up, it's up" and "when God wants me, he'll take me" often do not examine the risks associated with their activities. Consequently, they may unwittingly choose bad risks rather than good risks and thereby become involved in accidents.

Contrary to popular belief, freedom from risks does not imply safety. As previously mentioned, every activity in life involves some risk. Furthermore, many people in high-risk occupations, such as nuclear engineering and space exploration, are also the most "safety-minded" people in this country. For this reason, the following definition of safety will be used in this book: **Safety is the prevention of accidents and the mitigation of personal injury or property damage which may result from accidents.** According to this definition, safety has two distinct meanings. *First,* safety is "accident prevention." In this context safety deals with the *interruption* of the accident-producing sequence of events. For example, the application of adhesive decals to the bottom of the bathtub-shower unit is designed to provide a firm footing for the bather and thus interrupt the slipping events which lead to an accident. *Second,* safety is "accident mitigation." Safety in this context deals with an *alteration* of the accident-producing sequence of events. For example, since a bathtub or shower fall may occur even when adhesive decals are used, the installation of a safety-glass shower door, rather than an ordinary glass door, is designed to alter the final accident-producing events which lead to cuts and thus lessen or mitigate the severity of the injury.

Naturally, to function effectively, safety must contribute in a positive manner to the activities of everyday living. This is appropriately referred to as a "do" philosophy of safety. In this philosophy a person analyzes his activity and selects performance patterns that will reduce the inherent risk of the activity. In other words, he does not abandon an activity, such as fishing or snowmobiling, simply because it involves more risk than other activities, but instead, he plans positive steps which will lessen the probability of an accident occurring or the possibility of personal injury or property damage resulting. Consequently, a "do" philosophy of safety reduces risk while still maintaining the adventure and the excitement of life's activities. On the other hand, a "don't" philosophy of safety is a negative approach to life. According to this philosophy, a person avoids activities which involve an unusual amount of risk. Needless to say, if this philosophy were rigidly followed, an individual would certainly reduce risks to a minimum and thereby improve safety. However, without a certain level of risk, life becomes routine and unrewarding. For this reason, the "don't" philosophy of safety should whenever possible be discarded in favor of the "do" philosophy of safety.

Resource Materials

American Academy of Pediatrics
P.O. Box 1034
Evanston, Illinois 60204

National Safety Council
444 North Michigan Avenue
Chicago, Illinois 60611

Activities

1. Prepare a bulletin board display which illustrates each of the four components of an accident.

2. Write to the National Safety Council, and request the latest "Preliminary Condensed Edition of Accident Facts." Discuss the information with the class.

3. Prepare a scrapbook of newspaper articles which report local, alcohol-related traffic accidents. When at least thirty articles have been collected, write a two-page, statistical summary of the accidents.
4. Compile a list of ten safety rules which reflect the "do" philosophy of safety and ten safety rules which reflect the "don't" philosophy of safety. Discuss the philosophical implications of each rule with the class.
5. Select several classmates, and present a panel discussion on the topic of "A Philosophy of Safety."

Questions

1. How does Strasser's definition of an accident differ from the one given by Licht?
2. A driver lost control of his pick-up truck, and the vehicle ran off the road. However, the driver was not injured, and the truck was not damaged. According to Licht, was this an accident?
3. As defined by the author, what is the definition of an accident?
4. What are the five major classes of accidents?
5. According to the National Safety Council, what are the most frequent causes of traffic accidents?
6. What type of accident is the leading cause of death in the home?
7. Which jobs produce the most work deaths?
8. Why are people with such beliefs as "when your number's up, it's up" and "when God wants me, he'll take me" likely to become involved in accidents?
9. What is the definition of safety, and what two distinct meanings are apparent in the definition?
10. Why is the "do" philosophy of safety a much better approach to life than the "don't" philosophy of safety?

Selected References

Licht, Kenneth F. "Safety and Accidents—A Brief Conceptual Analysis, and A Point of View," *The Journal of School Health,* November, 1975, 530-32, 534.
National Safety Council. *Accident Facts—1977 Edition.* Chicago: NSC, 1977.
Painter, John H. Jr. (pub.) *Life and Health.* Del Mar, California: Communications Research Machines, Inc., 1972.
"Pioneer in Orbit," *Newsweek,* February 7, 1972, 8-9.
Strasser, Marland K. and others. *Fundamentals of Safety Education.* 2d ed.; New York: The Macmillan Company, 1973.

Accident Causation and Prevention/ Mitigation

2

In Memphis, Tennessee, a one-year-old boy drowned after accidentally falling into a bucket of water at his home. A thirty-year-old man in Jacksonville, Florida, playfully drew his pistol while kidding his wife about a nonexistent telephone call from another man and accidentally shot her in the stomach. In Cleveland, Ohio, two children died while sleeping in an overcrowded attic, and two others were burned critically when a fire of an undetermined origin destroyed their parents' frame home.

Why do people become involved in accidents? More important, how can accidents be prevented or, at least, how can the consequences of accidents be mitigated? Unfortunately, as the preceding accident reports show, there are no simple or easy answers to these questions. Every accident must be viewed as a highly complex problem in itself and must be analyzed within a broad conceptual framework.

Causes of Accidents

As the term was defined in Chapter 1, an accident is a sequence of sudden, unplanned events which has the potential for producing personal injury or property damage. Thus, according to this definition, an accident is always produced by a combination of factors. In a particular situation, this combination of factors is referred to as the cause of the accident.

In general, based on an epidemiological approach, accident causes may be classified under three headings: (1) human failures, (2) environmental hazards, and (3) defective agents.

Human Failures

Sometimes referred to as unsafe behavior, human failures are the principal cause of approximately 80 percent of all accidents. Psychological, physiological, and cultural factors are involved in most human failures.

Psychological Factors

According to numerous research studies, psychological factors are significant contributors to human failures. Perhaps the most important of these factors are the *emotions,* particularly anger, hatred, fear, anxiety, and joy.

Since emotions are altered psychological conditions, they often produce illogical, unpredictable behavior. As a result, a person who is experiencing a strong emotion may ignore safety precautions and act in a reckless manner, something he would not do under normal conditions. For example, a woman motorist who has just argued with her husband may unwittingly vent her anger by speeding, straddling lanes, taking needless chances, or driving in a manner entirely different from her usual driving behavior. Similarly, a workman who has just received notice of a salary increase and a promotion to foreman may in his excitement become temporarily inattentive and haphazardly perform his customary tasks. Since emotions are often triggered by existing events, such as a violent argument with a spouse, the loss of a job, a pay raise, a work promotion, or the death of a family member, they usually subside quickly, thus permitting the person to return to his normal behavioral patterns within a short period of time.

On the other hand, *attitudes* are relatively stable. Defined as predispositions to react in a certain manner to situations, attitudes are developed through repeated experiences. When these experiences are personally or socially undesirable, a person's attitudes may produce erratic and unpredictable behavior. As mentioned in the first chapter, persons with attitudes such as "when your number's up, it's up," and "when God wants me, he'll take me," often do not examine the risks associated with their activities. As a result, they frequently perform their activities in a careless manner and become involved in accidents.

Since most attitudes have developed over a period of many years, they are often interwoven with complex *personality traits.* One such trait is an exaggerated opinion of self-importance. Individuals with this personality trait tend to focus all their attention on themselves. Consequently, they often act irresponsibly and violate the rights of others. Overconfidence is another undesirable personality trait. Because they overestimate their abilities, persons with this characteristic often display inattention and a disregard for safety precautions. A third personality trait is an abnormal need for excitement. Individuals with this personal peculiarity frequently exercise poor judgment and attempt dangerous stunts, thereby becoming involved in accidents.

Like attitudes and personality traits, *habits* are formed through repeated experiences. However, in the performance of habits, conscious thought is not involved. Instead, habits are automatic responses to particular stimuli. For example, after fastening his safety belts for several weeks, a driver will probably discover that he has developed a habit. Similarly, a motorist who always signals before changing lanes will soon perform this action automatically. In these cases the habits promote safety and therefore are personally and socially acceptable. However, not all habits are desirable. For example, a man who gets out of his bed and walks into the bathroom every night without turning on the light has developed an undesirable habit. By performing this habit in the dark, the man is unable to deal with changes in the environment. Specifically, he may now fall over newly arranged furniture in his path. Thus, under normal conditions, undesirable habits may not be particularly dangerous, but with any change in the environment, they can result in accidents and injuries.

Unlike habits, conscious thought is always involved in the deliberate use of *knowledge*. However, when a person lacks a thorough knowledge of the hazards in an activity or when he lacks sufficient knowledge of the most desirable ways of performing the activity, his conscious thought is not always an effective deterrent to accidents. In fact, when a person possesses only partial knowledge of an activity, he is often filled with an unwarranted sense of security. For example, a camper may know that boiling an unopened can of food will heat the contents, but he may not know that a violent explosion could occur as the gases expand inside the can. Regardless of the degree of understanding, inadequate knowledge is often an important psychological contributor to human failures and, in turn, accidents.

Physiological Factors

Recently, research has shown that physiological factors may be almost as important in human failures as psychological factors. This is especially true for those persons at the extremes of the life cycle, since all of them possess numerous physical *impairments*.

Evidently, many of the physiological attributes which function for adults are not fully developed in children. For example, children do not possess an adult level of peripheral vision and peripheral hearing. Consequently, when they attempt to walk in traffic, children are physically unable to see or hear motor vehicles which are approaching them from the sides. On the other hand, many of the physiological processes in the elderly have been adversely affected by the aging process. For example, elderly persons cannot lift their feet as high as when they were younger. As a result, they frequently trip while walking or when climbing stairs. In addition, the elderly are often hampered by spells of dizziness and other equilibrium problems which may result in falls. For these reasons, the very young and the very old are often involved in more accidents than persons in other age groups.

Like age-related impairments, physiological *handicaps* may contribute abnormally to human failures and accidents. For example, while he is experiencing a seizure in deep water, a swimmer with epilepsy may drown. Similarly, a man with impaired hearing may unknowingly drive his pick-up truck into the path of an approaching train because he did not hear the engineer's warning whistles. However, not all persons with handicaps are highly susceptible to accidents. In fact, persons with known handicaps, such as color blindness, tunnel vision, hearing loss, and slow reflexes, often compensate for their disabilities and consequently perform their everyday activities more skillfully and more safely than persons with normal abilities.

Despite the absence of physical impairments and handicaps, some individuals may become involved in accidents because they attempt certain *skills* which are greatly beyond their normal capabilities. For example, since novice motorcyclists lack the skills needed for handling their newly acquired vehicles in traffic, they are frequently involved in motor-vehicle accidents. Likewise, while they are performing long distance swims, such as across ponds or lakes, swimmers may drown because they have not developed sufficient skill in the various resting strokes. However, when individuals possess adequate skills in an activity, they may still become involved in accidents when their normal physical skills are modified by other factors.

Besides altering moods, attention, perception, and judgment, *alcohol* interferes with many of the body's physiological processes. Typically, after consuming alcoholic beverages, persons exhibit slower reflexes, poorer coordination, impaired vision, and reduced sound discrimination. As accident reports show, these modifications of physical abilities are frequent factors in accidents, particularly traffic, boating, and snowmobiling mishaps.

Like alcohol, certain *medicinal drugs* may produce alterations in normal physical abilities. For example, cough syrups may cause sleepiness and impaired coordination; antihistamines and sedatives may induce drowsiness, as well as confusion and perceptual problems; tranquilizers may cause sleepiness, dizziness, blurred vision, and impaired coordination; and amphetamines may produce dizziness and hallucinations when their stimulating effects have worn off. Although the exact relationship between medicinal drugs and accidents is unclear, many safety experts believe that the physical problems created by drugs are frequent factors in traffic and home accidents.

In addition to hindering judgment and other mental processes, bodily *fatigue* may reduce the efficiency with which individuals normally perform certain physical acts. Typically, after long periods of mental or physical exertion, persons experience slower reflexes and poorer coordination. For example, when an individual has been driving for several hours on a long trip, he may not react quickly enough to avoid hitting a suddenly-braking automobile. Similarly, after returning home from a tiring day at work, a woman may shuffle her feet rather than lifting them and, as a result, trip over a slightly protruding throw rug in her living room. As these examples suggest, fatigued individuals are more likely to become involved in accidents than rested persons.

Cultural Factors

According to research studies, cultural factors, which are inherently related to both psychological and physiological factors, are often contributing elements in human failures. Specifically, in this country the *frontier heritage* is an important cultural factor in accident causation.

Paradoxically, despite contemporary society's vast industrialization and urbanization, our schools and the mass media still support and popularize the values of this nation's early frontier tradition. Consequently, rugged values, such as competitiveness, aggressiveness, initiative, and risk taking, become cultural demands. However, most individuals cannot meet these demands in their daily work situations, and as a result, they may try to demonstrate their ruggedness in traffic, at home, or in recreational activities. For example, because of his need for excitement or his desire to prove his bravery, a young motorist may attempt to pass other vehicles on curves or hills. Likewise, in an effort to protect his property and family against outsiders, a man may keep a loaded pistol or shotgun near his bed. Needless to say, frontier values were indispensable in the founding of this country. However, in today's modern society, values such as aggressiveness and unnecessary risk taking are often undesirable and may contribute in certain situations to accidents, injuries, and deaths.

At the other extreme, several modern cultural *trends* may also encourage human failures and accidents. One trend in this country is society's preoccupation with speed. In practically every mode of transportation, from cars to airplanes, daredevils have established speed records, surpassed them, and later reestablished them. However, few people have the opportunity to enjoy this particular type of excitement and adventure. Consequently, most individuals seek their thrills within the traffic setting. Thus, a motorist may deliberately speed in an effort to prevent another driver from passing him. Similarly, a young driver may attempt to beat a train to a railroad crossing, or he may drag race with friends on a city street or public highway. Ironically, automobile manufacturers actually encourage this type of activity by designing sporty-looking cars with 160 mph-marked speedometers, and by publicizing the thrills of owning and driving these sporty cars. Another cultural trend that may encourage human failures in this country is society's acceptance of the use of drugs, both prescription and nonprescription. However, like all good things, medicinal drugs can be abused. For example, individuals often take their medicines in excessive dosages or in combination with alcohol. Likewise, parents frequently leave or store their drugs within easy reach of their children. As a result, poisoning has become one of the most frequent types of accidents in this country.

Unlike trends, cultural *fads* are short-lived. However, during their popularity, fads may contribute significantly to accidents. In recent years two specific fads have produced an exceptionally large number of injuries.

One fad is the sport of skateboarding. Riding in a standing position on a small board equipped with roller-type wheels, the skateboarder performs his stunts on sidewalks, parking lots, streets, and highways. However, because the stunts are difficult to master, participants in the skateboarding fad are often thrown off their boards and onto the hard concrete or asphalt pavement, thus suffering cuts, bruises, or fractures. Strangely enough, unlike other fads, skateboarding tends to reappear every few years. Another fad which has produced numerous accidents in recent years is barrel jumping. Most often, after placing several garbage barrels side-by-side, a youngster will set a wooden ramp at one end of the line and then attempt to jump over the barrels with his bicycle. Because of the hazardous nature of the activity, the bicyclist is almost always injured when he does not successfully clear the barrels. Apparently, participation in barrel jumping has been stimulated by the recently publicized exploits of Evel Knievel and other motorcycle daredevils.

Environmental Hazards

Environmental hazards are the leading cause of approximately 15 percent of all accidents. In general, natural and man-made factors are responsible for all environmental hazards.

Natural Factors

Obviously, many hazards are inherently present in any environmental setting. However, in the traffic environment, natural factors are especially apparent in accident causation. For instance, because *rain, snow, sleet, dust,* or *sunlight* has reduced visibility, a driver may inadvertently cross the centerline of a highway and crash head-on into another vehicle. On the other hand, a motorcyclist may lose control of his bike after driving over a wet or icy patch in the road. Similarly, after he has been stung on the face by an *insect,* a motorist may lose control of his car and drive into the rear of a parked vehicle. In these instances, before an accident could occur, the naturally-created hazards had to alter or modify human behavior. However, not all environmental hazards of the natural type involve human interaction. For example, *lightning, floods, blizzards, tornadoes, hurricanes,* and *earthquakes* are not conditioned by human behavior, but they are still frequent causes of accidents.

Man-made Factors

A *disorderly situation* is a common source of man-made environmental hazards. In many cases poor housekeeping practices are responsible for creating the hazards. For example, instead of using his toy box, a youngster may leave his toys scattered on the living room floor, thus providing tripping hazards for the family. On the other hand, a woman may inappropriately rearrange the furniture and thereby create tripping obstacles near doorways or on normally traveled paths within the room. In other cases *improperly stored items* are factors in man-made environmental hazards. For instance, lacking adequate storage space, a housewife may permit old newspapers to accumulate near a basement furnace, thus creating a serious fire hazard. Similarly, a woman may create a poisoning hazard by storing bleach, drain cleaner, and other dangerous chemicals under the kitchen sink where her children can easily reach them.

Defective Agents

Approximately 5 percent of all accidents are caused primarily by defective agents. Apparently, design and mechanical factors are responsible for most defective agents.

Design Factors

Even in the most orderly environment, physical elements or agents may contain certain *inherent hazards*. Sometimes, the hazards are the result of the agent's specific design or function. For instance, a toy with sharp edges or pull-away parts can easily injure or kill a baby or young child. Likewise, because of the tremendous force generated by turning gears, a piece of work equipment may snag an operator's clothing and effortlessly pull the person's hand, foot, or head into the machinery. Fortunately, in recent years many of the hazards associated with the design and function of agents have been minimized or eliminated by the development of special safety features, particularly improved designs and protective guards.

Mechanical Factors

According to some safety experts, most defective agents are the product of mechanical or *structural failures*. For example, a rusted connection in the steering mechanism of an automobile may suddenly break, thereby creating steering difficulty and a loss of control by the driver. Similarly, the suction discs on a bath mat may slip and cause the bather to lose his balance and fall. Because of mechanical or structural breakdowns, even normally safe agents may become defective and thus hazardous.

Accident Prevention/Mitigation Model

Any conceptual model of accident prevention/mitigation must incorporate certain fundamental assumptions. In this textbook the following assumptions form the basis for an epidemiological accident prevention/mitigation model:

1. Accidents are produced by an aggregation of factors, each interacting in a sequence with the other factors. In a specific situation, this aggregation of factors is termed the cause of the accident.
2. Accident causes may be grouped under three headings: (1) human failures, (2) environmental hazards, and (3) defective agents.
3. Accidents can be prevented or mitigated by a modification of the accident-producing sequence of events. This modification may be directed at the person, the environment, or the agent.

When the epidemiological method is applied to the accident problem, the approach will identify specific causes of accidents and permit an assignment of effective countermeasures.

In Des Moines, Iowa, a twenty-two-year-old woman removed her clothes, stepped into the shower, and closed the sliding-glass door. As the water rushed from the shower nozzle, the woman suddenly jumped backward, lost her footing, and fell headfirst through the shower door. Several weeks later, she was still in the hospital suffering from severe cuts and bruises on her face.

In analyzing this accident, several questions can be formulated. First, why did the woman jump backward? Second, why did she lose her footing? Third, what was the injury-producing mechanism in the accident? Before effective countermeasures can be applied in similar situations, these questions must be answered in detail.

According to the woman, when the water sprayed from the shower nozzle, she jumped backward to avoid getting her hair wet. As she did this, her foot slipped on the smooth bottom of the bathtub-shower unit, and she lost her balance. While she was falling, the woman struck her head on the old-style shower door, and when the glass in the door broke into sharp fragments, she received several deep cuts on her face.

Based upon this additional information, the sequence of events in the accident can be analyzed in terms of the person, the environment, and the agent. Apparently, several factors were instrumental in either causing the fall or producing the facial injuries:

1. The woman was fearful of getting her hair wet. Influenced by her emotions, she acted suddenly and recklessly by jumping away from the spraying water. (**Human failure**)
2. The bottom of the bathtub-shower unit was smooth. In combination with the water, the smooth surface provided an extremely slippery footing for the woman. (**Environmental hazard**)
3. The shower door was constructed of ordinary glass. When the woman crashed through the door, the glass shattered and formed sharp, daggerlike pieces that sliced and punctured her face. (**Defective agent**)

ACCIDENT CAUSATION SUMMARY

I. **Human Failures**

   A. **Psychological factors**

      1. Emotions
      2. Poor attitudes
      3. Undesirable personality traits
      4. Undesirable habits
      5. Inadequate knowledge

   B. **Physiological factors**

      1. Age-related impairments
      2. Handicaps
      3. Inadequate skills (often modified by alcohol, medicinal drugs, or fatigue)

   C. **Cultural factors**

      1. Frontier heritage
      2. Cultural trends
      3. Cultural fads

II. **Environmental Hazards**

   A. **Natural factors**

      1. Rain, snow, sleet, dust, or sunlight
      2. Insects or animals
      3. Lightning, floods, blizzards, tornadoes, hurricanes, or earthquakes

   B. **Man-made factors**

      1. Disorderly situation
      2. Improperly stored items

III. **Defective Agents**

   A. **Design factors**

      1. Inherent hazards

   B. **Mechanical factors**

      1. Faulty mechanical or structural features

Figure 2.1   Causes of accidents.

Once the factors in an accident have been identified, countermeasures can be applied to the person, the environment, and/or the agent. Specifically, the following recommendations should be valuable in preventing similar bathtub-shower falls or mitigating the consequences of the falls:

1. In future showers the woman should wear a plastic shower cap to protect her hair from the water. (**Person**)
2. Strips or decals of nonslip material should be applied in a pattern on the bottom of the bathtub-shower unit to produce a slightly abrasive surface for better footing. (**Environment**)
3. To mitigate glass injuries a safety-glass shower door should be installed in the bathtub-shower unit. (**Agent**)

While the epidemiological accident prevention/mitigation model was applied to a specific accident in the preceding discussion, the approach can be readily expanded to include any potential accident location or situation. In such cases, the following steps should be taken by the individual:

1. List all of the types of accidents which may occur at the location or in the situation.
2. For each type of accident, identify and list all of the possible causative factors under the headings of human failures, environmental hazards, and defective agents.
3. Analyze each accident factor and assign a possible countermeasure which is directed at the person, the environment, or the agent.

Since its introduction over twenty-five years ago, the epidemiological model of accident prevention/mitigation has received widespread attention by safety experts. Today, the epidemiological approach is used by almost everyone who has an interest in preventing accidents or in mitigating their consequences.

Systems Safety Analysis

In recent years systems safety analysis, an approach which originated in the aerospace industry, has been applied to the accident problem. In analyzing the causes of accidents and applying countermeasures for their prevention/mitigation, the systems safety approach is quite similar in many aspects to the epidemiological model.

By definition, a system is an orderly arrangement of interrelated components which act and interact to perform some task or function under specific conditions. In systems safety analysis, emphasis is placed upon the interaction of three components: (1) man, (2) his machines, and (3) the environment. As parts of a system, the components usually complement each other. However, if a component fails and this failure affects the other components, an accident can result.

In simple terms, systems safety analysis is a logical, step-by-step approach for examining situations with accident potential. The components of the system—human, mechanical, and environmental—are placed in an orderly arrangement and then subjected to detailed analysis. Ideally, systems safety analysis will help identify accident causes which could be overlooked in a less detailed approach. However, while the systems safety approach has been highly successful in analyzing some very complex systems and in providing effective countermeasures against accidents, many problems still exist in quantifying the human influence as a system component.

Accident Repeaters and the Accident Prone

An accident repeater is a person who has been involved in several accidents of a particular type. As Strasser notes,

He may have this label because of statistical chance; that is, by chance alone a person may have more than his share of accidents; or he may have greater exposure. A cross-country salesman driving 100,000 miles or more per year has greater exposure and may, therefore, have more accidents than the average person who drives about 15,000 miles per year.[1]

On the other hand, an accident-prone individual is someone with an attraction for accidents.

Over the years the phenomenon of accident proneness has been the subject of much study. Originally, researchers felt that accident-prone individuals could be identified by certain psychological traits. However, all attempts to discover these characteristics have been unsuccessful. Apparently, accident-prone individuals cannot be identified by a single set of psychological traits.

Today, many researchers feel that the psychological traits which produce accident proneness are present in all individuals. Whether or not these psychological traits manifest themselves in accident proneness, however, is the function of a complex interaction among a multitude of factors within the individual. In simple terms, the accident susceptibility of the person is a reflection of his ability or inability to maintain a harmonious relationship among these innumerable internal factors.

---

1. Marland K. Strasser and others, *Fundamentals of Safety Education* (2d ed.; New York: The Macmillan Company, 1973), p. 93.

Naturally, at certain times in a person's life, this harmonious relationship may be temporarily upset by external stress factors. For example, research studies indicate that automobile drivers who are involved in divorce proceedings are more likely to become accident prone than other drivers. Similarly, women are inclined to be more accident prone during menstruation and the four preceding days than at other times in the monthly cycle. Characteristically, with the disappearance of the stress factors, the individual will return to a state of better adjustment, reestablish the harmonious relationship among the internal factors, and again become less susceptible to accidents.

The harmonious relationship may also be upset for relatively long periods of time at various stages in a person's life. As a result, the person may be more accident prone at one age than at another age. Generally, young people, despite their well-developed motor coordination and physical fitness, are inclined to be somewhat accident prone because of their immaturity and inexperience. On the other hand, middle-aged persons, because of their experience and their psychological and sociological maturity, are less likely to become consistently involved in accidents. Finally, older people, despite their maturity and substantial experience, are inclined to exhibit some degree of accident proneness because of the persistent deterioration of their mental and physical abilities.

According to most researchers, accident proneness is a matter of degree, ranging from the slightly-prone individual to the multiple offender. Furthermore, different types of accident proneness may be recognized. Some persons are susceptible to only a specific type of accident; others are vulnerable to all types of accidents. Moreover, some persons are especially susceptible to very serious or major accidents; other individuals are vulnerable primarily to minor accidents. Apparently, in different people the psychological traits for accident proneness may manifest themselves in different ways.

In summary, an endless number of factors are responsible for determining from time to time the accident potential of an individual. Accordingly, for accident proneness to possess any meaning, the concept must be viewed in a flexible manner, since the proneness may manifest itself in different ways, in different people, and for different reasons, and may change considerably over a period of time.

Safety and Consumer Protection

"Let the buyer beware!" For years this was the only protection that consumers had against hazardous products on the market. However, by the early 1970s, American users of goods and services, spurred by the efforts of consumer action groups, had become acutely aware of the need for product safety. With this awareness, consumers became more and more vocal in their discontentment. Finally, on May 14, 1973, the United States government activated the Consumer Product Safety Commission.

Designed to be independent of political pressures, the U.S. Consumer Product Safety Commission is charged with the following responsibilities: (1) protecting the public against unreasonable risks of injury associated with consumer products; (2) developing uniform safety standards for consumer products and minimizing conflicting local and state regulations; (3) assisting consumers in evaluating the comparative safety of market products; and (4) promoting investigation and research concerning the causes and prevention of product-related deaths, illnesses, and injuries. Members of the Commission are nominated by the President and confirmed by the Senate. According to federal law, no more than three members may belong to the same political party, and unless they are found guilty of malfeasance or neglect of duty, the members are permitted, after initial shorter appointments, to serve on the Commission for a term of seven years.

In protecting the public, the Consumer Product Safety Commission establishes mandatory safety standards for consumer products sold in the United States. To assure that manufacturers comply with the provisions of the standards, the Commission has the authority to enforce the standards in the courts. Manufacturers who are found guilty of violating the standards may be sentenced to one year in jail and may be fined slightly over one-half million dollars. In addition, the Commission has the authority to ban hazardous products from the market, as well as to require the recall, repair, replacement, or refund of products which are judged to be unreasonably hazardous.

As a part of its responsibility for educating the public, the Consumer Product Safety Commission provides information to consumers and manufacturers, conducts educational campaigns and training programs, and publishes studies and reports on product safety. Furthermore, to determine the causes of product-related deaths, illnesses, and injuries, the Commission maintains an injury information clearinghouse and operates the National Electronic Injury Surveillance System which monitors throughout the country over one hundred hospital emergency rooms for injuries and deaths associated with consumer products. The Commission also conducts studies, tests products, and contracts for outside research in an attempt to improve product safety.

Because of the vast number of items on the market, the Consumer Product Safety Commission welcomes consumer help in locating and identifying hazardous products. To report a product hazard or a product-related injury, consumers should write or call toll-free the Commission in Washington, D.C. (See "Resource Materials.")

Resource Materials

American Medical Association
535 North Dearborn Street
Chicago, Illinois 60610

National Safety Council
444 North Michigan Avenue
Chicago, Illinois 60611

U.S. Consumer Product Safety Commission
5401 Westbard Avenue
Washington, D.C. 20207
Toll-free: 800-638-2666 in the continental United States
800-492-2937 for Maryland residents only

Activities

1. Conduct a survey of twenty-five adults to determine what they believe are the most common causative factors in accidents. Summarize and discuss the results in a short paper.

2. Design a bulletin board display which illustrates in diagram form the various aspects of the epidemiological accident prevention/mitigation model.

3. Apply the epidemiological accident prevention/mitigation model to a specific location in the home. Distribute a copy of the analysis to each member of the class.

4. Write to the National Safety Council, and request a copy of *Systems Safety Analysis: A Modern Approach to Safety Problems* by J. L. Recht. Present a short, oral report to the class on the contents of the publication.

5. Based on the information presented in this chapter, write a short paper on the topic of "The Accident Proneness Concept—Does It Possess Any Value in the Prevention/Mitigation of Accidents?".

Questions

1. What are the three headings under which accident causes may be classified?
2. What are the five psychological factors which contribute to human failures and accidents?
3. What are the three factors that may modify normal physical skills and contribute to accidents?

4. What is the frontier heritage, and why is this heritage an important factor in accident causation?
5. What is the difference between cultural trends and cultural fads?
6. What factors are responsible for all environmental hazards?
7. What is the cause of most defective agents?
8. What are the three steps that should be taken by an individual in using the epidemiological accident prevention/mitigation model on a potential accident location or situation?
9. What is the difference between an accident repeater and an accident-prone individual?
10. What are the four responsibilities of the U.S. Consumer Product Safety Commission?

Selected References

Block, J. R. "Attention Failure—A Test That Tells Who Is Accident-Prone," *Psychology Today,* June, 1975, 84-85.

Englebardt, Stanley L. "Are You Accident Prone?" *The Reader's Digest,* September, 1969, 127-30.

Lykes, Norman Roberts. *A Psychological Approach to Accidents.* New York: Vantage Press, Inc., 1954.

Painter, John H., Jr. (pub.) *Life and Health.* Del Mar, California: Communications Research Machines, Inc., 1972.

Recht, J. L. *Systems Safety Analysis: A Modern Approach to Safety Problems.* Chicago: National Safety Council, n.d.

Schwenger, Cope W. "Injuries and Injury Control," *Canadian Journal of Public Health,* May-June, 1975, 221-33.

Shaw, Lynette, and Herbert S. Sichel. *Accident Proneness.* New York: Pergamon Press, 1971.

Strasser, Marland K. and others. *Fundamentals of Safety Education.* 2d ed.; New York: The Macmillan Company, 1973.

Wolaver, John H. "The Accident-Prone Patient—Are Accidents Ever Accidents?" *Journal of the Tennessee Medical Association,* September, 1975, 705-8.

Automobile Accidents

3

Near Lansing, Michigan, an automobile roaring along at seventy-five miles per hour struck a steel guardrail, hurtled into the air, and crashed in a series of end-over-end rollovers which tore up the ground for over two hundred feet. The crash was a "wipeout," usually resulting in certain death. Yet, to the astonishment of the police, the driver of the car survived the accident. Apparently, he had been saved by certain marvels of traffic engineering, a tapered guardrail and numerous automotive safety devices.

Although safer roads and automobiles have helped to reduce the traffic death toll in recent years, nearly forty-seven thousand persons still lose their lives every year in motor-vehicle accidents. For this reason, traffic safety experts stress that engineering, as well as enforcement, are only small parts in the solution to the motor-vehicle accident problem in this country. The most important factor is still the driver, since he must ultimately decide whether or not he is willing to take certain risks in the traffic environment.

Buckling-up for Safety

The term "safety belts," more than any other words, has become virtually synonymous with traffic safety in recent years. Interestingly enough, while the belts have been in existence for almost thirty years, they have not always been called safety belts. Originally, safety experts spoke of the protective devices as "seat belts." However, they soon learned that the term had a negative connotation for many drivers, as evidenced by the fact that people tended to leave the belts on the seat. Fortunately, with the introduction of the chest-restraint device or shoulder harness, "seat belts" was no longer an appropriate term for the devices. As a result, traffic safety experts wisely coined the term "safety belts" to describe the lap-restraint and chest-restraint belts.

While they initially had some difficulty in finding a suitable name for safety belts, traffic safety officials have never had any doubt about the value of the belts in saving lives. They have always agreed that the act of fastening safety belts is the single most important precaution which a driver and his passengers can take before entering traffic. Without safety belts, in a collision the front-seat occupants are thrown forward into the steering wheel, dashboard, or windshield, and the back-seat occupants are thrown forward into the back of the front seat or over the back seat into the front-seat occupants or the dashboard.

To understand better how safety belts work, a person should carefully examine the physics that are involved in a typical automobile accident. In any collision the force of impact is largely determined by the speed or velocity at which the car is traveling. For example, a car striking a solid, immovable object at thirty miles per hour will hit four times harder than a car striking the same object at fifteen miles per hour. Similarly, an automobile traveling at forty-five miles per hour and another automobile traveling at sixty miles per hour will strike the object nine and sixteen times harder, respectively, than an automobile traveling and striking the same object at fifteen miles per hour. The important point is that the impact forces do not increase proportionally, but rather they increase according to the squares of the speeds.[1] Consequently, the faster an automobile is traveling, the greater will be the impact forces in the event of a collision.

The impact forces, however, can be reduced considerably by increasing the automobile's stopping time. For example, driving into a concrete bridge abutment, by which the car is brought almost immediately to a stop, will result in a much greater force of impact than the impact which would result from striking a lawn hedge, in which the car is gradually brought to a stop. Thus, if a driver has the alternative of hitting either a sturdy object, such as an approaching automobile or a telephone pole, he should choose the weak object, since the impact of the latter crash will be less dangerous than the impact which would inevitably accompany the collision with a sturdy object.

Although at first this concept is somewhat difficult to understand, the same physics which pertain to the automobile during a collision also apply to the driver and his passengers. By their presence in the automobile, the occupants are traveling at the same speed or velocity as the vehicle. Consequently, the faster the occupants are traveling, the harder they will hit if they are thrown into the steering wheel, dashboard, or windshield during a collision. Yet, like the automobile, the impact forces can be reduced considerably if the occupants are gradually brought to a stop. This is the function of safety belts!

Because they are constructed of material which will lengthen under extreme stress, safety belts stretch gradually during a collision and bring the

---

1. For example, not $\frac{30 \text{ mph}}{15 \text{ mph}} = 2$ times, $\frac{45 \text{ mph}}{15 \text{ mph}} = 3$ times, and $\frac{60 \text{ mph}}{15 \text{ mph}} = 4$ times, but rather $\frac{(30 \text{ mph})^2}{(15 \text{ mph})^2} = 4$ times, $\frac{(45 \text{ mph})^2}{(15 \text{ mph})^2} = 9$ times, and $\frac{(60 \text{ mph})^2}{(15 \text{ mph})^2} = 16$ times.

wearer's body to a relatively slow stop. This action, in turn, prevents the driver and his passengers from striking the hard interior of the automobile or from being thrown out of the automobile onto the even harder pavement. However, if safety belts are to perform their function effectively, both the chest-restraint belt, which holds the person away from the interior of the car, and the lap-restraint belt, which holds the person inside the car, must be worn at all times by every occupant in the vehicle. Otherwise, safety belts cannot provide their fullest protection.

While safety belts conserve lives, as verified by the survival of three to four thousand individuals every year, most traffic safety officials are hesitant in admitting that the belts have another side: they sometimes cause injury. Yet, there is really no reason for concealing the fact, since numerous research studies on safety-belt injuries have actually supported the rationale for wearing safety belts . In a study by Hodson-Walker, the researcher concluded that lap-restraint belts have never been shown to worsen injury, and while producing injuries themselves, they have prevented more serious injuries.[2] In another study by Williams and Kirkpatrick, the researchers estimated that a majority of the injured victims would have been killed without a restraining device.[3] In still another study by Crosby and Costiloe which involved pregnant women, the researchers found that lap-restraint belts did not increase the mortality rate of either mothers or fetuses.[4] In fact, when the belts were not worn and the mothers were thrown out of the automobiles during the accidents, there was a significantly higher mortality rate for both the mothers and the unborn children. Thus, while safety belts can cause injury, the injury is almost always less severe than if the belts had not been worn. On the other hand, as the research by Williams and Kirkpatrick indicates, many safety-belt injuries could be avoided if the belts were used properly.[5] For example, the lap-restraint belt, either because it is worn above the hip bones or has moved above the hip bones during an accident, often produces injury to the abdomen, but this type of injury can be prevented by wearing the belt snugly and directly over the hip bones rather than over the stomach. Similarly, skeletal injuries to the ribs, breastbone, and vertebral column, caused by wearing only the chest-restraint belt, can be avoided by always wearing the chest-restraint belt in combination with the lap-restraint belt.

Contrary to popular belief, the prevention of serious or fatal injuries is

2. N. J. Hodson-Walker, "The Value of Safety Belts: A Review," *Canadian Medical Association Journal,* February, 1970, p. 393.

3. James S. Williams and John R. Kirkpatrick, "The Nature of Seat Belt Injuries," *The Journal of Trauma,* March, 1971, p. 218.

4. Warren M. Crosby and J. Paul Costiloe, "Safety of Lap-Belt Restraint for Pregnant Victims of Automobile Collisions," *The New England Journal of Medicine,* March 25, 1971, p. 636.

5. Williams and Kirkpatrick, p. 218

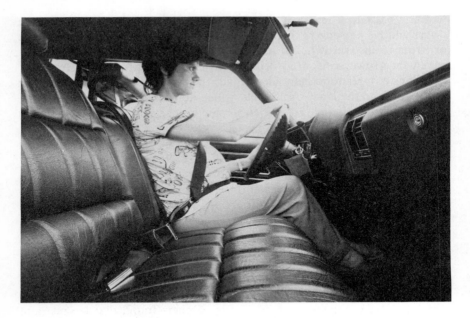

Figure 3.1   To protect both herself and her baby, an expectant mother should always wear safety belts.

not the only function performed by safety belts. Actually, the belts also play an important role in keeping drivers out of accidents. Because safety belts keep the driver fastened securely behind the steering wheel, a quick stop, sudden turn, hole or bump in the road, or minor collision cannot jostle the driver and thereby cause him to lose control of his vehicle. In turn, this enables the driver to use his skill to steer the automobile so as to avoid further trouble.

Why Safety Belts Are Not Worn

Although the National Safety Council estimates that safety belts can prevent as many as twelve thousand deaths every year, many individuals do not wear the belts regularly or, worse yet, do not wear the belts at all. According to some safety experts, the lap-restraint belt, which is now available to nearly all passenger car occupants, is used less than 40 percent of the time. The chest-restraint belt, on the other hand, is used even less or about 10 percent of the time by occupants in vehicles with the belts. Although many reasons are given for not wearing safety belts, such as "They are too much trouble to wear." or "They are too confining," most of the explanations are simply excuses! However, some individuals are sincerely fearful of wearing safety belts.

In many instances the individuals are afraid that they will be crushed to death during an accident. As a result, they mistakenly believe that they are much safer by being thrown out of the automobile than by remaining confined within the vehicle. Unfortunately, this belief is founded upon newspaper and television reports of infrequent cases in which the occupants have been thrown out of the automobiles into dense brush, muddy ditches, snowbanks, and other soft spots. Most people, however, are not as lucky and end up lying dead on the hard pavement or under the wheels of another vehicle. According to researchers at Cornell University, a driver's chances of being killed are five times greater if he is thrown from the automobile than if he is held inside the hard, protective shell of the vehicle.

In other cases the individuals are afraid that they will be trapped in the car by the safety belts while the vehicle burns or sinks in deep water. Consequently, they want to be able to get out of the automobile quickly in these types of accidents. In actuality, safety belts can be unfastened in a second. Furthermore, automobile accidents involving fire and water are relatively rare, occurring in less than 3 percent of all injury-producing collisions, but when they do occur, automobile occupants are undoubtedly better-off wearing safety belts.[6] Since safety belts keep the users firmly in position, the driver and his passengers are less likely to be stunned or knocked unconscious during an accident and are better able to escape the vehicle before the fire or the water can reach them.

In addition to fear, many individuals do not wear their safety belts because they believe that the belts are unnecessary at low speeds or on short trips in the community. The truth is that all driving is dangerous. Unfortunately, many persons believe that in a low-speed accident they can adequately protect themselves from being thrown forward by firmly bracing their hands against the dashboard or the steering wheel. Actually, in an abrupt stop at only thirty miles per hour, an individual would need to generate a force of nearly twenty-three hundred pounds to keep himself in place on the seat. Ironically, this requires as much strength as singlehandedly holding up an elephant. According to accident statistics, more than one-half of all injury-producing mishaps occur at speeds of less than forty miles per hour.[7] In addition, fatalities involving nonbelted occupants have been recorded at speeds as low as twelve miles per hour.[8] Other statistics show that three out of every four fatal accidents occur within twenty-five

---

6. *There Are Lots of Safety Belt Myths—Why Not Consider the Truths?* (Washington, D.C.: U.S. Government Printing Office, June, 1972), p. 6.
7. *Safety Belt Myths*, p. 2.
8. *Safety Belt Myths*, p. 2.

miles of home.[9] Thus, low speeds and short trips can be just as deadly as high speeds and long trips.

Selecting a Reliable Child Restraint System

The availability of safety belts to practically all passenger car occupants is an important first step in the prevention of serious injuries and deaths from traffic accidents. However, as mentioned earlier in this chapter, safety belts must be worn at all times by all occupants if the traffic death toll is to be reduced. Yet, while adults have the option of wearing or not wearing safety belts, small children are less fortunate. Because of their anatomical features, children are often unable to use the same safety belts that adults wear. As Alsever notes,

> The infant and young child have relatively larger and heavier heads than adults, with a higher center of gravity in both sitting and erect postures, and proportionately shorter lower extremities. Consequently, he tends to be top heavy and becomes airborne more readily than does the older child or adult. Thus if a child is prematurely placed in an adult seat belt, he may, in the event of sudden deceleration, be pulled up out of the belt and somersaulted toward the point of impact like a projectile.[10]

By the time children reach four years of age, most of them are able to wear adult safety belts, but since age is often a poor index of physical maturity, the best guide to whether or not a child over four years of age can use adult belts is his weight and his height. If he weighs at least fifty pounds, he can safely wear the lap-restraint belt; if he is at least fifty-five inches tall, he can safely wear the chest-restraint belt. As with adults, the chest-restraint belt should never be worn without the lap-restraint belt.

For children under four years of age, some special type of restraining device must be used. This becomes even more important when one considers that more than sixteen hundred children under the age of four years are killed in motor-vehicle accidents every year. Fortunately, the problem of selecting a reliable child restraint system has been greatly simplified by federal law. Under Safety Standard No. 213, "Every child car seat—built to seat and restrain the child—manufactured on or after April 1, 1971, must meet the performance requirements set by the safety standard."[11] This standard is designed to assure that child restraint devices will provide adequate protection for children.

---

9. *Safety Belt Myths,* p. 2.
10. William D. Alsever, "The Child's Place in the Car," *American Family Physician,* February, 1971, p. 168.
11. *What to Buy in Child Restraint Systems.* (Washington, D.C.: U.S. Government Printing Office, June, 1972), p. 9.

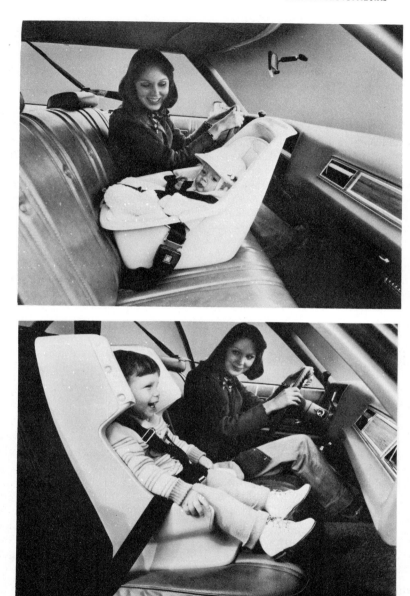

Figure 3.2   (Top) Infant Love Seat—designed for babies from birth to twenty pounds and (Bottom) Child Love Seat—designed for children between twenty-one and forty pounds and under forty inches in height. (Courtesy of the General Motors Corporation)

When purchasing a child restraint system, parents should always make certain that the device has met all of the requirements of the standard which were in effect on the date of its manufacture. This can be verified quite easily, in addition to determining the proper device for a child of a given weight and height, by reading the label on the system. By federal law a label must be attached to all child-restraint devices and must contain the following information:

> Month, year and place of manufacture, plus manufacturer's name.
>
> Manufacturer's recommendation for weight and height of child for whom the seat will give the required protection.
>
> The types of motor vehicles and all seating positions in the vehicle where the seat should be safely used.
>
> Displayed either on the child seat or on its container must be the manufacturer's certification that the child seat does comply with the requirements of Federal Motor Vehicle Standard No. 213.[12]

In addition to the label, Federal Safety Standard No. 213 requires that the manufacturer include a set of printed, step-by-step, installation instructions with each child restraint system. Parents should follow these instructions carefully. In providing full protection for the child, correct installation can be just as important as the design of the system.

Why Air Bags Have Been Introduced

Since safety belts were introduced as mandatory equipment in the late 1960s, traffic safety officials have been extremely confident that the belts could reduce the annual traffic death toll by as much as one-fourth. However, safety belts are designed to be an active restraint system. If automobile occupants fail to fasten the belts, the devices cannot protect them in a collision. Today, despite large-scale promotional efforts, only a small percentage of the drivers in this country are taking advantage of the protection afforded by safety belts. For this reason, the National Highway Traffic Safety Administration has established requirements for a passive restraint system, which does not demand the cooperation of automobile occupants, among the provisions in Federal Safety Standard No. 208.

Over the past few years, automotive designers and manufacturers have introduced numerous experimental passive restraint systems, such as blankets that deploy in front of the occupants, nets that drop from the roof in front of the occupants, belt systems that automatically enclose the occupants as they shut the doors of the vehicle, and air bags that inflate in front of the occupants. However, at present, only the air bags provide total body restraint for the driver and his passengers.

---

12. *What to Buy in Child Restraint Systems,* p. 9.

THE AIR BAG PASSIVE RESTRAINT SYSTEM

The air bag passive restraint system is composed of six basic parts: the front bumper detector, the dashboard sensor, the passenger's air bag and inflator assembly, the driver knee restraint, and the passenger's lap restraint system. Each of these components perform an important function in the injury prevention capabilities of the air bag during a crash.

When the ignition of the car is started, an indicator lamp on the instrument panel will glow for 4-6 seconds. This charges a capacitor which will fire the air bags even if the battery is destroyed in a crash. If the light goes out, the air bag system is operable. However, if the lamp continues to glow, fails to light up or lights up while you are driving, the system may have a malfunction and might not work properly in the event of a crash. Because there may be no air bag protection, the car should immediately be taken to the dealer for analysis and correction.

The GM air bag unit is a dual level system. When the car is involved in a crash with another vehicle or solid object at 11-17 miles per hour, the sudden deceleration causes the pendulum in the dashboard sensor to move forward and close a contact. The circuit then sends a signal to the air tanks and inflator assemblies where argon gas is stored. The gas expands and deploys the air bags at a low threshold level which restrains the occupants in a slow soft manner.

If the crash is over 17 miles per hour and the forces continue on the car, the air tanks continue to supply gas to the air bags and they are activated at a high threshold level. This provides faster protection as the occupants are thrown forward into the air bags.

The driver knee restraint functions to keep the driver from sliding under the deploying air bag during a crash if he is not wearing his lap belt. It holds the lower portion of the driver's body in place so the upper half of his torso is in the optimum position during deployment.

The front bumper detector is a backup system to the dashboard sensor. It is there to assure the dash detector that a real crash is taking place. It also reduces the inflation time needed to protect the occupants when the front bumper rather than the car body makes contact with an object. A sudden deceleration causes the leaf spring in the bumper detector to move forward and close a contact. This sends a signal to the dashboard sensor which completes the circuit and activates the inflators to deploy the air bags.

The passenger air bags have side vents which allow the gas to escape as they are being inflated. Thus, there is minimum rebound of the occupant as he moves forward into the air bags. It is comparable to striking a partially inflated beach ball.

The steering wheel air bag does not vent immediately, but rebound is controlled through the collapsible steering column shaft assembly.

Figure 3.3   Description of the air bag system. (Reproduced from *Automotive Air Bags—Questions and Answers,* 6th ed., August, 1974, n.p., courtesy of Allstate Insurance Companies)

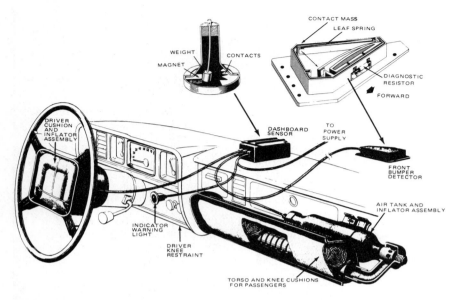

Figure 3.4   Diagram of the air bag system. (Reproduced from *Automotive Air Bags—Questions and Answers,* 6th ed., August, 1974, np., courtesy of Allstate Insurance Companies)

Air bags, officially called the Inflatable Occupant Restraint System for Automobile Vehicles, are not a recent innovation. Actually, several systems were patented in the early 1950's. The principle underlying air bags is simple: when the car is involved in a crash of a predetermined intensity, approximately eleven miles per hour, the bags will inflate automatically in a fraction of a second with argon gas, thus permitting the occupants to strike the soft bags rather than the hard interior of the car. Since the primary objective of air bags is to reduce or prevent injuries and deaths in frontal collisions, the bags do not provide the driver and his passengers with protection in low-speed crashes, side collisions, rear-end impacts, and rollovers. However, this problem can be easily solved. Automobile occupants should wear their lap-restraint belts at all times. As Martens explains,

> Air bags perform their safety function in frontal impacts, of which 70 percent of the crash modes involve frontal impact by at least one vehicle. Those 15-20 percent of the occupants presently wearing their lap belts would be protected in the remaining 30 percent of the crash modes. Air bags used in conjunction with lap belts offer the best protection possible for automobile occupants in all types of crashes.[13]

---

13. Jack E. Martens, *Why Your Best Life Insurance Is A Passive Restraint* (New York: Society of Automotive Engineers, Inc., 1975), p. 6.

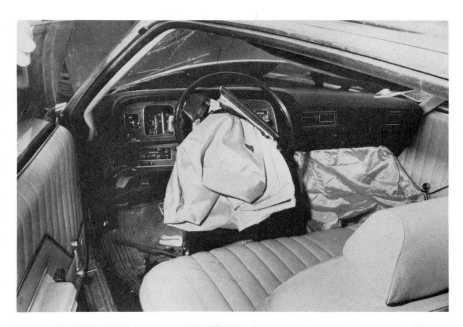

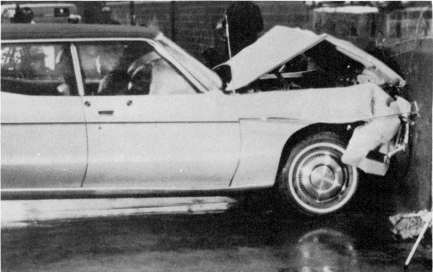

Figure 3.5   (Top) Deployed air bags in a wrecked car illustrate how the driver and the right-front passenger are protected during a collision. (Bottom) In a test situation, the air bag inflates in a fraction of a second to cushion the passenger as he hurtles toward the dash. (Courtesy of Allstate Insurance Companies)

In addition, the lap-restraint belt keeps the driver in position behind the wheel, thus permitting him to maintain control of his car during a sudden or sharp evasive maneuver.

Once the air bags have deployed in the vehicle, they cannot be repaired. The bags must be replaced by a skilled technician. Since they are replaced as a module, the replacement is similar to the replacement of a television picture tube. While new bags will normally cost approximately two hundred dollars, the automobile owner's insurance company will pay the charges as a part of its collision and comprehensive insurance coverage.

Although the effectiveness of air bags still must be proven over the years by large-scale public usage, traffic safety officials nevertheless are highly optimistic. They estimate that air bags can reduce deaths due to automobile accidents by one-third within ten years of their introduction.[14] However, the public is far less optimistic. Because people still know very little about the bags, many individuals naturally have doubts and fears about the presence of air bags in their vehicles.

In many cases the individuals are afraid that the air bags will inadvertently deploy, thus causing the driver to lose control of the automobile. However, this is not a problem, since the air bags are inflated for a maximum of one-half second or about the length of time that a sneezing driver has his eyes closed. As shown in a study by Ziperman and Smith, even drivers who are startled by the inadvertent deployment of the air bags are able to maintain good control of their vehicles.[15] In addition, the reliability of the sensors is such that accidental inflation or deployment is extremely remote. Based upon the computations of the Department of Transportation, ". . . every 6,000th driver might expect one such inadvertent deployment during his 54 driving years."[16]

In other cases the individuals are afraid that the rapid expansion of the air bags within the car will damage the eardrums of the occupants. In numerous tests by Allstate Insurance Companies, researchers found that the occupants did not experience any hearing change, damage, or discomfort.[17] Apparently, while scarred eardrums may be damaged, normal ears are not affected.

Choosing a Safer Car

For years the big car has been a status symbol for the American driver. However, views and values in this country are rapidly changing. Today, as

---

14. John D. States, "Air Bags: Some Myths Dispelled," *Journal of Trauma,* February, 1972, p. 178.
15. H. Haskell Ziperman and George R. Smith, "Startle Reaction to Air-Bag Restraints," *The Journal of the American Medical Association,* August 4, 1975, p. 436.
16. Allstate Insurance Companies, *Automotive Air Bags—Questions and Answers* (Northbrook, Illinois: Allstate, 6th ed., August, 1974), n.p.
17. Allstate Insurance Companies, np.

McCluggage notes, "No longer is it officially 'American' to buy the biggest car on the block."[18] Motivated by the rising cost of operating a car, millions of people have begun to reexamine their automotive needs. As a result, in recent years the small car has enjoyed tremendous popularity.

Obviously, the small car has many attractive features for potential buyers. For the price of a standard-size car without any optional accessories, the driver can purchase a small car with an automatic transmission, air-conditioning, a radio, and other options. In addition, compared to the big car, the small car is less expensive to operate, is easier to handle in tight spaces, and has greater maneuverability in emergencies. As a bonus, some insurance companies even offer discounts to small-car drivers.

On the other hand, the small car does have a few unattractive features. For a large-size person, the small car is awkwardly confining and generally uncomfortable on long trips. Furthermore, the small vehicle is not a good package or luggage hauler and does not possess the necessary power for towing trailers or easily passing other cars on the highway. More important, in comparison to the big car, the small car is not as safe for the driver and the occupants.

In studies by the University of North Carolina Highway Safety Research Center, the New York State Department of Motor Vehicles, the New Jersey Highway Authority, and the University of Michigan Highway Safety Research Institute, researchers found that a proportionately greater number of serious injuries and deaths occurred in the small cars than in the big cars—as much as three times greater in some small cars. Furthermore, in almost every accident between a big car and a small car, the occupants of the small car were more seriously injured than the occupants of the big car.

While the results of these studies apparently condemn the small vehicle, many questions about the safety of the small car still remain unanswered. As critics of the studies explain, most small-car drivers are in the under thirty age group, the most accident-involved segment of the driving population. Thus, the seriousness of small-car accidents may result because young people drive faster and take greater chances in traffic. In addition, in accidents between big cars and even bigger cars, the occupants of the big cars suffered a proportionally higher number of serious injuries and deaths, a ratio similar to the comparison between small cars and big cars. Thus, according to small-car proponents, the safety of any vehicle during an accident is dependent upon the relative sizes of the cars that are involved. As McCluggage quips, ". . . to come through a collision unscathed, one would best be driving a well-padded Sherman tank."[19]

Despite the controversy surrounding small-car safety, one statement remains unquestioned: by the laws of physics, in any collision the lighter vehi-

---

18. Denise McCluggage, "Big Car, Small Car—Which Is for You?," *American Home,* October, 1973, p. 23.
19. Denise McCluggage, p. 23.

cle must absorb more of the impact forces than the heavier vehicle. Consequently, "All other things being equal, small cars are not as safe as larger cars."[20] Before buying a small vehicle, the driver should consider certain fundamental facts about small-car safety: (1) in a two-vehicle collision, the small car is more likely to collide with a big car, since more of the big cars are on the road; and (2) when a small car collides with a big car, the driver and the passengers of the small vehicle are more likely to be seriously injured or killed than the occupants of the big car.

Maintaining a Safer Automobile

Mechanical failures are rarely publicized as causes of traffic accidents. One reason for this is that few victims live to tell about the failures. On a rural highway near Hannibal, Missouri, a car veered off the road and crashed into a tree. Apparently, as the police theorized, the driver had fallen asleep at the wheel. However, through the efforts of a local garage mechanic, the police soon learned the real reason for the accident. A small piece in the steering mechanism had snapped, and as a result, the driver was unable to control his vehicle.

According to some safety experts, approximately one out of every five cars on the road has a potentially dangerous defect. Even though the average driver is not trained to make mechanical repairs, he should learn to recognize the signs of impending problems and to seek professional help in correcting the situations. Better still, he should have his vehicle inspected at regular intervals by a qualified, reliable mechanic.

Steering Mechanism

Fortunately, a failure of the steering mechanism is extremely slight if the driver recognizes the early warning signs of the problem. These signs include a steering wheel that is difficult to turn, indicating poor lubrication and possibly excessive wear, a steering wheel that will turn several inches before the wheels begin to turn, indicating a loose steering mechanism, and a steering wheel that begins to "shimmy" or shake from side to side at normal driving speeds, also indicating a loose steering mechanism. When any of these signs appear, the driver should explain the problem to his mechanic and authorize a thorough tightening and lubrication of the entire steering mechanism.

Brakes

Brake problems, like steering problems, usually provide ample warning for the driver. If the brakes do not grip when the brake pedal has been

---

20. "Are Small Cars Safe?," *Changing Times,* October, 1973, p. 13.

depressed a short distance (one-half inch for power brakes or one inch for standard brakes), if they take hold violently, or if they cause the car to pull to the left or right, an adjustment of the brakes is needed. On the other hand, if a scratchy sound can be heard when the brakes are applied, new brake linings should be installed, since the old linings are worn completely away and the rivets are hitting the inside of the brake drum.

In addition, the hydraulic fluid in the braking system should be maintained at the proper level. A low-fluid level can easily lead to a complete brake failure. If the brake pedal must be "pumped" to obtain a braking effect, this is a sure sign that fluid needs to be added to the system.

While a qualified mechanic can easily and accurately test the brakes in his shop, the driver can obtain a rough estimate of the ability of the brakes to stop the car safely by depressing the brake pedal at a marked spot while traveling at twenty miles per hour. If the distance from the spot to the front of the stopped vehicle is greater than twenty-five feet, the brakes should be checked by a mechanic. However, for the results of the test to be accurate, the driver must conduct the test on a dry, smooth surface.

Tires

Although the brakes stop the wheels, the tires actually stop the car. Thus, if the tires are allowed to become badly worn or damaged, the driver's chances of becoming involved in an accident are greatly increased. For example, bald tires skid easier, require more stopping distance on wet surfaces, and blow easier than tires with good tread. For this reason, the driver should never allow the tread on a tire to become less than a minimum of one-sixteenth inch deep. To check the depth of the tread, the individual should insert the top edge of a penny into the grooves of the tire. If the tread does not cover at least the top edge of Lincoln's head, the tire should be replaced as soon as possible. (See Figure 3.6) On the other hand, any tire with "wear bars," bald lines across the surface of the tread, should be replaced immediately, since the bald spots can easily lead to stopping problems in certain situations. (See Figure 3.6)

Besides maintaining good tread depth on the tires, the driver should make certain that the tread wears evenly. New tires should always be balanced before they are installed, and thereafter, they should be rotated every five thousand miles. Furthermore, since underinflation and overinflation also affect how evenly tread wears, tires should be inflated to the pressure recommended by the automobile owner's manual. According to safety officials, underinflation of the tires will cause excessive wear on the outside of the tread, make the car more difficult to steer, and cause an excessive buildup of heat within the tires that may result in a blowout. On the other hand, overinflation of the tires will cause excessive wear on the middle of the tread, reduce traction by decreasing the area of the tires on the road surface, and produce strain on the tire sidewalls that may lead to a blowout.

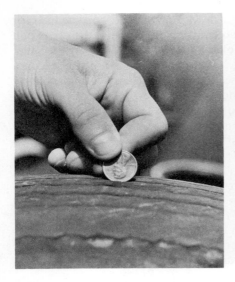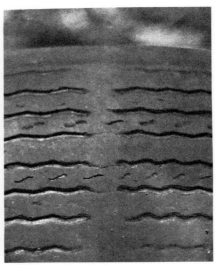

Figure 3.6   (Left) Lincoln-penny test for tread depth and (Right) wear bar on an automobile tire.

Lights

When the term "lights" is mentioned in connection with the automobile, most people automatically think of "headlights." However, the terms are far from synonymous, not only in meaning but also in importance. In addition to the headlights, automobile lights include turn signals, brake lights, parking lights, taillights, and back-up lights. Without this array of lights, the automobile driver could not communicate his intentions, such as turning and stopping, much less see or be seen at night.

Thus, before starting to drive in traffic, the driver should always check the lights. This can be accomplished quite easily by observing the reflections on the garage wall. Then, if a bulb has burned out or if a fuse has blown, it can be replaced before an accident can occur. Also, dirt and dried bugs should be periodically removed from the lights with soap and water. This is especially important for the headlights, since such accumulations may reduce illumination by as much as one-third.

The garage is also a good place to check the alignment of the headlights. With the lights on low beam, one-inch marks should be made on the garage wall, one at the center of each light spot. Three inches below these marks, two more marks should be made. The automobile should then be moved backward twenty-five feet, and the headlights should be switched to high beam. If the headlights are aligned, the second marks will be at the center of the new light spots. If either mark or both of the marks are not at the center, the driver should have the headlights realigned.

Exhaust System

Most people can easily understand how faulty steering mechanisms, brakes, tires, and lights can lead to accidents, but few people realize that a faulty exhaust system may be just as dangerous. Unfortunately, most persons mistakenly believe that a leaky exhaust system presents very little danger in a moving vehicle. (See Figure 3.7) Although most cases of carbon monoxide poisoning occur when cars are idled in closed garages, many people have died from carbon monoxide poisoning while traveling along highways. Undoubtedly, many single-car accidents in which drivers had fallen asleep at the wheel were actually caused by the loss of consciousness associated with carbon monoxide poisoning. For this reason, the driver should have the exhaust system checked periodically by a reliable mechanic and have any defective parts repaired or replaced.

Other Automotive Equipment

In addition to the "Critical Five" (steering mechanism, brakes, tires, lights, and exhaust system), other pieces of automotive equipment can readily lead to accidents if they are allowed to become defective. Consequently, windshield wipers should be refurbished with new blades and arms when they are needed; horns, defrosters, and mirrors should be maintained in proper working condition; and accelerators should be checked at the first sign of sticking.

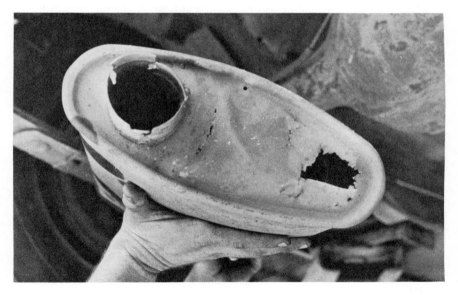

Figure 3.7   A faulty exhaust system can easily lead to carbon monoxide poisoning, even in a moving vehicle.

Driving Under the Influence of Alcohol or Drugs

That alcohol is a major problem for traffic safety officials can hardly be questioned! Drinking has been shown to be a factor in at least one-half of all fatal motor-vehicle accidents. In addition, statistics show that if a driver has consumed a drink, his chances of becoming involved in an accident are six times greater than if he had not consumed the drink.[21] On the other hand, if a person is driving while drunk, his chances of having an accident are increased twenty-five to fifty times.[22]

Strangely enough, alcoholics are not the primary problem on the streets and highways. Perhaps because the alcoholic is often greatly incapacitated by the liquor, he stays off the highway or gets off the highway before he can cause an accident. The real problem involves three distinct groups: problem drinkers (many of whom are not blatant alcoholics), teenagers, and heavy social drinkers. These groups comprise the overwhelming majority of the drinking drivers who are involved in alcohol-related accidents. The reason for their involvement is readily apparent: most people in these groups possess little knowledge about how alcohol affects the body.

Depending upon a person's body weight, the amount of food in his stomach, and the length of time in which the drinks are consumed, reactions to alcohol vary from person to person and from time to time in a given person. The less of any of the above factors, the greater are the effects of alcohol, especially on driving ability. Yet, regardless of these variations, traffic safety officials stress that as little as two to three ounces of whiskey or four twelve-ounce bottles of beer will significantly affect driving ability. A driver who has consumed this amount of alcohol has slower reflexes, poorer coordination and timing, decreased peripheral vision, reduced light and sound discrimination, and poorer judgment. Still, this amount of alcohol is approximately one-half of the quantity which is needed to produce the 0.10 percent blood alcohol level recognized in most states as an indication that a driver is intoxicated or driving under the influence.

Although the old saying "Don't drink and then drive." is still the best advice, sometimes this warning is not really practical. However, to drink and then expect cold showers, exercise, or hot coffee to hurry the sobering-up process is even more impractical, for time is the only way to remove alcohol from the body. Thus, to permit the effects of the alcohol to wear off, the driver should do his drinking early and then allow one hour of nondrinking time before driving for every ounce of whiskey or its equivalent that has been consumed.

---

21. Nicholas J. Chetta, "Alcohol, Drugs and Driving," *The Journal of the Louisiana State Medical Society,* September, 1967, p. 345.
22. Chetta, p. 345.

While alcohol is probably the only drug that is a frequent cause of automobile accidents, other drugs can easily impair a person's ability to operate a motor vehicle. For example, antihistamines, which are used to relieve nasal congestion and to fight colds, allergies, and motion sickness, and barbiturates, which are used to calm nervousness and induce sleep, may cause inattention, confusion, and drowsiness. Tranquilizers, which are used to relieve anxiety, may cause dizziness, drowsiness, double vision, and impaired dexterity, and amphetamines, which are used to increase alertness and efficiency for a short time, may cause dizziness, agitation, reduced concentration, fatigue, and hallucinations when the effects of the drug wear off. Since these drugs, as well as other medications frequently prescribed by physicians, can impair driving ability and lead to an accident, the individual should avoid taking any type of medicine before he drives. Better still, he should let another person drive.

Handling Driving Emergencies

Most driving emergencies cannot be practiced. However, advanced planning and knowledge about the proper reactions in emergencies can be beneficial. Even in situations which demand an immediate reaction, a driver with advanced knowledge about how to react is more likely to react properly than a driver with little or no knowledge. The following pages include some driving emergencies and the correct ways to react to them.

Skidding

Rain, snow, ice, or loose gravel can cause an automobile to skid, but the method of regaining control of the vehicle is the same regardless of the condition of the road surface. Quite simply, during a skid, the driver should always steer in the direction that he wants to travel. In other words, if the rear of the car skids to the right, he should turn the steering wheel to the right, but if the rear of the car skids to the left, he should turn the steering wheel to the left. In addition, the driver should avoid applying the brakes or removing his foot suddenly from the accelerator, since either action will intensify the skid.

Tire Blowout

While a tubeless tire will normally retain enough air to allow a safe stop after a sudden blowout, the driver will still encounter some difficulty in controlling the vehicle. As a rule, the blowout of a front tire will cause the car to pull toward the side of the blown tire, but the blowout of a back tire will cause the rear of the car to swerve from side to side. In either situation the driver should retain a firm grip on the steering wheel with both hands, depress the brake pedal gradually, and steer the vehicle slowly onto the shoulder of the road.

Brake Failure

A failure of the brakes, while extremely frightening for the driver, does not need to automatically result in an injury-producing accident. If the brake pedal moves all the way to the floor without activating the brakes, the driver should immediately "pump" the pedal. If this maneuver fails to build up sufficient pressure to restore the brakes, he should then shift into a lower gear and gradually apply the parking brake. If this maneuver also fails, the driver must then employ his last and most drastic method for stopping the vehicle: he should gently sideswipe "weak" objects, such as the curb, roadside embankment, bushes, or even parked cars.

Stuck Accelerator

A stuck accelerator can easily send a driver racing through heavy traffic at breakneck speeds. Fortunately, however, this situation is one of the easiest emergencies to handle. If there is no immediate danger or urgent need to stop, the driver should first attempt to pry up the accelerator pedal with his foot. If this fails or if the automobile must be stopped quickly, the driver should then switch the ignition key to the "off," not the "lock," position and apply the brakes. Although steering and braking will be more difficult in vehicles equipped with power steering and power brakes, even a small woman can usually manage to bring the vehicle to a stop in this situation.

Blinded by Oncoming Vehicle

A driver should never deliberately look into the headlights of an oncoming vehicle. However, if the vehicle's headlight beams are set on "high" or aimed abnormally high while they are set on "low," the driver may still find himself momentarily blinded by the sudden brightness. If this occurs, he should immediately look toward the right edge of the road, reduce speed, and steer the car as far to the right as possible without leaving the roadway. Even while looking away from the approaching car, the driver will be able to see the vehicle with his side or peripheral vision.

Sudden Vision Obstruction

A piece of paper which suddenly blows onto the windshield or a hood which suddenly opens can easily obstruct the view of a driver and lead to an injury-producing accident. Sometimes, as in the case of the paper, the driver will be able to see around or under the obstruction until he can stop the car and remove the item. At other times, as in the case of the hood, he will be forced to look through the side windows until he can slow the vehicle sufficiently to steer off the roadway and onto the shoulder. In either situation the driver should judge his position on the roadway by looking at the center line or the lane-dividing line.

Wrong-lane Driver

An encounter with a wrong-lane driver is one of the most frightening emergencies that any driver can experience. Needless to say, the primary goal in this situation is to avoid a head-on collision. As a rule, the person should first try to attract the driver's attention by blowing the horn without interruption and by rapidly switching the headlights from low beam to high beam. If these actions are unsuccessful, the individual should then begin braking and steering the automobile toward the right shoulder of the highway. Since the wrong-lane driver may suddenly steer back into his lane, the person should never attempt to outguess the driver by steering across his lane toward the left shoulder of the highway.

Passing Emergency

In attempting to pass cars, drivers sometimes misjudge the speed or the distance of oncoming vehicles and, as a result, find themselves in the wrong lanes and in danger of becoming involved in head-on collisions. Obviously, in this situation the driver should brake gently and return to the right-hand lane. However, if the vehicle being passed suddenly slows, he should accelerate, pass the car, and then steer into the right-hand lane again. If neither maneuver can be accomplished quickly, the driver should immediately steer for the right-hand lane, even though this action may force the car being passed off the highway. As in the preceding emergency, the primary goal in this situation is to avoid a head-on collision.

Impending Rear-end Collision

Besides producing whiplash injury, a rear-end collision can easily push the car into the path of an oncoming vehicle or into a group of pedestrians. As a rule, while the car is stopped for a left-hand turn, the driver should keep the wheels straight so the vehicle will be pushed forward, rather than left into the lane of oncoming traffic, if it is struck from the rear. On the other hand, when approaching a crosswalk, the driver should stop at least ten feet behind the nearest line so the vehicle will not be pushed into pedestrians if it is struck from the rear. In either situation, upon seeing an impending rear-ender, the driver should grasp the steering wheel securely with both hands and depress the brake pedal firmly.

Fire Under the Hood

Most fires under hoods start in the cars' electrical systems and, as a result, are relatively minor in both size and severity. While a portable fire extinguisher can easily put out this type of fire, most people do not carry extinguishers in their automobiles. In this situation the driver should secure the jack handle from the trunk and pry loose the battery cables. Then, he can easily smother the fire with heavy clothing, snow, mud, or dirt. However, if the fire spreads out of control, the driver should close the hood and quickly move at least fifty feet away from the car, since the gas tank may explode.

Sinking in Water

Accidents involving water are extremely rare, but when they do occur, the accidents almost always catch the driver and his passengers unprepared. In cooperation with the American National Red Cross, the Michigan State Highway Department, and the Indiana University Department of Health and Safety, the Michigan State Police conducted a study on vehicle submersion.[23] A two-door compact, a standard two-door sedan, a four-door sedan, and a four-door station wagon were repeatedly plunged right-side up, upside down, and sideways into a water-filled pit with combinations of all windows closed, one window open, and more than one window open.

The results of this study revealed that a vehicle will float for three to ten minutes after it hits the water. Normally, during this period of time, the driver and his passengers can open the windows and swim toward shore. However, if the automobile begins to sink, the occupants will have to wait until the vehicle settles on the bottom, since the windows and the doors cannot be opened against the pressure of the water. Fortunately, regardless of the position in which the vehicle enters the water, the automobile will settle in a wheels-down position about 85 percent of the time. Using the ever-present trapped bubble of air which is usually located at the highest point of the passenger compartment, the occupants can breathe easily until they are ready to open the windows or the doors and push for the surface.

Determining a Safe Following Distance

For many years traffic safety experts have recommended the "one-for-ten" rule as a guide for determining a safe following distance. According to this rule, the driver should remain at least one car length behind the vehicle he is following for every ten miles per hour of speed. However, since the one-for-ten rule provides only a minimum safe following distance, some experts have even suggested "two-for-ten" and "three-for-ten" rules.

---

23. "What to Do If Your Car Goes into Water," *Popular Mechanics,* August, 1970, pp. 92-95, 182.

Actually, all of these rules are quite limited in practicality, since few drivers can accurately judge following distance, particularly at night. For this reason, the National Safety Council has endorsed the "Second Interval Concept" as an aid in determining a safe following distance.

A relatively simple notion, the Second Interval Concept is explained as follows:

> Briefly, the "Second" Interval concept is based on the travel time in seconds needed to cover the length of a safe following distance. At any speed, this is about 1.1/3 seconds—the time it takes the motorist to say "one-thousand-one, one thousand . . . ." To determine a safe following distance, the motorist watches the vehicle ahead of him passing some definite spot or object, such as a light post, tar strip, etc. He then counts normally to himself "one-thousand-one, one-thousand-two." If the motorist passes the spot before finishing the first six syllables, he knows he is too close.[24]

By design the Second Interval Concept is equivalent to one and one-half vehicle lengths for every ten miles per hour of speed, thus providing an even safer following distance than that provided by the popular one-for-ten rule.

For drivers of trucks and buses, the two seconds will not provide a safe following distance, since their vehicles are longer than the automobile. However, the truck or bus driver can easily devise his own unique second interval. Simply, he should divide the length in feet of his vehicle by ten and then, rounding any fraction to the next highest whole number, use this number instead of the normal two seconds. This extra time will provide plenty of stopping distance for the longer vehicle.

Naturally, like the one-for-ten rule, the Second Interval Concept is calculated to provide a safe following distance in good weather, that is, when the roadway surface is dry. In bad weather, such as when the roadway is wet or icy, the number of seconds which is normally used in the concept will not provide adequate stopping distance in an emergency. Thus, to assure a safe following distance in bad weather, the driver should double or even triple the second interval.

Resource Materials

Allstate Insurance Companies
Allstate Plaza
Northbrook, Illinois 60062

American Association of Motor Vehicle Administrators
1828 L Street, N.W.
Washington, D.C. 20036

24. "National Safety Council Position on the 'Second' Interval Concept," November 20, 1967.

American Association of State Highway
and Transportation Officials
341 National Press Building
Washington, D.C. 20004

American Automobile Association
1712 G Street, N.W.
Washington, D.C. 20006

American Driver and Traffic Safety
Education Association
1201 16th Street, N.W.
Washington, D.C. 20036

American Medical Association
Committee on Medical Aspects of
Automotive Safety
535 North Dearborn Street
Chicago, Illinois 60610

American Society for Safety Engineers
850 Busse Highway
New York City, New York 10017

Cocoon Club
51 Weaver Street
Greenwich, Connecticut 06380
(See Chapter 15—Maintaining Interest
in Safety—Recognition organizations)

Drunk Driver
Box 2345
Rockville, Maryland 20852

Employers Mutual of Wausau
Safety Engineering Department
407 Grant Street
Wausau, Wisconsin 55402

Eno Foundation for Highway Traffic
Control
Westport, Connecticut 06880

Ford Safety Seats
Ford Motor Company
P.O. Box 3000
Livonia, Michigan 48151

G.M. Love Seats
P.O. Box 1973
Northend Station
Detroit, Michigan 48202

Highway Research Board
2101 Constitution Avenue
Washington, D.C. 20418

Highway Traffic Safety Center
Michigan State University
East Lansing, Michigan 48823

Highway Users Federation for Safety
and Mobility
1776 Massachusetts Avenue, N.W.
Washington, D.C. 20036

Institute of Traffic Engineers
2029 K Street, N.W.
Washington, D.C. 20006

Insurance Institute of Highway Safety
Watergate 600
Washington, D.C. 20037

Kangaroo Club International
P.O. Box 950
Coatesville, Pennsylvania 19320
(See Chapter 15—Maintaining Interest
in Safety—Recognition organiza-
tions)

Motor Vehicle Manufacturers Association of the United States, Inc.
320 New Center Building
Detroit, Michigan 48202

National Committee on Traffic Law
Enforcement
744 Broad Street
Newark, New Jersey 07100

National Committee on Traffic Training
700 Hill Building
Washington, D.C. 20006

National Committee on Uniform Laws
and Ordinances
Suite 430
1776 Massachusetts Avenue, N.Y.
Washington, D.C. 20036

National Safety Council
444 North Michigan Avenue
Chicago, Illinois 60611

North American Association of Alcoholism Programs
1611 Deveonshire Drive
Columbia, South Carolina 29204

Northwestern University Traffic Institute
405 Church Street
Evanston, Illinois 60204

Safe Winter Driving League
625 North Michigan Avenue
Chicago, Illinois 60611

Society of Automotive Engineers, Inc.
Two Pennsylvania Plaza
New York City, New York 10001

State and Local Officials' National Highway Safety Committee
912 Barr Building
Washington, D.C. 20006

U.S. Department of Transportation
National Highway Traffic Safety Administration
Washington, D.C. 20590
Toll-free Auto Safety Hot Line: 800-424-9393

Activities

1. Develop an instrument to show how safety belts work, and prepare a demonstration before the class.

2. Prepare and submit to a local newspaper a short article on the importance of restraining children in the automobile. (Be sure to stress the use of approved child restraint devices.)

3. Compile a list of ten articles on the topic of air bags. Distribute a copy of the list to each member in the class.

4. Write a position paper "For" *or* "Against" buying and driving a small car.

5. Invite the mechanic from a local garage to speak to the class about the proper care of the automobile.

Questions

1. Why has the term "safety belts" replaced the old term "seat belts?"
2. "Safety belts have another side: they can cause injury." How does this statement actually reinforce the importance of wearing safety belts?
3. What are three reasons why some individuals are sincerely fearful of wearing safety belts?
4. Why are small children unable to wear the same safety belts that adults use?
5. What is the purpose of Federal Safety Standard No. 213?
6. Why have air bags been introduced into automotive design?

7. What two facts about small-car safety should always be considered before a person purchases a small vehicle?
8. What three groups of people make up the overwhelming majority of drinking drivers who are involved in alcohol-related crashes?
9. Why does the "one-for-ten" rule for determining a safe following distance lack practicality?
10. How can the Second Interval Concept be utilized in bad weather?

Selected References

Alsever, William D. "The Child's Place in the Car," *American Family Physician.* February, 1971, 167-70.

Allstate Insurance Companies. 6th ed. *Automotive Air Bags.* Northbrook, Illinois: Allstate, August, 1974.

"Are Small Cars Safe?" *Changing Times.* October, 1973, 11-13.

Chetta, Nicholas J. "Alcohol, Drugs and Driving," *The Journal of the Louisiana State Medical Society.* September, 1967, 344-47.

Crosby, Warren M., and J. Paul Costiloe. "Safety of Lap-Belt Restraint for Pregnant Victims of Automobile Collisions," *The New England Journal of Medicine.* March 25, 1971, 632-36.

Douglass, John M. "Protection of Automobile Occupants," *American Family Physician.* December, 1971, 117-24.

Finch, Alfred C. "A Following Distance You Can Count On," *Traffic Safety.* November, 1967, 12-14, 34-35.

Hames, Lee N. "Air Bags," *The Journal of the American Medical Association.* November 9, 1970, 1109.

Hodson-Walker, N. J. "The Value of Safety Belts: A Review," *Canadian Medical Association Journal.* February, 1970, 391-93.

"How to Cope with the Worst Driving Crises," *Good Housekeeping.* May, 1971, 188-89.

Martens, Jack E. *Why Your Best Life Insurance Is a Passive Restraint.* New York: Society of Automotive Engineers, Inc., 1975.

McCluggage, Denise. "Big Car, Small Car—Which Is for You?" *American Home.* October, 1973, 23-24, 26.

National Safety Council. *NSC Position Paper on the "Second" Interval Concept.* Chicago: NSC, November 20, 1967.

Shuldiner, Herbert. "Is Your Small Car Really More Dangerous?" *Popular Science.* May, 1971, 47-49, 118.

States, John D. "Air Bags: Some Myths Dispelled," *Journal of Trauma.* February, 1972, 178-79.

There Are Lots of Safety Belt Myths—Why Not Consider the Truths? Washington, D.C.: U.S. Government Printing Office, June, 1972.

Waller, Julian A. "Truths, Traps, and Tactics Concerning Alcohol, Other Drugs and Highway Safety," *California Medicine.* February, 1972, 10-15.

What to Buy in Child Restraint Systems. Washington, D.C.: U.S. Government Printing Office, June, 1972.

"What to Do If Your Car Goes Into the Water," *Popular Mechanics.* August, 1970, 92-95, 182.

Williams, James S., and John R. Kirkpatrick, "The Nature of Seat Belt Injuries," *Journal of Trauma.* March, 1971, 207-18.

Ziperman, H. Haskell, and George R. Smith. "Startle Reaction to Air-Bag Restraints," *The Journal of the American Medical Association.* August 4, 1975, 436-40.

Motorcycle Accidents

4

Every year more than three thousand Americans are killed in motorcycle accidents. According to the National Safety Council, the death rate for all motor vehicles is 3.3 per one hundred million miles of travel; for motorcycles the death rate is 13 per one hundred million miles of travel or almost four times greater.

However, some traffic safety officials feel that death rates do not reflect the true problem, since eight out of every ten motorcycle accidents result in injury or death, as compared to only one out of every ten automobile accidents. They estimate that a person's chances of being injured or killed are at least fifteen times greater on a motorcycle than in an automobile. As one expert quipped, "You're safer roller skating in a buffalo herd than riding on a motorcycle."

Attacking the Problem

Obviously, motorcycle driving can never be as safe as automobile driving, since the motorcyclist receives little or no protection from his vehicle. In a typical accident the motorcycle driver is catapulted over the handlebars into another vehicle or onto the hard pavement. If he survives the accident, his injuries usually resemble limb-shattering war wounds which often plague the person for the rest of his life.

Of all persons, physicians are naturally most familiar with the many types of injuries which are commonly sustained in motorcycle accidents. Consequently, with few exceptions, physicians do not recommend the motorcycle as a safe mode of transportation. As one surgeon explained, "My brain is monitored to live, live, live. I had to cut two legs off last week because of motorcycles. I regard the human machine as beautiful, and I destroyed part of it. I hated it. But to make them well, I had to take their legs. That is why I am so against motorcycles."

Still, motorcycling has been gaining in popularity at a phenomenal rate. While the total number of motor vehicles has increased by approximately 48 percent over the last ten years, the number of motorcycles has increased by almost 192 percent. Today, more than five million motorcycles are being operated on the roads. Undoubtedly, the leading factor in the motorcycle's surging popularity has been the changing image of the cycle and its driver. As a recent article notes,

> No longer does a motorcycle automatically conjure up a picture of the "Hell's Angels" gangs. Now the motorcycle is billed as a unique, slightly adventurous way for businessmen, families, campers, and college students to get around. [1]

With the leading cycle manufacturers pursuing an advertising policy of reaching the entire family, this new image will not change much in the near future. Fortunately or unfortunately, depending upon an individual's particular viewpoint, the motorcycle is and will continue to be an integral part of the traffic picture for many years.

Consequently, traffic safety officials are faced with a paradoxical situation. While the cycle is undoubtedly more dangerous to drive than an automobile, more and more people are purchasing and driving motorcycles every year. Obviously, the motorcycle driver's chances of avoiding serious injury or death will never approach those of the automobile driver, but they can be improved considerably if he chooses an appropriate cycle, wears protective equipment, and learns to drive properly. When combined with the automobile driver's acceptance of the motorcycle as a legitimate mode of travel, these precautions will help to make motorcycling as safe as possible.

Choosing an Appropriate Cycle

With the great variety of types, sizes, and brands of motorcycles on the market, choosing an appropriate cycle is often a complex problem, especially for the new cyclist. Sometimes, the decisions which must be made are quite confusing. However, certain general guidelines can simplify the process considerably.

Generally, the person must first decide which type of motorcycle will best meet his particular needs. For one who is interested in driving only on dirt roads and wooded trails, the most appropriate cycle is the dirt or trail bike. Designed to meet problems associated with off-road driving, the dirt bike is normally equipped with raised fenders, a high-mounted exhaust pipe, and knobbies, special tires with a block-type tread pattern that produces better traction on dirt surfaces. However, because of these special features, the dirt bike is unsuitable for on-road driving. The high exhaust pipe, which is unnecessary for on-road driving, exposes the motorcyclist to a needless

---

1. "Can Cycling Be Safe?," *Better Homes and Gardens,* May, 1972, p. 76.

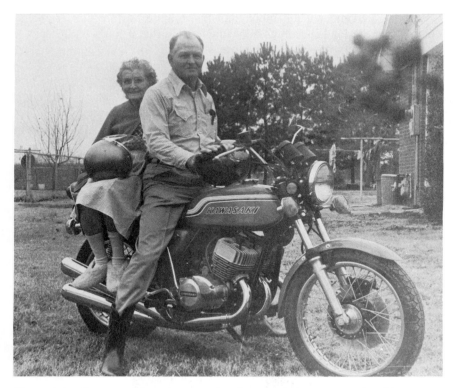

Figure 4.1   Demonstrating the changing image of the motorcycle, this woman celebrated her ninetieth birthday by taking her first ride on a motorcycle. (Courtesy of James Cortese, Memphis, Tennessee)

burn hazard, even when a heat shield is used. In addition, the knobbies, compared to conventional tread tires, produce poorer traction on paved roads and thus permit cornering spills on wet surfaces. Consequently, for the person who is interested in driving only on streets and highways, the most appropriate cycle is the street bike.

After deciding upon the type of motorcycle, the individual must determine which size engine is most suitable for his needs. As a rule, dirt bikes should be selected according to the driver's experience. For an inexperienced motorcyclist, a 125 cc cycle is probably the most appropriate. Only an experienced driver can control a larger cycle on rough terrain. On the other hand, street bikes should be slected according to the intended type of driving. For use in city traffic, a 125 cc cycle is most suitable for an inexperienced driver. However, for use on highways and expressways, at least a 250 cc cycle is needed, since smaller cycles cannot keep up with the higher speed traffic.

After determining the type and the size of the motorcycle, the person has only one remaining decision: he must choose which brand to purchase. Fortunately, this is the simplest of the three decisions. Although some brands are slightly better than others, the major manufacturers produce machines which are all basically comparable in quality. Thus, for the new motorcylist, a brand which is commonly sold in the neighborhood is a good selection, since repair parts are more likely to be available for the cycle. However, where several brands are commonly sold, the motorcyclist should select a brand from the dealer who will give the best deal and offer the best service after the sale.

Avoiding the Minibike

No discussion about the selection of a motorcycle would ever be complete without mentioning the smallest and fastest selling of the cycles, the minibikes. Because of their comparatively small cost, these miniature motorcycles are selling at an even faster pace than their larger counterparts. With sales reaching considerably over one-half million each year, minibikes are now owned by almost two and one-half million individuals in this country.

Although no technical or legal definition of a minibike is generally recognized throughout the United States, the membership of the Motorcycle Industry Council accepts the following definition:

A two-wheeled vehicle with wheel rims of less than 10 inches diameter . . . or with hub-to-hub wheelbase of less than 40 inches . . . or an engine rated at less than 45 cubic centimeters . . . or a seat-height of less than 25 inches from the ground.[2]

Sold strictly for off-road use, the minibike does not meet the safety requirements for registration as a vehicle in most states. In fact, nearly all states have outlawed minibikes for street use. Yet, over one-fourth of all minibikes are being used on streets and highways.[3] More important, two-thirds of all minibikes are being driven by children between the ages of ten and fourteen.[4]

Because of its small size and cost, many parents consider the minibike to be an ideal gift for their children, but safety officials all agree that the minibike is no toy. Capable of reaching a speed of nearly forty-five miles per hour, minibikes are generally condemned for several reasons: they are

---

2. "Minibikes—What Every Parent Should Know," *NHTSA Fact Sheet: Department of Transportation News,* October, 1971, p. 4.
3. "Minibikes," p. 2.
4. "Minibikes," p. 1.

unstable, many have poor brakes, and the steering is often inadequate. Therefore, regardless of where the minibike is driven, it is dangerous for children of any age to use. Yet, many children, as well as adults, place themselves in even more danger by driving their minibikes on streets and highways.

Each year accident statistics continue to support the fact that most minibike injuries and deaths occur when the minibikes are driven in traffic and are subsequently struck by other vehicles. The reason is simple:

> Minibikes provide a low profile and small size. Together with usually inadequate lights, the young rider is hard to spot in traffic and often unseen by the motorist in time to avoid a collision.[5]

From this explanation one can easily understand why minibikes are designed strictly for off-road use. Obviously, driving a minibike in traffic is not only dangerous but also foolish!

Regardless of where the cycle will be driven, the best advice for a person who is considering the purchase of a minibike, especially for a child, is "DON'T." For a person who already owns a minibike, the best advice is to use the cycle only on wooded trails or on private property with the owner's consent, never on streets and highways.

Wearing Protective Equipment

During a motorcycle-automobile accident, the motorcycle driver, because of the nature of his vehicle, will inevitably come into direct contact with the automobile, the highway pavement, or a fixed object. However, while the cyclist cannot prevent this contact, he can alter its effects by wearing protective equipment.

When the motorcyclist is thrown from his cycle during an accident, one of the most common types of injuries is the deep skin abrasion. Caused by the cyclist's sliding over the rough pavement, skin abrasions can usually be prevented by wearing heavy footgear and vinyl or leather clothing. Fortunately for the modern cyclist, motorcycle clothing is no longer symbolic of the motorcycle gang. Manufacturers now offer brightly colored pants and jackets that are not only attractive but also highly visible in traffic.

Since most cycles are not equipped with windshields, the motorcyclist is constantly subjected to dust, insects, and small flying objects. Even the wind can cause the eyes to tear and thereby blur the vision. For this reason, the cyclist should always wear goggles, glasses with plastic or safety lenses, or a face shield.

Unquestionably, the most important piece of protective equipment is the helmet. Accident statistics show that three-fourths of all motorcycle deaths

---

5. "Minibikes," p. 4.

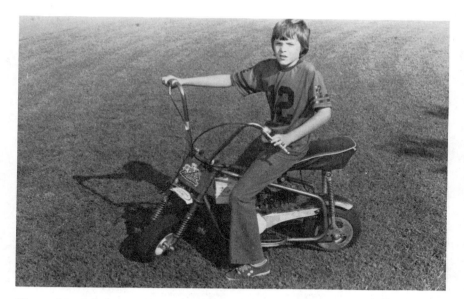

Figure 4.2   Inherently dangerous, a minibike is never a toy for a child.

are caused by head injuries. However, according to some experts, helmets can reduce the risk of head injury by about two-thirds and the risk of death by almost three-fourths. Yet, unfortunately, not all helmets provide the same degree of protection. In fact, some helmets are so poorly constructed that they are practically worthless.

Helmets are constructed of two basic materials. Until recently, fiberglass was the only material used, but now, polycarbonate, a plastic material, is available. Of the two materials, polycarbonate is the stronger. However, the polycarbonate has a disadvantage in that strong chemicals and gasoline can weaken or dissolve it. Thus, as a rule, when purchasing a new helmet, the average motorcyclist should select the fiberglass helmet rather than the polycarbonate. However, if the cyclist already owns a polycarbonate helmet, certain precautions should be taken:

> Polycarbonate helmets should not be painted or decorated by the user except with paints that the manufacturer certifies as compatible with the helmet material; incompatible paints could cause a destructive chemical reaction. The safest way to clean any helmet is with a damp rag. Solvents or cleaning materials, unless certified by the helmet manufacturer as compatible, should not be used.[6]

Yet, not all fiberglass helmets are constructed equally well by the manufacturers.

---

6. "Motorcycles," *Consumer Reports,* January, 1973, p. 40.

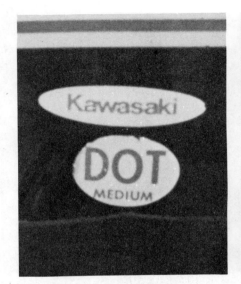
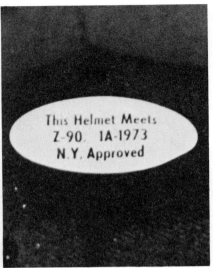

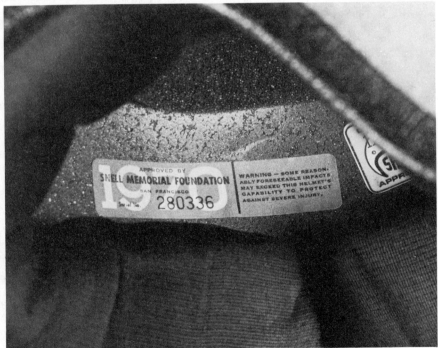

Figure 4.3   DOT, ANSI, AND SNELL seals indicate that the helmets conform to acceptable safety standards.

When purchasing any helmet, the motorcylist should always look for evidence that the helmet conforms to acceptable safety standards. Under Motor Vehicle Safety Standard No. 218, motorcyle helmets designed for on-road use must meet certain performance requirements set by the standard. The symbol DOT (Department of Transportation), constituting the manufacturer's certification that the helmet conforms to the applicable federal requirements, will be located on the outer surface of the helmet. (See Figure 4.3.) Since helmets designed for competitive events and off-road sports are not covered by Standard No. 218, the DOT symbol is not a reliable guide for the dirt or off-road cyclist. However, the ANSI-Z90.1 (American National Standards Institute) and the SNELL MEMORIAL FOUNDATION seals are excellent guides to the reliability of off-road helmets. (See Figure 4.3.) Each seal indicates that the helmet has passed test requirements for impact absorption, resistance to penetration, and retention on the wearer's head, as well as other critiera. However, used helmets, even if they do still display the DOT, ANSI, or SNELL seal, should be avoided, since they may no longer provide adequate protection for the wearer.

Once a helmet has suffered a good "shock," it should be refurbished or replaced immediately. While the outer shell may not be damaged, the inner liner, which really protects the wearer, is usually weakened. However, regardless of whether or not a helmet has received a shock, the average cyclist should replace or refurbish his helmet every two years, since dirt, perspiration, and hair oil will cause disintegration of the liner, thus reducing the helmet's protective properties.

Learning to Drive Properly

Manufacturers, dealers, professional race-drivers, traffic safety officials, and others associated with motorcycling agree that one of the leading causes of motorcycle accidents is lack of experience. According to a recent study, three situations most frequently lead to injuries and fatalities among motorcycle drivers and their passengers:

(1) many new riders lack adequate training and experience in controlling their vehicles (2) riders have not been well enough informed of the inherent dangers of motorcycle riding and are unprepared to cope with hazardous traffic situations (3) pedestrians and operators of other motor vehicles are either unprepared or unwilling to recognize and face the traffic problems created by motorcyles.[7]

---

7. Davis W. Clark and John H. Morton, "The Motorcycle Accident," *Journal of Trauma,* March, 1971, p. 233.

Unfortunately, most beginning cyclists believe that because they can drive an automobile safely they can also drive a motorcycle safely. Needless to say, statistics on motorcycle accidents show the fallacy of such thinking. As experienced cyclists know, the motorcycle is a completely different type of vehicle and requires different skills and a different outlook on what constitutes safe driving. Only an awareness of the problems associated with motorcycle driving and practice under a variety of driving conditions will enable the inexperienced cyclist to operate his new vehicle safely.

Acquiring the Skills

The first few hours of driving are by far the most dangerous for the beginning cyclist, since during this period he will be making a great number of mistakes. Therefore, the new driver should always practice where he will not have to contend with the additional problems posed by other vehicles. Besides the many skills which are common to automobile driving, the cyclist must learn certain other skills which are peculiar to the motorcycle. The most important of these skills are steering and braking.

Unlike the automobile, steering the motorcycle requires the use of the driver's entire body. Yet, contrary to what many people think, the motorcyclist does not deliberately lean when turning a corner or changing directions. Rather, when the handlebars are turned, the angle of the fork automatically leans the motorcycle to the proper degree. All the cyclist does is sit naturally and ride with the cycle.

Braking is another skill which is completely different from its counterpart in the automobile. The motorcycle has two separate brakes, one for the front wheel and one for the rear wheel. To stop the cycle, the driver should always apply the rear brake first and then, if additional stopping power is needed, the front brake. Using only the front brake or using it before the rear brake can easily lead the motorcycle into an uncontrollable skid.

Driving to Be Seen

Outnumbered twenty-eight to one by automobile drivers, the motorcyclist is constantly faced with a problem which safety officials refer to as "invisibility." Because of the comparatively small number of cycles on the road, automobile drivers naturally direct their attention to spotting and avoiding other automobiles. Thus, the automobile driver is not expecting to see a small vehicle, and when the slim silhouette of the motorcycle does appear, he may not see it. However, there are ways for the cyclist to make his vehicle and himself more visible to other drivers.

One of these is for the motorcyclist to drive with his headlight on even during the day. In fact, this is required by law in many states. In states which recently passed such headlight laws, the number of daytime motorcycle accidents has dropped by nearly 4 percent. Wearing bright clothing is another way for the cyclist to make himself more visible during the day, especially when the color is fluorescent orange. Bright colors are normally not found in the traffic environment, and when they do appear, they immediately attract the attention of other drivers.

Bright clothing, particularly white trimmed with retroreflective material, is also excellent for nighttime driving. The reflective quality of the material enables the wearer to be seen at night by other drivers almost twice as far away as a motorcyclist who is not wearing retroreflective material. For greater safety the motorcyclist should also apply strips of reflective tape to his helmet and motorcycle, since the tape will significantly add to the effect already produced by the retroreflectorized clothing.

Traveling in the Lane

Because of the size of his vehicle, the motorcylist has a choice concerning where he will travel in the traffic lane. However, generally, he should drive in the left part of the lane for several reasons: first, this position allows the cyclist to avoid the rocks, oil drippings, old automobile parts, and other debris which tends to accumulate in the center of the lane; second, the position prevents overtaking automobiles from crowding the cyclist on the left and thereby forcing him off the road; third, the position permits the automobile driver to see the cycle in his rearview mirror; and fourth, the position protects the cyclist in city traffic from suddenly-opening car doors. Yet, there are some exceptions to the "left-part-of-the-lane" rule.

For example, when the motorcyclist is traveling in the left lane of a multilane roadway, he should drive in the right part of the lane, since this position prevents overtaking automobiles from squeezing into the lane, but when the cyclist is traveling in the right lane, he should drive in the left part of the lane, since this position offers the same advantages which were mentioned in the preceding paragraph. If a middle lane exists, the motorcycle driver should avoid using it, since cars can easily squeeze into the lane on either side of the cyclist. On the other hand, when motorcyclists are traveling in pairs, one cyclist should drive in the left part of the lane, and the other cyclist should drive in the right part of the lane. Furthermore, since gusts of wind or irregular road surfaces can suddenly cause the cycles to deviate from a straight path, one of the cyclists should travel slightly ahead of the other. This arrangement will provide adequate space for quick maneuvering.

Preventing Spills

Since a two-wheeled vehicle is inherently less stable than a four-wheeled vehicle, some road conditions which may have little effect upon the automobile can easily cause the motorcycle to spill. This is why the motorcyclist must use extreme caution when driving on any surface which departs from the normal.

Even for the automobile, snow, ice, and water are substances which can make road conditions extremely hazardous. Yet, for the motorcyclist, driving safely on snow and ice is next to impossible because of the reduction in friction between these surfaces and the tires. Water, on the other hand, presents fewer problems for the cylist, but it can still make the road surface quite slippery. As a rule, paved surfaces are more slippery just after the start of a rain, since the water mixes with the oil on the roadway to form an oily film, but after a period of hard rain, the surface becomes less slippery, since the oily film is washed away. Painted lines, metal inserts in the road, and metal bridge gratings, however, remain quite slippery regardless of the amount of rain, while loose sand and gravel are always slippery, even when dry. Consequently, when driving on any abnormal surface, the motorcyclist should avoid sudden stops, sharp turns, and quick accelerations, since these maneuvers can easily lead to uncontrolled skidding.

Unfortunately, slippery surfaces are not the only road conditions which may present problems for the motorcycle driver. Ruts, potholes, rocks, and railroad tracks are all obstacles which can cause the motorcycle to spill. By staying an ample distance behind the vehicle in front, the cyclist can usually spot most obstacles and steer around them. However, when he cannot avoid the obstruction, which is obviously the case with railroad tracks, the cyclist should try to hit the obstacle at a right angle, that is, head-on.

Yet, even this advice is useless when the motorcycle driver is confronted by "moving obstacles." Because dogs are unpredictable, they present a special hazard for the cyclist. In many cases the motorcyclist can scare the dog by shouting an angry command, but most often, the only action a cyclist can take is to keep driving and hope the dog abandons his pursuit. Fortunately, most dogs, while they may bark loudly, never attempt to bite. For this reason, the cyclist should avoid kicking at the dog, since this action will only make the animal angry and may cause the cyclist to lose his balance and fall.

Sharing the Responsibility

Most people believe that the motorcyclist should accept the major responsibility for avoiding accidents with automobiles. However, accident statistics show the fallacy of such thinking. Without exception, research studies on motorcycle-automobile accidents reveal that the automobile driver is usually at fault. Needless to say, this fact dramatically points out the need for automobile drivers to share with motorcylists the responsibility for preventing accidents. As a recent article notes, "Unless motorists make special efforts to avoid running over cyclists, the collison problem won't be solved."[8]

Because of its size, an approaching motorcycle is extremely hard to see, but traffic safety officials agree that the cycle can be seen if the automobile driver makes a special effort to look for it, especially when entering the traffic flow from a side street or when crossing a lane of traffic during a left-hand turn. However, motorcycles approaching from the rear require even more effort by the automobile driver, since many cyclists travel in the automobile driver's blind spot. Thus, before changing lanes or passing, the automobile driver should quickly look over his shoulder to make certain that no motorcycle is behind him to interfere with the movement. The same visual check is also essential when emerging from a parked vehicle on the traffic side, since many cyclists wrongly drive on the right part of the lane and can easily collide with an opening door.

Naturally, not all motorcycle-automobile accidents result because the automobile drivers failed to see the cyclists. Many accidents occur because the automobile drivers are unfamiliar with the dangers and inherent features of the motorcycle. For example, few drivers realize that motorcycles can stop faster on dry pavement than automobiles. Consequently, even when the driver uses the normal two seconds in the "Second Interval Concept," he can easily strike a quick-stopping cyclist from behind. For this reason, the automobile driver should allow extra seconds, and thereby extra distance, when following any motorcycle.

Resource Materials

American Automobile Association
1712 G. Street, N.W.
Washington, D.C. 20006

American Motorcycle Association
5655 North High Street
Worthington, Ohio 43086

American National Standards Institute
1430 Broadway
New York City, New York 10019

Bell Helmets
2850 East 29th Street
Long Beach, California 90806

Motorcycle Industry Council, Inc.
1001 Connecticut Avenue, N.W.
Washington, D.C. 20036

Motorcycle Safety Foundation
6755 Elkridge Landing Road
Linthicum, Maryland 21090

National Safety Council
444 North Michigan Avenue
Chicago, Illinois 60611

National Technical Information Service
5285 Port Royal Road
Springfield, Virginia 22151

---

8. "Can Cycling Be Safe," *Better Homes and Gardens,* May, 1972, p. 76.

Snell Memorial Foundation
761 Laurel Drive
Sacramento, California 95825

U.S. Department of Transportation
National Highway Traffic Safety Administration
Washington, D.C. 20590

United States Suzuki Motor Corporation
13767 Freeway Drive
Santa Fe Springs, California 90670

Yamaha International Corporation
Box 5450
Los Angeles, California 90054

Activities

1. Survey twenty adults to determine their attitudes toward the motorcycle and the motorcyclist. Discuss the results in a short paper.

2. Invite a local motorcycle dealer to speak to the class about choosing a proper cycle and helmet.

3. Write to a major manufacturer of minibikes, and request information about their use by children. Present the reply to the class, and discuss its implications for the parent who is considering the purchase of a minibike for his children.

4. Write to the American Automobile Association, and request information on motorcycle safety. Using this material, develop a list of safe-driving habits.

5. Prepare a twenty-five question true or false test over the material in this chapter. Administer the test to fifteen automobile drivers and fifteen motorcycle drivers. Discuss the results of the test with the class.

Questions

1. What is the reason for the motorcycle's surging popularity in recent years?
2. Why is the dirt or trail bike unsuited for road use?
3. What is the best size motorcycle for an inexperienced driver who intends to use the cycle only in city traffic?
4. Why do many parents consider the minibike to be an ideal gift for their children?
5. Why do safety officials generally condemn the minibike as being unsafe?
6. What is the most important piece of protective equipment that a motorcycle driver can utilize?
7. Why should a helmet that has suffered a good shock be refurbished or replaced immediately?

8. Why should the motorcyclist drive with his headlight on even during the day?
9. Generally, where is the safest place for the cyclist to travel when driving in the traffic lane?
10. What are "moving obstacles?"

Selected References

American Automobile Association. *Guide to Safe Motorcycling.* Washington, D.C.: AAA, 1971.

"Can Cycling Be Safe," *Better Homes and Gardens.* May, 1972, 76.

Clark, Davis W., and John H. Morton. "The Motorcycle Accident," *Journal of Trauma.* March, 1971, 230-37.

Dodson, C. Frank, Jr. "Motorcycle Injuries: Problem Without Solution," *The Journal of the Arkansas Medical Society.* July, 1976, 115-19.

Hodgdon, T. A. *You and Your Motorcycle.* Worthington, Ohio: Motorcycle, Scooter and Allied Trades Association, 1968.

Kelly, Albert Benjamin. "Commentary—Motorcycles and Public Apathy," *American Journal of Public Health.* May, 1976, 475-76.

"Minibikes: Supertoys or Safety Hazards?," *Good Housekeeping.* September, 1970, 159.

"Motorcycles," *Consumer Reports.* January, 1973, 40-44.

National Safety Council. *Motorcycle Facts.* Chicago: NSC, 1976.

"Save Your Head," *Senior Scholastic.* December 11, 1972, 34.

Speca, John M., and Henry R. Cowell. "Minibike and Motorcycle Accidents in Adolescents—A New Epidemic," *The Journal of the American Medical Association.* April 7, 1975, 55-56.

U.S. Department of Transportation, National Highway Traffic Safety Administration. *A Motorcycle Safety Helmet Study.* DOT-HS-801 137. Washington, D.C.: DOT-HS, March, 1974.

———. *For Your Information Concerning Federal Motor Vehicle Safety Standard No. 218, Motorcycle Helmets.* Washington, D.C.: DOT-HS, September, 1974.

———. *Motorcycle Safety.* Washington, D.C.: DOT-HS, July, 1976.

———. *Motorcycle Safety—Program Memorandum,* DOT-HS-802 099. Washington, D.C.: DOT-HS, November, 1976.

———. *Motorcycle Safety—The Case for Helmet Use.* DOT-HS-801 836. Washington, D.C.: DOT-HS, February, 1976.

———. "Minibikes—What Every Parent Should Know," *NHTSA Fact Sheet: Department of Transportation News.* October, 1971.

Warshofsky, Fred. "Death Rides on Two Wheels," *Reader's Digest.* October, 1967, 151-52, 154, 156.

Pedestrian Accidents

5

A crowd of Christmas shoppers in San Francisco, California, quietly stood on a pedestrian island and mentally prepared themselves for the holiday season. Sadly enough, at least six of the shoppers never lived to see another day. Within seconds a runaway fire truck hurdled into the group and, as observers screamed, sent bodies flying through the air. Except for this story and similar accounts of unusual violence and mayhem, pedestrian accidents rarely attract attention. This is an unfortunate situation, since approximately eighty-three hundred pedestrians are killed every year in traffic accidents.

Vulnerability of the Young and the Old

Children are unpredictable! Any parent will verify this statement. Yet, parents and other adults are frequently guilty of teaching pedestrian safety rules to children and then expecting them to walk predictably in traffic. Needless to say, children are frequent victims of traffic accidents. In fact, approximately one-fourth of all pedestrian deaths involve children.

In recent years several studies have dealt with child pedestrians, not only in this country but also in Great Britain. However, one of the more interesting and still relevant investigations of this subject was made almost ten years ago in Stockholm, Sweden. After studying the traffic maturity of children between the ages of four and ten, researchers at the Research Institute of Child Psychology concluded that adults overestimate children's abilities as pedestrians and cyclists.[1] Apparently, children under the age of approximately ten years do not possess the sensory and cognitive abilities which are necessary for coping with modern traffic situations.

Specifically, children have not yet developed an adult level of peripheral vision and hearing. Consequently, they are physically unable to see or hear motor vehicles which are approaching them from the sides. Furthermore, children lack experience and cannot comprehend abstractions. Thus, they frequently misinterpret the meaning of words which they see on traffic signs

---

1. "The Child Pedestrian," *School Safety,* March-April, 1970, pp. 4-6.

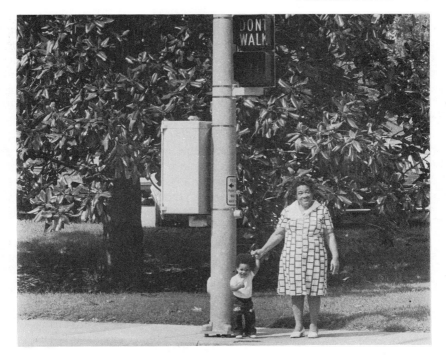

Figure 5.1   The very young and the very old account for nearly one-half of all pedestrian deaths.

and signals. A typical example of this behavior was seen recently in Memphis, Tennessee. A six-year-old boy approached a pedestrian crosswalk at an intersection, and when the signal flashed "DON'T WALK," he started across the street. About fifteen feet from the curb, the boy was struck by a car. Miraculously, he was not severely injured. Later, when his mother scolded him for disobeying the traffic signal, the boy announced, "But, Momma, I did what the sign said. It said 'don't walk,' so I ran." Undoubtedly, both physical and mental immaturity are frequent causes of child-pedestrian accidents and deaths.

However, children are not the only age group which contributes abnormally to the pedestrian death toll. Despite their fewer numbers, the elderly account for approximately one-fourth of all pedestrian deaths.

In an effort to determine why elderly pedestrians are frequently involved in traffic accidents, a study was conducted by Wiener and his colleagues at the University of Miami.[2] According to the researchers' observations,

2. Barbara Ford, "Traffic Safety's Mystery Man," *Science Digest,* December, 1969, pp. 66-67.

elderly pedestrians are not timid. On the contrary, when they are walking in traffic, oldsters are often brazen and aggressive. Perhaps this is because they formed their attitudes and habits many years ago when the traffic problem was less complicated. Regardless of the reason, the elderly frequently take unnecessary risks in traffic and then become confused in threatening situations. In addition, elderly pedestrians are more likely to base their walking decisions on the movement of traffic rather than on traffic signs and signals. However, even when oldsters do rely on traffic signals, they often make fatal decisions. For example, when elderly pedestrians are waiting at intersections, they often mistakenly watch the side of the signal rather than the front. Consequently, when a green light appears on the side of the signal, they obey this light rather than the red light which is directly in front of them and then walk directly into the path of oncoming traffic. This mistake is often referred to as the "error of perpendicular green."

Obviously, not all elderly-pedestrian deaths can be attributed to personality or mental factors. In many cases elderly persons simply cannot react quickly enough to avoid accidents. Unlike younger pedestrians, older persons are often handicapped by inadequate vision, deficient hearing, poor reflexes, and reduced agility. Furthermore, when they are struck by motor vehicles, the elderly are especially susceptible to shock, a frequent cause of pedestrian deaths.

According to most safety officials, education is only a small part of the solution to the problem of pedestrian deaths among the young and the old. Because of peculiar mental and physical characteristics, children and elderly persons can never walk as safely in traffic as persons of other ages. For this reason, some safety experts recommend that the transport system in this country be designed with maximum consideration for pedestrians. Specifically, pedestrian paths should be situated in convenient locations. Needless to say, when pedestrians must walk several hundred feet to overpasses and underpasses, they are more likely to risk accidents at other locations. In addition, intersections should be equipped with painted crosswalks and pedestrian signals.

Walking Under the Influence of Alcohol

In numerous studies dealing with alcohol and traffic accidents, researchers have found that intoxicated persons account for an unusually large number of pedestrian deaths. Although the exact percentage is unknown, most safety officials estimate the figure at somewhere between 40 and 75 percent.

Undoubtedly, the wide range of estimates is the result of the difficulty involved in determining whether or not pedestrians had been intoxicated. Due to the exceptional violence encountered in pedestrian-motor-vehicle accidents, most pedestrians lose a large amount of blood. Consequently, even though they had been drinking heavily prior to their deaths, the pedestrians will show negative blood-alcohol levels during laboratory tests.

Although the magnitude of the pedestrian-alcohol problem in this country is unknown, traffic safety experts are in agreement about the way in which alcohol affects pedestrian behavior. It dulls reaction time, adversely affects judgment, reduces muscular coordination, hinders perception, and, worst of all, causes pedestrians to make mistakes which often result in death. In short, alcohol makes every pedestrian an easy target for fast-moving vehicles.

Because of the danger of drinking and driving, safety experts have coined the phrase "Don't drink and then drive." However, drinkers should not become pedestrians. In short, the best advice for a drinker is to ride home with a nondrinking friend. However, when this is not possible, the person should do his drinking early and then allow several hours for the effects of the alcohol to wear off. He can then walk or drive home by himself.

Walking Safely in Traffic

While the very young, the very old, and the intoxicated account for most pedestrian deaths, no one is absolutely safe while walking in traffic. However, certain measures can be taken to reduce the risk.

Of all pedestrian habits, the most important are those employed when crossing streets, highways, and roads. Before entering a street or roadway, the pedestrian should always double-check to the left and to the right for traffic. Then, since a slow-moving car or truck may suddenly increase its speed or a vehicle may be traveling faster than it appears, he should periodically look to both sides for approaching traffic as he walks. Furthermore, since dodging fast-moving vehicles between intersections is both difficult and dangerous, the pedestrian, whenever and wherever possible, should obey all pedestrian signs and signals and should cross roads and streets only at marked crosswalks.

According to safety experts, the best protection for the pedestrian is to walk where the automobile driver expects him to be. This place is on the sidewalk, not in the roadway. However, where sidewalks are not available, the pedestrian should walk on the left side of the shoulder or roadway and thus face the oncoming traffic. Besides enabling him easily to see approaching vehicles, the habit of walking on the left allows the pedestrian to step off the roadway whenever necessary. In addition, since turned-up collars, scarves, hats, and ski masks may easily hinder vision, he should avoid wearing such items. In practice, the pedestrian's only effective defense against fast-approaching vehicles is his eyes!

Improving the Pedestrian's Visibility

Although pedestrian activity is much greater during the daytime, more than one-half of all pedestrian deaths occur at night. The reason for this is simple: nighttime drivers cannot see pedestrians well enough to avoid hitting them.

Without question, dark colors are the worst attire for the night pedestrian. On the other hand, fluorescent-colored clothing is the best. However, for practical reasons safety experts usually recommend that pedestrians wear light-colored clothing, particularly white, which has been supplemented with retroreflective material.

In an effort to evaluate the effectiveness of retroreflective material, researchers covered dummies with various types of materials and then recorded the ability of nighttime, drinking drivers to see and avoid hitting the dummies. They discovered:

> . . . that despite the driver's alcohol-slowed reflexes, he was still usually able to avoid the dummy covered by retroreflective material. With a blood alcohol level between .06 percent and .10 percent, the driver saw a reflectorized dummy in time to stop at 70 miles per hour, 100 percent of the time. If the dummy material were white, but not retroreflectorized, the driver could stop 100 percent of the time at 30 miles per hour. The speeds fell to 20 miles per hour if the dummy was gray and even less when the dummy was black.[3]

Retroreflective material is effective because it returns light directly to the source, no matter at what angle the light strikes the material. Consequently, pedestrians with retroreflective apparel can be seen almost twice as far away at night as pedestrians with ordinary clothing.

Although reflectorized materials can be purchased in many different forms, some items are undoubtedly more useful for the pedestrian than others. Especially valuable are sew-on or iron-on patches and trim which can be permanently attached to clothing. Besides being decorative, retroreflective patches and trim are indispensable for young children. However, for adults, clothing with permanently attached retroreflective material is rarely practical. In such cases the adult pedestrian can make himself more visible at night by wearing "dangle tags," pieces of cardboard covered with reflective tape or sprayed with fluorescent paint. Attached to

---

3. John M. Douglass and Frederick D. Burg, "The Physician's Role in Protecting Pedestrians and Cyclists," *American Family Physician,* February, 1970, pp. 156-57.

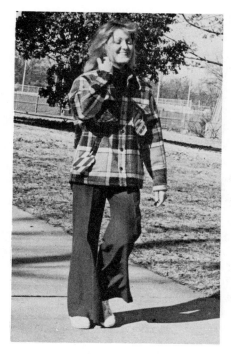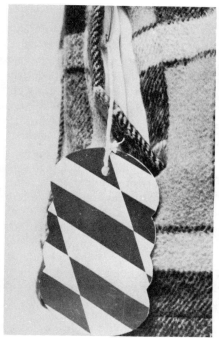

Figure 5.2 Dangle tags can be used by the pedestrian to make himself more visible to nighttime drivers.

strings and then carried inside the pockets, the tags are flipped outside and allowed to dangle as the pedestrian walks in the dark. (See Figure 5.2.)

Surviving in the Streets

Believe it or not, some people do not own motor vehicles. Besides those persons who cannot afford cars or motorcycles, there are the very young, the very old, and the incapacitated. All of them must normally rely on their feet for transportation. Furthermore, for shopping and business reasons, everyone must walk in urban areas. Yet, not all pedestrians walk because they want to get from one place to another.

Specifically, all people who are afoot may be classified as pedestrians. This group includes motorists who are working on stalled cars, persons who are hitchhiking along highways, individuals who are walking or jogging for recreational purposes, and children who are playing in the streets. For the safety of all of these road users, special precautions must be taken at all times.

Nightlighting the Stalled Vehicle

Undoubtedly, the most irritated pedestrian is the motorist who has been forced afoot by mechanical problems. However, since flat tires and engine breakdowns are frequent occurrences, every driver should prepare himself for the role of a temporary pedestrian.

In some cases the driver may want to spray the inside of his trunk lid with orange or yellow fluorescent paint, or trim the inside of the lid with patterns of reflective tape. During a breakdown at night, the raised lid will glow as a warning to other motorists. In other cases the driver may spray an old sheet on one side with fluorescent paint. When the sheet is draped over the raised trunk lid, it will serve the same warning function as the painted lid. In all cases the driver should carry several flares in his vehicle.

In an emergency situation the driver-turned-pedestrian should activate his flasher lights, raise his trunk lid, and then place one lighted flare near his stalled car and another lighted flare at least three hundred feet behind his car, thus warning approaching vehicles of his stopped car and his activity near the vehicle. If the car cannot be repaired, the person should never stand in the roadway and attempt to stop other motorists. Instead, he should wait for help from a passing police car or a highway emergency truck.

Getting a Ride Without Injury

For persons who do not own motor vehicles, hitchhiking has become a popular form of transportation in recent years. Besides being a cheap way to travel, hitching rides with motorists is both exciting and educational. However, the practice is also extremely dangerous.

Although almost everyone has read newspaper accounts of rapes and other physical violence perpetrated on young hitchhikers by obliging motorists, few people realize that hitchhiking is the most dangerous form of pedestrian behavior. Because he must attract a driver's attention, the hitch-hiker will usually position himself on the roadway or at least several feet from it. However, with an inattentive driver, the hitchhiker is viewed as just another part of the traffic environment.

Although light-colored clothing is undoubtedly more visible to drivers than darker clothing, even white is not the safest color for traveling attire. According to safety experts, the hitchhiker should always wear a fluorescent orange outfit which has been supplemented by dangle tags or reflective trim. Besides being extremely visible in the dark, the fluorescent orange color is distinguishable in the daylight traffic environment.

Exercising with Visibility

In an age when many people live in apartments and work at sedentary jobs, walking and jogging have become popular recreational pastimes. Furthermore, because of the nature of these activities, walking and jogging can be enjoyed at the same time by all members of the family. However, for many health-conscious participants, the results of these recreational pursuits have actually proven to be detrimental to health and life.

In Chicago, Illinois, a thirty-three-year-old man, his thirty-year-old wife, and their ten-year-old son were jogging on a sidewalk next to a busy street. Suddenly, the father started across the street, followed by his wife and his son. All three were struck by a truck and killed. According to the truck's driver, the three joggers suddenly appeared out of nowhere from a space between two parked delivery vans.

Like all pedestrians, walkers and joggers may blend into the background of the traffic environment. For this reason, they should always wear some type of fluorescent orange outfit and obey all pedestrian regulations, signs, and signals. In addition, wherever possible, the participants should perform their recreational walking and jogging on sidewalks, not in the streets.

Watching for Children

As most drivers will verify, roads and streets are favorite playgrounds for youngsters. In fact, in many congested urban areas, the streets are the only places where children can play with any freedom. Furthermore, even where yards and playgrounds are available, children may suddenly dart into the roadway after balls or during the course of their play.

Obviously, parents should try to provide suitable play areas, as well as supervision, for their children. However, this is not always practical or possible. In addition, youngsters are unpredictable. For these reasons, while he is driving, the motorist should constantly remain alert and watch for children in or near the streets and roadways.

Resource Materials

American Automobile Association
1712 G. Street, N.W.
Washington, D.C. 20006

American Driver and Traffic Safety Education Association
1201 16th Street, N.W.
Washington, D.C. 20036

National Safety Council
444 North Michigan Avenue
Chicago, Illinois 60611

Activities

1. Write to the American Automobile Association, and request information on pedestrian safety. Using this material, develop a list of safe-walking habits.

2. Develop a checklist of illegal and/or dangerous practices of pedestrians. Using this list, observe the actions of pedestrians at a busy intersection, and prepare a short report on their behavior.

3. Invite a policeman to speak to the class about his department's enforcement of pedestrian traffic laws and regulations.

4. Prepare five dangle tags, and demonstrate their reflective qualities to the class.

5. Write a short article on "Pedestrian Safety," and submit it to a local newspaper for publication.

Questions

1. Why are children unable to walk as safely in traffic as adults?
2. What is the "error of perpendicular green?"
3. What three groups account for most pedestrian deaths?
4. Why are blood-alcohol tests on dead pedestrians often unreliable?
5. What are the effects of alcohol on pedestrian behavior?
6. What is the secret behind the effectiveness of retroreflective material?
7. What are dangle tags, and how are they constructed?
8. Why should a motorist spray the inside of his trunk lid with fluorescent paint?
9. What is the safest color for a hitchhiker's clothes?
10. What is the safest color for a jogger's outfit?

Selected References

American Automobile Association. *Older Adult Pedestrian Safety*. Washington, D.C.: AAA, 1970.

———. *The Young Pedestrian*. Washington, D.C.: American Automobile Association, 1972.

Douglass, John M., and Frederick D. Burg. "The Physician's Role in Protecting Pedestrians and Cyclists," *American Family Physician*. February, 1970, 155-57.

Ford, Barbara. "Traffic Safety's Mystery Man," *Science Digest*. December, 1969, 64-68.

Howarth, C. I.; D. A. Routledge; and R. Repetto-Wright. "An Analysis of Road Accidents Involving Child Pedestrians," *Ergonomics*. May, 1974, 319-30.

———. "The Exposure of Young Children to Accident Risk as Pedestrians," *Ergonomics*. July, 1974, 457-80.

"Let's Light Up Night Walkers," *School Safety*. September-October, 1969, 18-19.

"Needed: Pedestrian Safeguards for Ambling Oldsters," *Today's Health*. February, 1970, 64-65.

Pignataro, L. J. *Traffic Engineering—Theory and Practice*. Englewood Cliffs, New Jersey: Prentice-Hall, Inc., 1973.

Sleight, Robert B. "The Pedestrian," *Human Factors in Highway Traffic Safety Research*. ed. T. W. Forbes, New York: Wiley-Interscience, 1972.

"The Child Pedestrian," *School Safety*. March-April, 1970, 4-6.

Thistle, Franklin L. "Let's Put An End to Pedestrian Slaughter," *Today's Health*. March, 1976, 6-8.

Bicycle Accidents

6

A Houston, Texas, youth worked on odd jobs for his parents and his neighbors for nearly two years. Finally, on the morning of his tenth birthday, he had saved enough money to buy a new red bicycle. By that afternoon the youngster had run a stop light and had been struck by a delivery truck; by that night he had been pronounced dead by his doctor. According to the National Safety Council, the youth is just one of approximately nine hundred persons who are killed each year in bicycle accidents. In addition, nearly one million bicyclists are injured seriously enough every year to require medical attention.

Operating the Bicycle as a Vehicle

Bicycles have long been a favorite mode of transportation among children, but in recent years the bicycle's popularity has spread to all age groups. With the sale of over fifteen million new bicycles annually, this country is evidently in the midst of a bicycling boom. Today, approximately one-hundred million persons enjoy the thrill of bicycling.

Undoubtedly, the increasing popularity of the bicycle stems from many different roots. Some owners use the bicycle as a cheap means of transportation or as a way to reduce the pollution problem. Most people, however, simply operate the bicycle for fun and wholesome exercise. Regardless of the reason, with the increased use of the bicycle, more and more bicyclists are driving on city streets without recognizing or assuming full responsibility for their actions. The result is an increasing number of bicycle-motor-vehicle accidents.

What few drivers realize is that their bicycles, unless excluded by a local ordinance, are legally considered to be vehicles and must obey the same laws that pertain to motor vehicles. As shown in numerous studies, when traffic laws are broken, accidents occur. In fact, in approximately four out of every five bicycle-motor-vehicle accidents, the bicyclist is legally at fault. Apparently, six violations of traffic laws by the bicycle driver are the most frequent causes of accidents. They include failure to yield the right-of-way,

76

improper turning, failure to obey stop signs or signals, reckless weaving in and out of traffic, riding in the center of the street, and riding against traffic. To blend safely into the traffic flow, the bicyclist should realize that he is operating a vehicle, just like the automobile, and that he must obey all traffic laws.

Naturally, the bicycle driver should never automatically assume that every automobile driver will instantly view the bicycle as a vehicle and grant it all the rights specified by traffic law. Many drivers will not! Therefore, the most important rule in bicycle safety is that the bicyclist should always be prepared to give up his legal right-of-way to the automobile driver. After all, in any confrontation between a bicycle and a motor vehicle, the bicycle and the bicycle driver will always turn out to be the losers.

While they are not required by law, bicyclists should also follow other rules that are designed to further the safety of their driving in traffic. These rules include: driving at the far right side of the roadway or street so that faster moving vehicles can pass without moving into the path of oncoming traffic;[1] dismounting at busy intersections and crossing at crosswalks; listening for vehicles approaching from behind; driving single file, rather than abreast, when in a group; and utilizing bicycle paths wherever they are available.

Providing a Safe Place to Play

Despite the recent tremendous interest in bicycles among adults, the two-wheeled vehicles will always remain "playthings" for some children. In fact, according to many safety officials, the largest portion of a child's riding time on a bicycle is devoted to playing games, and only a small portion is devoted to using the bicycle for transportation.

Understandably, "racing" is the most popular bicycle game among children. It is also the most dangerous, since streets, highways, and sidewalks are most often used as the racetracks. Next to racing in popularity is "trick riding." Of the various tricks that are frequently performed on bicycles, only one, called the "wheelie" (riding only on the back wheel), has resulted in a disproportionate number of injuries in recent years. Perhaps this is associated with the great popularity of the high-rise bicycles among youngsters. Because of their design, the high-risers are difficult to maneuver and can easily topple backward whenever their riders attempt wheelies.

---

1. Although this practice is much safer than driving in the middle of the traffic lane, it does present additional problems for the bicyclist. Because he is driving at the far right side of the roadway, the bicyclist must be constantly alert for automobile drivers who are opening doors and leaving parking spaces.

With the recent national coverage of Evel Knievel and other motorcycle daredevils, another bicycle game has suddenly developed and grown in popularity. Depending on the particular region of the country, the game and its variations are referred to as "gully jumping," "creek jumping," and "barrel jumping." Of the three variations, barrel jumping is the most dangerous. In Denver, Colorado, a thirteen-year-old boy placed four garbage cans (barrels) side-by-side and a wooden ramp at one end of the line. He then prepared to jump over the cans with his bike. Unfortunately, he did not succeed. His front wheel struck the space between the last and the second-to-last cans, and he was thrown headfirst over the handlebars. Luckily, the youngster suffered only a broken collarbone and minor cuts on his face.

While bicycles are becoming more and more expensive every year, games of fear and violence are still extremely popular among children. The most commonly played games of this type are "chicken," "demolition derby," and "terror." In the "chicken" game two bicyclists drive directly toward each other, and each bicyclist waits for the other to swerve or "chicken out" first. In many cases neither of the participants swerve, and a head-on collision results. Naturally, in "chicken" such collisions are unintentional, but in "demolition derby" repeated collisions are exactly what the bicyclists

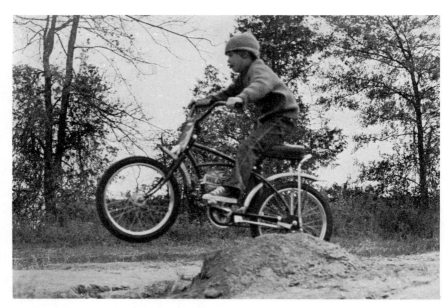

Figure 6.1   Gully jumping is one of the newest and fastest growing bicycle games in this country.

want. During the demolition game, the bicyclists drive into each other and deliberately attempt to destroy the other participants' bicycles. The winner is the youngster with the last operative bicycle. Finally, in the "terror" game the bicyclist drives toward a pedestrian, usually a woman or an elderly person, and attempts to frighten him. Most often, the bicyclist and the pedestrian never touch each other. However, if both the pedestrian and the bicyclist move quickly in the same direction at the last instant, a collision may result. In such cases the pedestrian is usually more seriously injured than the bicyclist.

Since many bicycle games are played on streets and highways, parents cannot rely simply on teaching their children traffic laws and bicycle safety rules. Most bicycle games, particularly those mentioned in this section, cause children to violate laws and safety rules. For this reason, parents should either attempt to change the types of bicycle games that their children play or, more realistically, they should provide a location where their children can play the various bicycle games away from traffic.

Relearning to Drive

As most of the adults who reenter the world of bicycling soon discover, modern bicycles are much more sophisticated than those of ten to fifteen years ago. Multispeed gears, hand-operated brakes, and narrow tires are standard features on many of today's bicycles. Ten to fifteen years ago, middleweight bicycles with balloon tires and coaster brakes were popular among children.

Needless to say, most of today's adult bicyclists learned to drive while they were youngsters, using middleweight bikes. However, modern bicycles require a different set of skills for safe handling, and unless today's adult bicyclists learn these new skills, accidents will inevitably occur.

Although shifting gears while pedaling is a common problem at first, with a little practice most bicyclists are usually able to master the technique. Braking, however, requires more practice and greater skill. A bicycle which is stopped by the driver's hands has two separate brakes, one for the front wheel and one for the back wheel. To slow or stop the bicycle safely, the person should always apply the back brake first. If more stopping power is needed, he can then apply the front brake. Applying the front brake alone, or applying it before the back brake, can easily lead the bicyclist into an uncontrollable skid or even throw him over the handlebars.

Oddly enough, narrow tires may also cause the driver to be tossed off his bicycle. In many cities storm sewer gratings with wide openings are located along the sides of the streets. If a person drives over the sewer gratings with his bicycle, the narrow tire may slip into the space between the metal gratings, and the front of the bicycle will stop abruptly. When the bicyclist has been traveling at a normal speed or faster, this sudden stop will toss the person headfirst over the handlebars and onto the hard street. In recent years several people have been killed in this type of accident. When driving in cities with storm sewer gratings, the bicyclist should stay at least five feet away from the curbs, since most gratings are located in this area.

Selecting an Appropriate Bicycle

With the tremendous increase in bicycle sales in recent years, the number of bicycle-related injuries and deaths has also risen substantially. Consequently, bicycle safety has become a high-priority item for safety officials.

Since the latter part of 1975, all new two-wheeled bicycles, except racing bikes and "one-of-a-kind" custom models, sold in interstate commerce must comply with federal safety standards. These standards set minimum strength and performance requirements for brakes, wheels, frames, steering systems, and other bicycle parts. They also require protection from sharp metal edges, chain-guards or derailleur guards, and clamps from seats, handlebars, and handlebar stems. To increase the visibility of the bicycle at night, the standards also require reflectors on the front, back, and sides of the bicycle and on the pedals.

Unless a person buys from a bike shop, he will probably discover that most bicycles are sold disassembled in cartons. In such cases the person must either assemble the bicycle himself or pay the store to assemble it. Yet, when the bicycle is completely assembled, it will still need minor adjustment of the brakes, alignment of the wheels, adjustment of the seat height, and lubrication of various parts. For this reason, an individual should, whenever possible, purchase a new bicycle from an established bike store, preferably one that sells and services only bicycles.

Naturally, every bicycle should meet the needs of the user. For youngsters the middleweight bicycle, with balloon tires and a coaster brake, is ideal. Besides being sturdy, dependable, and easy to maintain, the middleweight bicycle is easy to drive and very stable. Unfortunately, however, most children prefer the high-rise bicycle which is difficult to control and quite unstable. For adults the recreational bicycle is probably the most practical. Equipped with narrow tires and hand-operated brakes, this type of bicycle is enjoyable to drive because it has different gears for easy pedaling. On the other hand, for adventurous adults the lightweight bicycle may be more attractive than the recreational bicycle. Possessing handlever brakes, dropped-down handlebars, and usually ten gears, the lightweight bicycle is ideal for racing and for driving on long trips.

Regardless of the type of bike, a person should make certain that the bicycle is the correct size for the user. Generally, when the bicyclist is seated with the ball of his foot on the pedal in its lowest position, his leg should not be fully extended. Furthermore, the person should be able to stand while he is straddling the bicycle frame.

Making the Bicycle Safer

Although the violation of traffic laws by bicyclists is the primary cause of bicycle-motor-vehicle accidents, the operating condition of the bicycle should not be overlooked. As many as 15 percent of all bicycle accidents may be caused primarily by some mechanical defect, and this does not include many accidents which could have been avoided if all bicycles were equipped with warning devices and protective seating for passengers. Undoubtedly, the operating condition of the bicycle plays a larger role in the accident picture than is generally recognized.

Without a mechanically sound vehicle, the bicyclist risks his life every time he drives in traffic. In Rockford, Illinois, a thirty-year-old man was driving a bicycle down a steep hill when his chain suddenly snapped. Without the chain the bicycle's coaster brake was inoperative, and the man was carried directly into a busy intersection. Fortunately, the man was not hit, and he was finally able to stop the bicycle. After pushing the bicycle home and performing a makeshift repair on the chain, the man went for another drive. On the same hill the bicycle chain broke again, and the man was carried into the intersection. This time, however, he was not as lucky. The man was struck by a truck and was killed instantly. Because of the danger presented by a mechanically defective bicycle, the operator should periodically inspect and repair any defective parts, particularly brakes, tires, chain, seat, and handlebars. For information on bicycles, the bicyclist should write to The Bicycle Institute of America. (See Resource Materials at the end of this chapter.)

Besides being mechanically sound, the bicycle should also be equipped with reliable warning devices, both visual and audible. This is especially important in nighttime driving, since the bicyclist will blend into the darkness and become invisible to the automobile driver. A bike flag, reflective trim, a horn or bell which is audible for at least one hundred feet, a headlight which is visible for at least five hundred feet, and numerous reflectors which are visible for at least three hundred feet, are all essential equipment items for the bicycle. Furthermore, when children are frequently carried on the bicycle, protective seating should also be included. Far too often, youngsters stick their feet into the spokes of the wheel or they lose their balance,

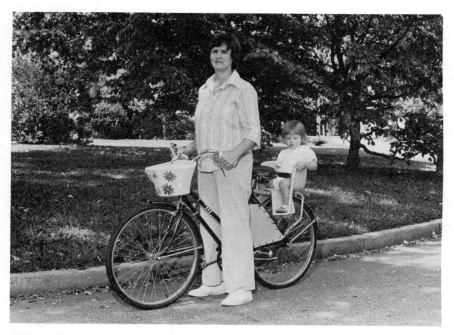

Figure 6.2   Bicycle child carrier with seat belt and leg guards.

thereby causing the driver to lose control of the bicycle and fall in traffic. For this reason, bicycles should be fitted with specially designed carriers which have seat belts to keep the children in place and shields to guard their feet against the spokes. (See Figure 6.2.) However, these carriers should be used only for children between the ages of one and five years, since younger children cannot be properly restrained and older children are too big for the carriers.

Resource Materials

American Association of State Highway
and Transportation Officials
341 National Press Building
Washington, D.C. 20004

American Automobile Association
1712 G. Street, N.W.
Washington, D.C. 20006

Bell Helmets
2850 East 29th Street
Long Beach, California 90806

The Bicycle Institute of America, Inc.
122 East 42nd Street
New York, New York 10017

The Bicycle Manufacturers Association
1101 15th Street, N.W.
Washington, D.C. 20005

Consumer Information
Public Documents Center
Pueblo, Colorado 81009

National Safety Council
444 North Michigan Avenue
Chicago, Illinois 60611

U.S. Consumer Product Safety Commission
5401 Westbard Avenue
Washington, D.C. 20207
Toll-free: 800-638-2666 in the continental United States
800-492-2937 for Maryland residents only

U.S. Department of Transportation
National Highway Traffic Safety Administration
Traffic Safety Programs
Washington, D.C. 20590

Activities

1. Develop a checklist of illegal and/or dangerous practices of bicyclists. Using this list, observe the actions of bicyclists in your community, and write a short paper on the results.

2. Check with local traffic officials, and inquire as to whether or not your community has a bicycle ordinance. If it does, obtain a copy of the ordinance, and present a short report to the class on its provisions.

3. Using the material in the section titled "Providing a Safe Place to Play," survey at least fifty children, and report on the frequency with which they play the various bicycle games.

4. Obtain a "recreational type" bicycle, and demonstrate to the class the various problems faced by an adult in relearning to drive a modern bicycle.

5. Invite the owner of a local bicycle shop to speak to the class about the selection and care of a new bicycle.

Questions

1. Why has the popularity of the bicycle increased in recent years?
2. Why is the bicycle considered to be a vehicle?
3. Which violations of traffic law are the most frequent causes of bicycle-motor-vehicle accidents?
4. What is the most important rule of bicycle safety?

5. What is a "wheelie," and why does it often lead to bicycle accidents?
6. What is "gully jumping," and why has it suddenly developed and grown in popularity?
7. Why are today's bicycles more difficult to drive than those of ten to fifteen years ago?
8. What is the best type of bicycle for children?
9. Why should an individual purchase a new bicycle from an established bike store rather than from a department store?
10. Why should a child be transported on a bicycle only in a specially designed carrier?

Selected References

"A Helmet for the 'Ordinary' Cyclist," *Consumers' Research Magazine.* September, 1976, 2.

Berry, Teresa and others. "The Toddler as a Bicycle Passenger," *Pediatrics.* March, 1972, 443-46.

"Bikes Are Like Cars, Obey the Same Rules," *School Safety.* September-October, 1967, 15-18.

Brooks, Thomas R. "Bike Boom—And Boomerang," *Family Safety.* Summer, 1974, 24-27.

———. "Safety-First for Cyclists," *Reader's Digest.* August, 1974, 35-38.

"Children's Bicycles," *Consumer Reports.* November, 1971, 649-55.

Daven, Joel; J. F. O'Conner; and Roy Briggs. "The Consequences of Imitative Behavior in Children: The 'Evel Knievel Syndrome', " *Pediatrics.* March, 1976, 418-19

"High-Rise Bikes," *Consumer Reports.* January, 1975, 8-16.

Horwitz, J. and others. "Dangers of Stunt Riding," *The New England Journal of Medicine.* November 28, 1974, 1194-95.

"How to Find the Bicycle Built for You," *Good Housekeeping.* June, 1976, 220, 222.

"How to Shop for a Bicycle," *Changing Times.* March, 1972, 45-47.

"Pedal Power—Is It Time You Taught Your Parents How to Ride a Bike?" *Senior Scholastic.* February 14, 1974, 20-21.

Schildkraut, Midge Lasky. "Be Sure You Know These Bike Safety Rules," *Good Housekeeping.* March, 1976, 183.

Stahnke, Carl J. "Bike Safety for Beginners," *Parent's Magazine.* August, 1975, 44-45.

Falls

7

Claiming approximately seventy-seven hundred lives each year, falls rank as the leading cause of accidental deaths in the home. Of those persons who die from falls, nearly 80 percent are included in the over-sixty-five age group. On the other hand, almost 50 percent of the disabling injuries involve persons under fifteen years of age. Apparently, while persons of all ages are susceptible to falls, the elderly are most likely to be killed. Yet, even oldsters who survive their falls and recover completely are never the same individuals again. Most will live with the fear of falling for the rest of their lives. As one elderly woman explains, "No one knows what it's like to fear just walking in your own home. Every step is a nightmare. I know if I make one mistake I'll end up on the floor again. Still, I have to live with it. My home's the only thing I've got left now that my husband's dead."

Preventing Falls from Different Levels

Generally, just as many falls occur inside the home as occur outside on the home premises. However, the types of falls vary slightly. Inside the home, over two-thirds of all falls are from different levels, such as from stairs and ladders. Outside the home, on the other hand, only one-half of all falls are from different levels.

Avoiding Stairway Accidents

Of the various locations where falls may occur, most people, especially the elderly, find stairways the most frightening. Nothing can cause more fear than the thought of tumbling down a long flight of stairs! Fortunately, stairways can be relatively safe if they are maintained and used in a proper manner.

Making the Stairs Safe

To ascend and descend stairs safely, an individual must be able to see where he is going. Accordingly, the first effort to make stairways safer should be directed at providing proper lighting. This entails the installation of either a large fluorescent lamp above the center of the stairs or two high-watt, nonglare light bulbs, one near each end of the stairway. When the light is installed properly, the person can switch it on at either end of the stairway before even placing his foot on the first step.

If the stairway is wooden or concrete, a further effort can be made to assure that the steps will be well seen by painting a white or luminescent color along the edge of each step. If for some reason paint is undesirable, strips of reflective tape can be set down to serve the same purpose. Furthermore, since many people fall because they think the lowest step is the floor level, the homeowner may want to paint the last step white or a luminescent color. This will serve as a warning that it is the last step and not the floor.

However, high visibility is often not enough, since anyone can easily fall on the best lighted stairways if they are poorly surfaced. For this reason, the homeowner should make certain that stairs are finished with a surface which will minimize the danger of foot-slippage. Contrary to what one might expect, of all surfaces, bare or painted wood does this the best. This is particularly true for painted stairs, where an abrasive surface has been obtained by mixing a little sand with the paint before it is applied. (See Figure 7.1 for paint-sand formula.) Less safe surfaces include varnish, bare concrete, rubber mats, and carpeting.

Varnish and bare concrete both produce smooth, slick surfaces. Concrete, however, can be made safer by applying a paint-sand mixture or strips of adhesive-backed, nonskid tape to make the surface somewhat abrasive. Of course, roughly finished concrete has its own abrasive surface. While rubber mats and carpeting are safer than either varnish or concrete surfaces, they are frequently the cause of falls because they are worn smooth and/or fastened down poorly. Yet, if these surfaces are properly secured and replaced before they become badly worn, they can be both attractive and relatively safe.

Naturally, falls can occur even on the safest surfaces. Therefore, every stairway should have at least one handrail that can be used by a person to maintain his balance when he is walking up or down the stairs. Open stairways should have two handrails, one on each side. Furthermore, when small children are present in the home, an expansion gate should be installed at the top of the stairs. On the other hand, in homes having stairways with doors at the top, the doors should open away from the stairs, since a door opening onto the stairs can easily strike anyone on the stairway and cause a fall.

Keeping Stairways Safe

Proper lighting, nonskid stairway surfaces, and sturdy handrails are not an absolute guarantee against falls, especially when poor housekeeping practices are tolerated. Stairways can be exceptionally safe in design and

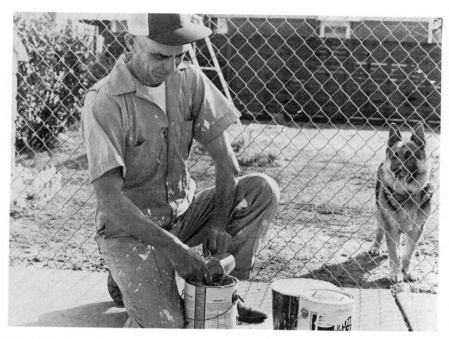

Figure 7.1   A mixture of one-half cup of sand and one gallon of paint will provide an abrasive surface on wooden or concrete stairs.

still be extremely dangerous if the homeowner fails to constantly guard against permitting and even creating stairway-related hazards.

Of all poor housekeeping practices, one of the most dangerous is using the stairway for storage purposes. Yet, this practice is also one of the most common. Since brooms, mops, buckets, and other cleaning items can be hidden from view behind a closed door, they are often stored on stairway steps leading to the basement. Obviously, a person can easily trip over such items and fall. For this reason, all household cleaning items should be stored only in cabinets or closets. However, where storage space is limited, the person can easily construct a small closet on the back of the stairway door. When it is built properly, this door closet can hold brooms, mops, detergents, and other narrow household items. Naturally, buckets and other wide items must be stored elsewhere.

Another housekeeping practice that can easily lead to stairway falls is placing a throw rug at the top of the stairs. Although it is placed in this location to prevent basement dirt from being tracked throughout the home, the rug can easily slip as an individual starts to descend the stairs, thereby causing a fall. While the best precaution is to eliminate all rugs at the top of stairways, the homeowner can still use with minimal hazard a rug with a rubber, nonslip backing. Naturally, while it will not easily slip, the rug can never be absolutely safe, since an edge can still catch a person's foot and cause a fall down the stairs.

Using Stairways Properly

Stairway maintenance is extremely important, but it is not the final step in the prevention of stairway falls. Equally important is the proper use of the stairways. Unless the safety items in the stairway design are utilized, stairway falls will still occur with frightening regularity.

One of the most frequent abuses is starting to use the stairs before switching on the light. Naturally, in the dark an individual can easily miss the first step and fall. Therefore, the person should always switch on the light before stepping onto the first step. Then, to help maintain balance while walking, he should use the handrail. This is especially important for elderly persons who may have lost much of their sense of balance. In addition, since the elderly do not lift their feet as high as when they were younger, they should watch where they place each foot to avoid tripping up the stairs.

Another common abuse, which is often used to save time, is running up and down stairs or taking two steps at a time. While this may save time and be good exercise for the heart, the practice may also result in serious injury if the person stumbles or hooks his toes on the edge of a step. The little time that is saved by the person rarely justifies the risk, and undoubtedly, jogging is much better for the heart than falling down a flight of stairs.

Safeguarding High Places

Guided by natural curiosity and a compulsion to climb, children are forever exploring their environment. While this activity is essential for normal growth and development, it can be extremely dangerous. In fact, several hundred youngsters are killed every year in falls from high places.

Quite often, a baby is placed on a bed, dresser, or table while his mother or father changes his diaper. Since a baby can easily wiggle his way off the structure in a matter of seconds, the child should be guarded at all times. Thus, if the telephone or doorbell rings, the parent should either take the baby along, or he should put him back in his crib.

Since a baby learns to stand and climb in his crib at an early age, parents should also make certain that the sides of the crib remain in a raised position. In addition, since an object may give the child a boost over the side of the crib, parents should remove stuffed animals and other large toys from the crib whenever the baby is left alone.

Surprisingly, numerous falls are associated with high chairs. Sometimes youngsters will stand on the seats and then topple over the sides of the chair, or they will slip out of the seat and then wiggle under the tray. At other times the youngsters will fall out of the chairs simply because the trays were inadvertently disengaged or were not used. As would be expected, most high-chair falls can be easily prevented. Simply, the parent should always fasten the tray securely in front of the child and then supervise the youngster as long as he is sitting in the high chair.

Without question, open windows, porches, and stairways present the greatest threat to toddlers. Because of this danger, parents should always install gates, screens, bars, or other protective devices wherever possible. Of course, all of the devices should be installed in such a manner that they can be easily removed by an adult during a fire.

Using Ladders Safely

When a job requires a ladder, an individual should always use one. Depending on a makeshift climbing device can easily result in a serious fall.

Undoubtedly, the most important factor in ladder safety is the condition of the ladder. Since paint may hide cracks and other defects, a ladder should always be finished with linseed oil, wood stain, or another clear nonslippery finish. Furthermore, a ladder should always be stored in a dry place, since dampness can easily cause deterioration of the wood. If a crack or break should appear, the individual should immediately purchase a new ladder or have the old ladder repaired by a professional.

Because the feet of the ladder may easily slip on hard, smooth surfaces, especially tile or concrete, rubber-faced shoes should always be attached to the feet of a ladder. Similarly, to keep the ends of the ladder head from slipping on a smooth wall, several pieces of an old innertube may be tacked securely to the ends.

When using a ladder on soft surfaces, a person should always place a wooden plank under the ladder feet to prevent sinking and slipping. Likewise, on uneven surfaces the lower foot of the ladder should be raised with a large block. While these suggestions also apply to self-supporting stepladders, an additional precaution is necessary. Since an unlocked stepladder can easily fold and cause its user to fall, an individual should invariably check a ladder of this type to make certain the feet are locked in place.

Because straight ladders are somewhat difficult to manipulate, certain precautions should also be taken. As a general rule, the ladder should be four feet longer than the height to be reached. When a straight ladder is used to reach a roof, the ladder should be propped against the roof so that it extends at least three feet above the roof. This will serve as a railing on which to hold and as an extension on which to lean.

When propping up a straight ladder against a wall, the user should make sure that the horizontal distance from the wall to the ladder feet is approximately one-fourth the vertical distance from the ground to the point where the ladder rests against the wall—a safe position which is neither too far from or too close to the wall. If the ladder is too far from the wall, the ladder feet can easily slip; if it is too close, the ladder can topple backward under the person's weight.

Regardless of the type of ladder, whether straight or step, certain climbing and usage rules should always be followed. When ascending a ladder, the user should always face the wall or ladder, since this position allows the person to use his toes in maintaining balance. Moreover, to keep both hands available for gripping the ladder, the user should place all of his tools in his pockets or clip them onto his belt. However, if the tools are too large or bulky for this or if a load of supplies must be taken up the ladder, he should attach a rope to the items, secure the rope to his wrist, and then climb the ladder. Once he is on the roof or other work platform, the person can then haul the tools or supplies upward with the rope.

While standing on a ladder and working, the user should always remain at least three rungs from the top, since this position provides for the best balance. In addition, the person should avoid excessive reaching which could cause him to lose his balance and fall. Ideally, at frequent intervals he should move the ladder into more suitable positions.

Eliminating Falls on the Same Level

Approximately 40 percent of all home falls, both inside the home and outside on the home premises, occur on the same level. From the standpoint of falls, the bathroom and the bedroom are the most dangerous rooms in the home.

Fallproofing the Bathroom

Of the various locations in the home where falls occur, many take place in the bathroom. Obviously, nothing can cause a fall quicker than water on tile or enamel! However, the problem is more complex than most people realize. Like all falls, bathroom falls can easily cause severe injury and even death if the person strikes his head on a hard surface, but unlike other falls, bathroom falls can also lead to death by drowning if the person is knocked unconscious and comes to rest with his nose and mouth in the bathwater.

Apparently much of the hazard can be eliminated by providing a firm footing where it is needed the most, in the bathtub and shower. In recent years special tubs with embossed bottoms have been introduced as safety innovations. Except for their attractively textured bottom surfaces, these embossed bathtubs are indistinguishable from ordinary tubs. However, an embossed bathtub may actually be hazardous for the average homeowner.

According to some safety experts, soap scum may accumulate in the indentations and eventually make the surface dangerously slippery.

Fortunately, an ordinary bathtub can still be equipped with a nonslip bottom. On the market are strips or decals of nonskid material, which can be applied in a pattern on the bottom of the bathtub or shower, and mats with an adhesive backing and a slightly abrasive top. Both devices are inexpensive and easy to install. (See Figure 7.2.) Unfortunately, the most popular device on the market is a mat constructed of rubber with suction discs on the underside. (See Figure 7.2.) However, since the suction discs frequently lose contact with the tub or shower bottom, the mats are not reliable and may cause the bather to fall. For this reason, rubber suction disc mats are not recommended for the homeowner.

Surprisingly, not only the feet can easily slip in the tub. Because the water makes the enamel slick, the hands can easily slide if they are placed on the rim of the bathtub as an aid in getting into and out of the water. However, this problem can be eliminated by affixing several strips or decals of nonskid material on the top of the bathtub rim. As an additional aid, firmly anchored grab-bars should be located along the sides of the bathtub and shower. Since the bather can grip entirely around the bars, his hands are less likely to slip.

Although the bars are an excellent safety precaution for everyone, grab-bars are essential equipment for the elderly, since they often experience difficulty in sitting, rising, and standing for long periods of time. In recent

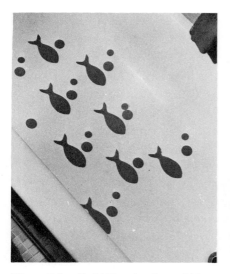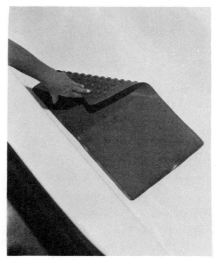

Figure 7.2 (Left) Decals of nonskid material and (Right) rubber suction disc mat.

years a special grab-bar that can be fastened to the front rim of the bathtub has been introduced. Because of its position on the bathtub rim, the bar is an excellent aid for the elderly bather. In addition, the homeowner should also provide the elderly person with an adjustable vinyl bath seat which hooks on the bathtub rim. Besides allowing the oldster to sit at a comfortable height while he is bathing, the seat, because of its higher position, reduces the difficulty that the person would normally experience in rising from the tub and thus lessens his chances of falling.

Unfortunately, even with nonslip material, grab-bars, and other bathtub aids, falls can still occur. However, the homeowner can take certain steps to reduce the severity of the falls. Since a bather will instinctively grab for the nearest support when he feels himself falling, towel and shower curtain rods should be anchored firmly so they can support a person's weight. Although the shower curtain will usually tear free, a firmly supported rod will help reduce the impact of the fall. Also, if a sliding glass door, instead of a curtain, encloses the shower, the door should always be made of safety glass, since a fall through a regular glass door will almost always result in severe injury or death.

Naturally, not all bathroom falls occur in the bathtub or shower. Because water is often splashed onto the floor, some of these accidents occur in the area adjacent to the tub or shower. These falls can usually be prevented by drying off as much as possible while still in the bathtub and then stepping onto a nonslip rug located near the tub to finish drying off. Of course, the bather should immediately wipe up any water that does splash onto the floor.

While most bathroom falls result directly or indirectly from bathing, some do occur for other reasons. A common causative factor in falls among the elderly is that they have difficulty in getting on and off the toilet because the seat is too low. Fortunately, this problem can be easily solved by installing a special attachment to make the seat higher and by installing sturdy grab-bars along the sides of the toilet to help them get on and off easier. However, if such precautions cannot be taken, the homeowner should at least purchase a portable toilet for the elderly person. Specially designed to be higher off the floor, the toilet has its own built-in grab-bars. (See Figure 7.3.)

Stopping Bedroom Falls

Perhaps the most deceiving location in the home where falls may occur is the bedroom. Although it appears to be relatively safe, the bedroom is actually the scene of many falls, especially by the elderly.

As one would expect, most oldsters fall in the vicinity of the bed. To help an elderly person maintain his balance while he is climbing into or out of the bed, a handrail can be installed either on the wall near the bed or on a special support connected to the side of the bed. Furthermore, as many

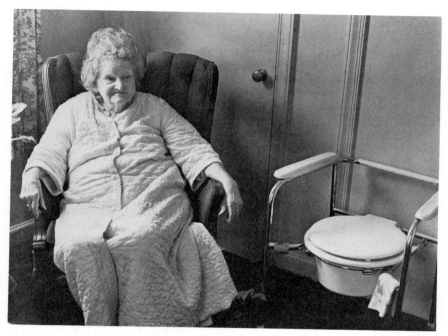

Figure 7.3 A portable toilet is an excellent fall-prevention aid for the elderly person.

elderly persons accidentally fall out of their beds during the night, a guard should be installed on each side of the bed. Similar to the sides of a hospital bed, the guards can be raised at night and lowered in the morning. While bed guards are an excellent safety precaution for all elderly individuals, the devices are indispensable to older persons who sleep on one side of the bed in order to be within easy reach of water or medicine on a nearby night-stand.

Undoubtedly, many falls by elderly persons are caused by dizziness. Since their bodies can no longer adjust quickly to changes in position, the elderly frequently become dizzy upon standing and fall as a result. However, such accidents can be prevented. When getting out of bed, the elderly individual should first sit on the edge of the bed for a few minutes so his body can slowly adjust to its new position. After this period of time, the person can slowly stand and begin walking without becoming dizzy.

Naturally, many bedroom falls occur because the elderly, as well as persons of all ages, cannot see where they are walking at night. Typically, without turning on the light, they will attempt to leave the bedroom to get a drink of water or to go to the bathroom. As a result, they will often stumble in the dark over furniture and other bedroom items. To prevent such falls, the individual should keep a large flashlight on a stand near the bed for use at night. However, in the bedroom of a young child or an elderly person, the flashlight should always be supplemented with a nightlight.

Creating a Fallproof Living Room

Falls in the living room are not overly common, but when they do occur, they are often serious. Generally, most living-room falls are the result of poor household planning.

One of the most frequent causes of living-room falls, especially for the elderly, is the failure to secure small throw rugs. Tacking down the edges of the rugs may provide a solution to the problem in many homes, but there are differing opinions on this subject. As Fales notes:

> An untacked rug sometimes turns up and trips you. But unless a rug can be so neatly tacked that there is not the slightest chance of catching your toe or heel, some safety men say it is better to leave it untacked. Catching your foot on a section of tacked rug might cause a fall that might have been avoided if the rug could yield.[1]

Perhaps the best solution is to buy only throw rugs with a nonslip rubber backing. These rugs will prevent slipping and yet will yield enough to reduce the possibility of tripping.

The blocking of normal traffic patterns with furniture is another frequent cause of falls in the living room. Since many falls occur as people absent-mindedly walk into poorly arranged furniture, the homeowner should make certain that chairs, end tables, and other living-room items are placed well away from hallways and doors. In addition, after furniture has been rearranged, the person should familiarize everyone with the new grouping, since a family member can easily fall over furniture which suddenly appears in a different place.

Like living-room furniture, extension cords may also present a hazard when they are poorly located. For this reason, all cords should be laid along the base of the walls to the electrical outlets. Since constant walking over electrical wiring may wear away the insulation and cause a fire, the homeowner should never place electrical cords under rugs or carpeting.

Another leading cause of falls in the living room is the improper waxing of floors. When wax is applied sparingly, it produces a hard, nonslippery finish. However, when it is applied excessively or when it is not polished properly, wax causes an extremely slippery floor. The best way to solve this problem is to use one of the nonslip floor finishes which are now on the market. However, if wax is preferred, the homeowner should apply a light

---

1. E. D. Fales, Jr., "Falls: Threat to Oldsters," *Today's Health,* February, 1959, p. 59.

coat and then buff the floor to a hard shine. Furthermore, since an oily mop will break down the wax and leave a slippery surface, the person should dust the floor only with a dry mop.

As a final note, two additional housekeeping hints may help prevent living-room falls. First, family members should immediately wipe up spilled drinks and foodstuff, and pick up rubber bands, pencils, and other small objects which have fallen onto the floor. Second, since long robes can easily cause a serious fall, the housewife should change into a dress or a pair of slacks before starting the morning chores.

Making Play Areas Fall-safe

Perhaps the most numerous and often the most serious falls by children occur while they are playing normally around the home. Since many youngsters fall over their own toys, parents should provide a large toy box in the home and require children to keep all their toys in the box. In addition, parents should limit children to three or four toys at a time. Even the youngest child should thoroughly understand these rules, and the parents must make certain that the rules are obeyed!

Another helpful precaution that parents should take is to establish a "no running in the house" rule and make sure that the rule is obeyed. Many serious head injuries occur each year as children fall while running and strike their heads on doors, tables, lamps, and other household fixtures. In an extreme case, a four-year-old boy in New York City was playing tag with his sister in the living room when he tripped and plunged headfirst into the television; the boy was killed when the vacuum tube in the set imploded and spewed daggerlike pieces of glass into his face and neck.

Naturally, regardless of safety rules, normal, healthy children are going to fall during play. However, parents can significantly reduce the possibility of serious injury by installing a thick rug where the children play most frequently.

Averting Sidewalk Falls

One of the surest ways to guard against slips and falls on sidewalks is the elimination of unsafe surfaces. When combined with careful and attentive sidewalk use, safe surfaces will considerably reduce the incidence of home sidewalk falls.

Whenever possible, snow and slush should be removed from sidewalks, as well as outside stairways, before the material can become trampled by pedestrians and then frozen into a solid mass of ice. Nevertheless, if ice does form and it cannot be removed immediately, the homeowner should sprinkle sand, fine cinders, or gravel on the icy surface. When used alone, each material provides a more abrasive surface, but when used in conjunction with rock salt, the new combination also helps to melt the ice. For the best results, the homeowner should mix the abrasive material with the rock salt in a three to one ratio.

When sidewalks are slippery, the best advice is to stay indoors. If this is not possible, the person should use a flat-footed shuffle and keep his weight forward, since the greatest danger of falling results when the body weight rests over the heels. Furthermore, before entering a building, the individual should clean his shoes thoroughly to remove any traces of water, slush, snow, or ice. Even the slightest trace of water on the soles of the shoes can form a slippery surface and cause a serious fall.

While slippery surfaces are probably the most frequent cause of sidewalk falls, holes and uneven surfaces may also cause an unwary pedestrian to fall. Whenever possible, sidewalk irregularities should be corrected immediately. However, if the conditions must be reported to authorities first, the homeowner should erect warning signs near the trouble areas and keep the signs in position until the problem has been corrected. Besides eliminating holes and uneven surfaces, the person should keep the sidewalk clear of foreign objects, such as rocks, twigs, cans, and toys.

Resource Materials

American Academy of Pediatrics
P.O. Box 1034
Evanston, Illinois 60204

American Hospital Association
840 North Lake Shore Drive
Chicago, Illinois 60611

National Safety Council
444 North Michigan Avenue
Chicago, Illinois 60611

U.S. Consumer Product Safety Commission
5401 Westbard Avenue
Washington, D.C. 20207
Toll-free: 800-638-2666 in the continental United States
800-492-2937 for Maryland residents only

Activities

1. Develop a checklist of conditions that can cause falls in the home. Use this checklist to survey your home.

2. Write a short paper on the importance of "keeping stairways safe."

3. Obtain information from a local department store about the relative popularity, in terms of sales, of both the rubber suction disc mat and the nonskid material that can be placed on the bottom of the bathtub. Report to the class on your findings.

4. Design a bedside tray that the elderly can reach while lying in the center of the bed. The tray should have space for a water pitcher, a glass, medicine, tissues, and other necessary items.

5. Obtain information from a local hospital about the frequency of head injuries to children caused by falls while running in the home.

Questions

1. Why is bare wood or plain paint on wooden steps much safer than steps finished with varnish or covered with rubber mats?
2. What unique problem must the elderly face when climbing stairs?
3. Why should ladders be finished with a clear, nonslippery finish instead of paint?
4. Why are rubber suction disc mats not recommended for use in bathtubs or showers?
5. Why should bath shower curtains and towel rods be firmly anchored?
6. When getting out of bed, how can the elderly person prevent dizziness and falls?
7. Why are nonslip throw rugs better for use in the living room than tacked-down rugs?
8. When waxing a floor, what steps should be taken to make sure that the wax produces a hard, nonslippery finish?
9. What rules should children obey when playing in the home?
10. When putting an abrasive material on snow or ice-covered sidewalks, why should the homeowner first mix the material with rock salt?

Selected References

Bergner, Lawrence and others. "Falls from Heights: A Childhood Epidemic in an Urban Area," *American Journal of Public Health*. January, 1971, 90-96.

Carper, Jean. *Stay Alive!* Garden City, New York: Doubleday & Company, Inc., 1965.

Fales, E. D., Jr. "Falls: Threat to Oldsters," *Today's Health*. February, 1959, 14-15, 58-61.

Gladstone, Bernard. "How to Stay Alive on a Ladder," *Popular Mechanics*. August, 1963, 166-69.

Grove, M. "Bad Case of Common Sense," *Good Housekeeping*. August, 1969, 36.

Higdon, Hal. "How to Make Yourself Fall-Safe," *Today's Health*. April, 1964, 72-76.

"Home Is Where Accidents Happen," *Changing Times*. December, 1971, 37-38.

"Improving Bathroom Safety," *Good Housekeeping*. September, 1968, 160.

Kinard, Epsie. "Safe at Home," *House Beautiful*. April, 1967, 30, 32, 34, 36.

Michaelson, Mike. "Are You Heading for a Fall?" *Today's Health*. October, 1969, 52-55, 73.

Nader, Ralph. "Home Unsafe Home," *Ladies' Home Journal*. January, 1972, 70, 72, 74, 121.

———. "Ralph Nader Reports: Rub-a-dub-dub, it can be unsafe in the tub. . .," *Ladies' Home Journal*. June, 1975, 41.

Peszczynski, Mieczyslow. "Why Old People Fall," *American Journal of Nursing*. May, 1965, 86-88.

"Safety Tips for Do-It-Yourselfers," *Good Housekeeping*. March, 1969, 198.

Solomon, Goody L. "Safeguarding Your Home—II. Help for House Hazards," *Reader's Digest*. March, 1975, 177-78, 180.

Speers, James F. "Accidental Falls in Infancy," *The Journal of the Iowa Medical Society*. December, 1968, 1256-58.

Fires

8

As the woman began to talk, tears rolled down her cheeks. "The smoke was thick and black. I could hear my daughter crying, but I couldn't reach her. She was calling, 'Mommy, where are you?' 'I can't see you.' Then, there was silence." That was all the woman could remember. Her four-year-old daughter had died in the fire that destroyed their home.

Every year home fires claim approximately fifty-one hundred lives. Almost one-fourth of the victims are children under fourteen years of age. Naturally, the sight of dense smoke and roaring flames is frightening for everyone, but for persons who are unaware of the dangers presented by a fire, the sight is especially horrifying. Fortunately, even the slightest knowledge about the dangers of fire can significantly increase a person's chances of survival.

Anatomy and Spread of a Fire

Many people mistakenly believe that fire spreads throughout a home by burning along the floor, up the walls, and then across the ceiling. Consequently, they cannot accept the fact that a home can be completely engulfed in flames within a matter of minutes. Actually, combustible material in the home may ignite without even being touched by the fire.

As a fire increases in size, the surrounding air becomes tremendously hot and rushes upward. When it is finally stopped by the ceiling, the air spreads outward and then downward to bathe the entire room in heat. If it is hot enough, the air will ignite any combustible material that it touches. As a result, various parts of the home may be simultaneously exploding into flames. One can easily visualize the effect of this superheated air on any person who has the misfortune of being in the home at the time of the fire. Even a single lungful of hot air will instantly cause death!

Surprisingly, however, heat and flames are not the major threats to life in a fire; actually, the real killer is the accompanying smoke which claims an overwhelming majority of the victims. According to fire officials, few people burn to death: most of the victims, approximately 80 percent, are asphyxiated by the smoke long before the flames ever touch them.

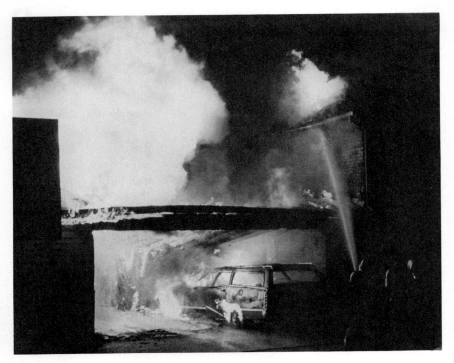

Figure 8.1   A raging fire completely engulfs a two-story home. (Courtesy of Dennis Wolf, Memphis, Tennessee)

Smoke consists of small liquid and solid particles suspended in various gases, many of which are toxic. Among the toxic gases most commonly found in smoke are carbon monoxide and carbon dioxide. Other gases which are no less deadly include the various nitrogen oxides, hydrogen chloride, hydrogen cyanide, hydrogen sulfide, sulfur dioxide, ammonia, formaldehyde, and phosgene. Although some are more toxic than others, the important factor in a fire is the concentration of the gases. Some gases are extremely toxic, but they may be produced in only small quantities. Other gases are only slightly toxic, but they may be produced in large quantities. In general, the type and quantity of gas which is produced in a fire will depend upon the nature of the burning materials.

Obviously, the danger presented by smoke is not solely a function of any particular gas. Rather, the gases work together in different ways to subdue their victims. Some gases, such as carbon monoxide, have no odor and are impossible to detect. Other gases which do have an odor prevent their detection by anesthetizing the victim's sense of smell. In such cases the victim is slowly poisoned without being aware of it. However, even when the victim perceives the smoke, he is often at the mercy of the toxic gases. Some gases, such as carbon dioxide, stimulate respiration and, as a result, cause the victim to inhale greater and greater amounts of the toxic gases. Other gases function in the opposite manner by depressing respiration to the point of respiratory failure. Perhaps the most frightening way in which gases work together, however, is that they combine to produce a far more toxic effect than the sum of their toxicities would suggest. Unfortunately, a person cannot accurately determine when the toxic gases in smoke are present in large quantities and thus when the smoke is most dangerous. In reality, thin, light-gray smoke may be just as deadly as thick, black smoke.

On the other hand, a person can easily ascertain the most dangerous locations in the burning home. Governed by a simple law of physics, the toxic gases in smoke will always rise because they are hot. As a result, the top floors of a building are always the most perilous. Moreover, the height to which a gas rises is a function of its temperature and density. Consequently, within each room during a fire, the smoke gases will stratify or form layers. Some gases are so heavy that they rise only slightly and thus settle close to the floor. Other gases which are lighter rise more and form layers higher above the floor. In a fire, layers of gases will reach all the way from the floor to the ceiling. Fortunately, for a person trying to flee from a fire, a relatively gas-free or smoke-free layer exists about eighteen inches above the floor.

Obtaining an Early Warning

Most of the home fire deaths in this country occur during the night. The reason is evident: at night the victims are asleep and thus unaware of the danger. Yet, many such deaths could be prevented by an early-warning system.

Of the various early-warning systems on the market, the automatic fire-alarm system is the oldest. In general, fire-alarm systems operate on the principle that a sustained high temperature and/or a given rate of rise in temperature will trigger the alarm system. However, fire-alarm systems detect heat, not smoke. Consequently, since fires are revealed faster by smoke than by heat, fire-alarm systems are no longer considered by fire officials to be the best type of early-warning systems for homes.

In recent years smoke detectors have grown remarkably in popularity. In fact, a few insurance companies now offer discounts to homeowners with smoke-detector systems. In the home two types of smoke detectors are commonly used. Each has its strengths and weaknesses.[1]

---

1. "Smoke Detectors," *Consumer Reports,* October, 1976, p. 555.

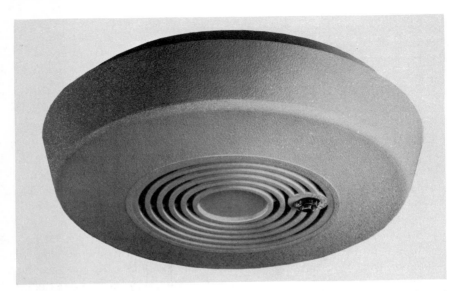

Figure 8.2   Ionization smoke detector. (Courtesy of BRK Electronics, Division of Pittway Corporation)

The photoelectric detector is designed with a small lamp that directs a beam of light into a chamber. Within the chamber is a light-sensitive photocell, normally placed out of the way of the lamp's direct beam. When smoke enters the chamber during a fire, the particles in the smoke scatter the light beam. Then, detecting the scattered light, the photocell activates the alarm. As a rule, the photoelectric smoke detector is relatively sensitive to smoke produced by smoldering fires. However, in the presence of flaming fires, the photoelectric detector will usually react rather slowly.

Using a harmless amount of radioactive material to transform air within the unit into a conductor, the ionization smoke detector has a small electrical current passing through the "ionized-air" chamber. (See Figure 8.2.) When smoke enters the chamber, the particles in the smoke disrupt the flow of the electrical current. When the current is sufficiently disrupted, electronic circuitry in the detector senses the reduction in current and activates the alarm. Generally, the ionization detector will respond exceptionally well to the slight smoke generated by a flaming fire. On the other hand, the ionization detector is less sensitive to smoke from a smoldering fire.

Before purchasing a smoke-alarm system, the homeowner should carefully consider several factors. *First,* how many single station detector units are needed in a home smoke-alarm system? In a single-level home, a minimum of two smoke detectors are essential. However, if the bedrooms are located at both ends of the home, at least three detectors may be needed for adequate protection. In a multilevel home, a smoke detector should be purchased for each floor of the building. *Second,* which type of smoke detector will provide the best protection? Apparently, both types of detectors offer certain advantages. For example, smoldering fires are the most deadly, and photoelectric detectors are especially sensitive to this type of smoke. On the other hand, flaming fires are the most damaging to the home, and ionization detectors are exceptionally responsive to this type of smoke. Therefore, a smoke-alarm system with both types of detectors will furnish the homeowner with maximum protection. *Third,* what type of power source is recommended for a smoke detector? All smoke detectors are powered by either batteries or a house wiring system. Each power source has its advantages and disadvantages. For example, because of the battery, the battery-powered detector will function even during an electrical failure. However, the battery must be replaced approximately once every year. Unless the battery is replaced, the detector cannot provide protection for the homeowner. On the other hand, because of its plug-in design, the electrically-powered detector will function inexpensively on normal household current. However, in the case of a blown fuse, tripped circuit breaker, or general power failure, the detector is useless for sensing smoke and warning the homeowner. For the best protection, a home smoke-alarm system should include both battery-powered and electrically-powered detectors. *Fourth,* which brand of smoke detector is the most reliable? Actually, most brands of smoke detectors are comparable in quality. To verify the reliability of a particular brand, the homeowner should check the detector for the seal of the Underwriters' Laboratories (UL). (See Figure 8.3.) If the unit has the UL label, the smoke detector is reliable under certain conditions stated by the Laboratories.

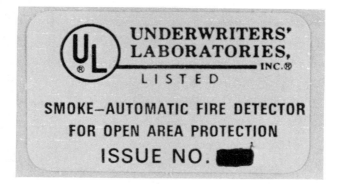

Figure 8.3   The UL label indicates that the equipment has been tested and meets the requirements established by Underwriters' Laboratories, an independent, not-for-profit organization which tests for public safety. (Courtesy of Underwriters' Laboratories, Inc.)

As the manufacturers of early-warning devices specify on their products, the smoke detectors must be installed in certain locations for the best protection. Ordinarily, a detector should be placed on the ceiling of a corridor or hallway just outside of the entrance to the bedrooms. In this position the unit can be most easily heard at night. If the bedrooms are located at both ends of the home, at least one detector is needed in each location. Preferably, this smoke detector should be an ionization model, since it reacts faster to flaming fires in which the smoke rises rapidly and travels along the ceiling. In a two-story home, another detector should be installed on the wall or ceiling near the stairway leading to the bedrooms; in a single-level home, the detector should be installed some distance away from the bedrooms, preferably in the living room. Ideally, this detector should be a photoelectric model, since it responds quicker to smoke from smoldering fires.

With practically all of the different brands of smoke detectors, the manufacturers include a suggestion that members of a family can increase their chances of escape by sleeping with the bedroom doors closed. Besides slowing the progress of the smoke, each door may impede the fire for approximately three to ten minutes. However, with modern smoke detectors, this advice may not be appropriate. According to *Consumer Reports,*

> . . . a recent study for the National Bureau of Standards notes that such traditional reasoning is questionable if you install a smoke detector. An open door lets sleepers hear the alarm more easily, affording extra time for escape. And should a fire start in a bedroom itself, the detector will respond more quickly if the door is open and will alert other occupants of the house faster.[2]

Apparently, individuals who are protected by smoke detectors should always sleep with their bedroom doors open, not closed.

Protecting the Exceptionally Vulnerable

Any escape from a fire may be difficult. As a thirty-two-year-old fireman from Memphis, Tennessee, related from a personal experience, "Dense, black smoke engulfed me. I felt as if I had crawled into a black oven and closed the door on myself. The heat was fierce, like a blast furnace. I found a doorknob, yanked it open, and rushed through the door. It was only a clothes closet. Finally, I found a window and dived out." As this account suggests, everyone is susceptible to smoke, flames, and heat. However, of the various family members, children and invalids are the most vulnerable in a home fire.

---

2. "Smoke Detectors," p. 558.

Paradoxically, unless they are properly trained, most children will not even attempt to escape from the home during a fire. In many cases the youngsters, apparently believing that they are safe from the fire if they cannot see it, will hide under a bed or in a closet. In other cases, screaming hysterically for their parents, the youngsters will run from one smoke-filled room into the next. For this reason, fire officials in recent years have been stressing the need for parents to identify children's bedrooms. In many communities parents can obtain fluorescent or retroreflective "C" (C = children) stickers from the fire department. (See Figure 8.4.) The stickers are designed to assist the firemen in locating children during a blaze. Generally, for each youngster who normally sleeps in the room, one "C" sticker should be affixed to the bedroom window.

With few exceptions, invalids cannot escape from a fire by themselves. Consequently, because of their illnesses or disabilities, they must either be carried from the burning home or be transported in wheelchairs or on stretchers. In many instances husky firemen who are trained in such rescues are needed to help the invalid escape. Therefore, like children's rooms, the bedrooms of invalids should be identified by fluorescent or retroreflective "I" stickers. (I = invalid, See Figure 8.4.) In addition, the homeowner should provide the invalid person with a downstairs bedroom, thereby simplifying the escape or rescue procedure.

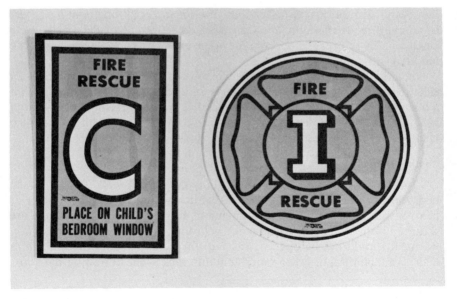

Figure 8.4   Fluorescent or retroreflective stickers identify for firemen the bedrooms of persons who require assistance in escaping from a fire.

Planning for Escape

Too often escape is viewed as something that will occur naturally and does not need to be practiced. Actually, escape is strange and difficult, not natural. As mentioned in the preceding section, unless they are properly trained, children will try to hide from a fire by crawling under a bed or into a closet, or they will rush through smoke-filled rooms while searching hysterically for their parents. Even adults have been known to stay in their homes too long to escape safely. According to fire officials, members of the family should be systematically trained not to panic during a fire.

When planning for an escape from a home fire, the head of the family should make sure that everyone, including the youngest child, thoroughly understands the various steps in the escape procedure. These steps include: (1) turning on the lights; (2) testing the door; (3) determining the escape route; (4) getting out of the home fast; (5) meeting outside in a pre-arranged spot; and (6) calling the fire department.

Turning on the Lights

If he is awakened at night by the early-warning system or by smoke or fire, the person should immediately switch on the nearest bedroom light. This simple action will alleviate many of the fears which are fostered by darkness and will reveal instantly the amount of smoke which has entered the room. In addition, the action may disclose information about the severity of the fire. If the light does not work, the fire has made considerable headway. Therefore, escape from the home by an appropriate route must be initiated without delay.

Since the bedroom light will not work if a fire has reached the house's electrical wiring system and since light is an invaluable aid in escaping from a burning home, the homeowner should always keep a flashlight on a stand near each bed. As noted in the preceding chapter, the flashlight can also help prevent falls as the person walks across the dark bedroom floor.

Testing the Door[3]

After turning on the light, the individual should walk to the closed bedroom door and feel its entire surface. Since wood is a poor conductor of heat, a warm door means that tremendous heat and poisonous smoke are waiting on the other side to enter the bedroom. If the door is even slightly warm, it should not be opened. Instead, the person should place a rug, a bedspread, clothes, or other material in the crack at the bottom of the door.

---

3. Families who are protected by smoke detectors should always sleep with their bedroom doors open, not closed. However, since family members may occasionally sleep overnight at friends and relatives' homes that are not protected by early-warning systems, the "testing the door" step should never be omitted in planning the escape procedure.

This material will help keep smoke out of the bedroom. Then the person can escape through the bedroom window, or after opening the window for air, he can wait in the room to be rescued by firemen.

Even when the surface is cool, the door should be opened cautiously, since heat and flames may be on the other side. Before opening the door, the individual should place his right hand on the doorknob, his right shoulder and right foot against the door, and his left hand along the door opening. If a fire is present on the other side, this "braced" stance will enable the person to slam the door shut before the pressure of the gases can force the door open. In addition, to prevent the inhalation of smoke, the individual should turn his face away from the door opening.

If no smoke or heat, or very little of either, enters the bedroom, the person should walk to the remaining bedrooms and awaken the other family members. Then he can search the home for other signs of smoke and fire. However, if smoke and heat seep into the room, he should close the door and seal the crack under the door with material. The individual can then escape through the bedroom window, or he can wait in the room to be rescued.

Determining the Escape Route

After deciding to leave the house because of the danger of smoke and fire, the individual should select the most suitable route from the room to the outside of the home. Normally, the most appropriate route will be the primary escape route, which is through the rooms, hallways, and doors to the outside. Unless smoke and fire conditions dictate otherwise, the person should always consider this route first. However, if the primary escape route is blocked, he should then choose the secondary escape route, which is through the window to the outside of the home. (See Figure 8.5.)

Compared to an escape through a door, a window escape is always difficult. However, when the window is located on an upper floor, the escape is even more complicated. Ideally, the homeowner should purchase several folding ladders or similar devices that will allow the family members easily to reach the ground. One device should be stored in each bedroom, and every member of the family should be able to use the device. However, in the absence of an escape ladder or similar device, other steps can be taken to lessen the impact of jumping. First, to cushion his landing, the person should quickly gather clothing, blankets, pillows, and other soft materials and drop them on the ground directly under the window. Next, he should ease the lower part of his body over the window sill and then hang against the outside of the house with his hands. This technique decreases the distance to the ground and thus allows a softer drop onto the pile of materials. Finally, to help cushion the impact of landing, the person should allow his knees to bend when his feet contact the ground.

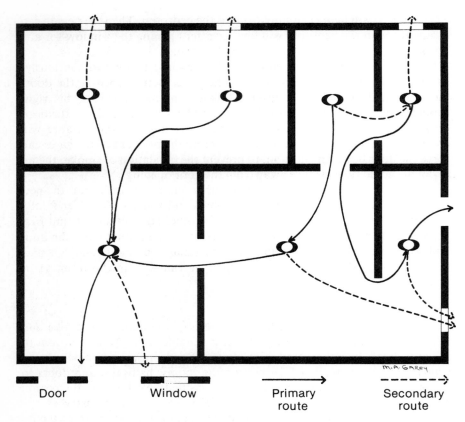

Figure 8.5   Two escape routes, preferably a primary and a secondary, should be planned for each room in the home.

Getting Out of the Home Fast

When using the primary escape route, the individual should always remember that smoke, not flames, is the real killer in a fire. Consequently, if he is to escape by moving through the rooms and hallways to the outside, the person must take certain steps to fight the toxic effects of the smoke. Specifically, he should hold or tie a damp washcloth or other piece of wet, thick material over his mouth and nose. Although the material will not filter out the toxic gases in smoke, the mask will help to alleviate many of the irritating effects which are normally caused by the inhalation of the smoke.

In addition, when moving through the rooms and hallways, the person should remember that smoke gases form layers, but that a relatively smoke-free layer exists about eighteen inches above the floor. To breathe the air in this layer, he should either crawl on his hands and knees or duck walk toward the door. Regardless of which method is used, the most critical factor for the person is to get out of the burning home before the toxic gases in the smoke can render him helpless.

Meeting Outside in a Prearranged Spot

After escaping from the burning home, the members of the family should assemble at a prearranged spot some distance from the home. This is especially important, since the members may have left the home by different routes. Only in this way can the head of the family reassure himself that everyone is outside and safe. In addition, by meeting at a considerable distance from the building, the family members will not become lost in the crowd of onlookers which normally gathers in front of the burning house.

After escaping from a fire, the person should never reenter the burning home, since his chances of escaping a second time are considerably reduced. Besides the possibility of becoming hysterical and exercising foolish judgment, the individual will encounter even more abundant smoke, flames, and heat during his second escape attempt. For this reason, only professional fire fighters should perform search and rescue operations.

Calling the Fire Department

After everyone is safely outside the home, the individual should notify the fire department immediately. Ideally, because of the danger of becoming trapped in the burning house, he should telephone from a neighbor's home. However, if he is forced to telephone from the burning home, the person should always make certain that the other family members have safely escaped. In addition, he should leave himself an unobstructed escape route.

When reporting a fire, the individual should always give the family name and street address and explain what has happened. After providing this information, he should not immediately hang up the telephone, but should wait to make sure that all the information has been understood. Unfortunately, many persons in their excitement will simply yell "Help, there's a fire here," and then hang up the phone. Other persons will become angry at the fire department and, as a result, will waste valuable fire-fighting time. As a Memphis, Tennessee, fire official explains, "You're in trouble as soon as the fire alarm phone rings. You ask the person where the fire is, the nearest cross street, and so on, and he screams into the phone, 'Why in the hell are you asking me all these stupid questions? Just come and put out the damn fire.' "

Practicing the Escape

After the head of the family has called everyone together and is reasonably certain that they understand the various parts of the escape procedure, he should establish a regular plan for practicing the home escape. At first, the practice sessions should be kept relatively simple. Fire drills should be announced beforehand, and family members should be instructed to use only the primary escape routes. Later, surprise fire drills should be conducted, and whenever the primary routes are designated as blocked by the head of the family, family members should be instructed to use the secondary escape routes.

For the first two or three months, the homeowner should conduct a fire drill at least once every week. Thereafter, he should plan two drills, both announced and unannounced, every month.

Fighting the Fire

While the emphasis up to this point has been on safely escaping from the home, in certain situations the homeowner should attempt to extinguish the fire to prevent its spread. Normally, these situations occur while the fire is still small or while it is still confined to a limited area. If the individual decides to fight the fire, he should always take at least two precautions. First, he should immediately evacuate everyone from the home. Tragically, many people have been asphyxiated by smoke while a family member fought a "small" fire. As Carper illustrates,

> After unsuccessfully trying to extinguish a smoldering chair, a housewife ran to a neighbor's for aid. The two women lugged the chair out-of-doors safely and complimented themselves on their quick action. Later, when the mother went upstairs to awaken her two napping children, she found them dead—asphyxiated by the toxic fumes that had risen up the stairway.[4]

Second, the person should always leave himself an escape route and never allow himself to become trapped because of his preoccupation with fighting the fire. Possessions can be replaced; human life cannot.

In home fire fighting one factor will always determine success or failure: preparedness. To extinguish a fire quickly, the person must be able to rapidly reach fire-fighting equipment. Using pans of water from the sink to extinguish a fire will usually result in failure. In fact, in some types of fires, water will only create additional problems. For example, throwing water on an electrical fire may cause a severe shock if the person has forgotten to turn off the electricity. Similarly, splashing water on flammable liquids will only spatter the fire. For small electrical and flammable-liquid fires, a five-pound box of baking soda will serve as an excellent extinguisher. The box should be stored where the person can easily reach it, preferably in the kitchen cabinet. For small, ordinary combustible fires, special fire blankets

4. Jean Carper, *Stay Alive!* (Garden City, New York: Doubleday & Company, Inc., 1965), p. 15.

can be prepared and stored in easily accessible locations in the home. Each blanket should be flameproofed by dipping it in a solution which is composed of nine ounces of borax, four ounces of boric acid, and one gallon of water. For their protection all family members should practice extinguishing clothing fires by rolling up in the blanket or by rolling on the ground or floor. Naturally, for large fires a commercial fire extinguisher is usually required.

While numerous types of fire extinguishers are available, some are more suitable for home use than others. In general, fire extinguishers are identified by letters that indicate the class or the classes of fires which the instruments are designed to extinguish. Class A fires involve ordinary combustible materials; Class B fires involve flammable liquids, greases, and gases; Class C fires involve electrical equipment; and Class D fires involve combustible metals. Of the four classes of fires, A, B, and C are commonly encountered in the home. In addition to the class of fire, extinguishers are identified by numbers that indicate the approximate size of the fire which the instruments can extinguish. As a rule, for use throughout the home, the individual should select a fire extinguisher with a minimum 2-A:10-B:C rating. This multipurpose dry chemical extinguisher is suitable for combating the sizes and classes of fires most commonly encountered in the home. In addition, when purchasing a commercial fire extinguisher, the homeowner should always select an instrument which is listed by Underwriters' Laboratories, Inc.

For ordinary combustible fires (Class A), the best extinguishing substance is still a large quantity of water. In fact, according to fire officials, an ordinary garden hose installed under the bathroom or kitchen sink is the best piece of fire-fighting equipment that a person can install in his home. During a fire, the hose can be quickly unrolled to reach almost any room in the home.

Preventing Home Fires

Of the various fire hazards in the home, the most innocent looking is the ordinary kitchen stove. Yet, almost one-half of all home fires occur while homeowners are cooking with stoves. In some cases the individuals accidentally touch their clothing to the stove burner; in other instances the individuals inadvertently permit grease or food to burn. To prevent clothing fires, the homeowner should always wear short sleeves or tight-fitting long sleeves. Because of their long, loose-fitting sleeves, bathrobes and dressing gowns are especially hazardous clothing for the person who is cooking on a stove burner. Furthermore, to prevent food fires, the homeowner should supervise oven and stove-top cooking at all times, as well as avoid "high heat" cooking that could spatter grease onto the burner.

As would be expected, the most treacherous home fire hazard is the common cigarette. Because it is treated with a special chemical, the cigarette will keep burning until it consumes itself. Consequently, when it is dropped in a bed or in an overstuffed piece of furniture, the cigarette has ample time to start a major fire. More important, a smoldering bed or sofa can easily generate enough smoke to asphyxiate everyone sleeping in the home, long before the flames ever reach them. To prevent cigarette fires, the individual should avoid smoking in bed or in chairs when he is extremely tired and sleepy. Also, before retiring for the night, he should conduct a thorough search to make certain that a lighted cigarette butt has not fallen unnoticed into a furniture crevice.

Another hazard which may be overlooked by adults is a child's natural fascination with fire. When children are left unattended, they will often start fires by striking matches or by igniting pieces of paper on the burner of the kitchen stove. In Panama City, Florida, a young mother walked to a neighborhood market to buy a loaf of bread for lunch. On her return she saw smoke and flames issuing from the window of her second-floor apartment. Despite rescue attempts by local firemen, her three young children

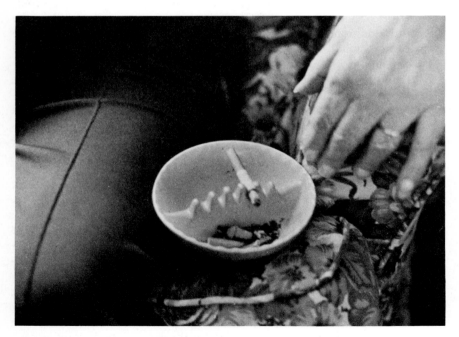

Figure 8.6   The cigarette, because it is treated with a special chemical, will keep burning until it consumes itself or ignites an overstuffed piece of furniture.

were later pronounced dead at the hospital. In the ten minutes that the mother had left her children alone, the youngsters had started fires in the bathroom, bedroom, and living room with matches that they had taken from a desk drawer. Obviously, matches and lighters should always be kept out of the reach of children. However, since children can often obtain these devices from other youngsters or from visitors' handbags without the parents' knowledge, the best precaution is never to leave children unattended. When leaving the home even for a few minutes, parents should always secure a responsible babysitter for the children.

Since heating equipment is a frequent cause of fires in the home, special efforts should be directed toward making the furnace, portable heater, and fireplace as safe as possible. Furnaces should be checked before every heating season by a reputable serviceman, combustible materials should be kept away from portable heaters, and fireplaces should be equipped with screens to prevent sparks from falling onto the carpeting.

Another source of fire hazards in the home can be attributed to poor housekeeping. When rags saturated with cleaning fluids, certain paints, furniture polish, and other petroleum-base products are left exposed to the air, spontaneous combustion can easily occur. For this reason, the individual should always destroy oily or greasy rags, or store them in closed, metal containers.

As one may expect, misuses of electricity are frequent causes of fire hazards in the home. Although electrical wiring in the walls is insulated and safe under normal conditions, overloading the circuits may cause the wires to burn their insulation, short-circuit, and give off sparks. Therefore, the continual blowing of fuses or circuit breakers is the best warning that overloading has occurred. When overloading is suspected, the homeowner should immediately remove excess appliances from the circuits to reduce the load on the wires. He should never tamper with fuses or breakers in an attempt to keep them from blowing, since they are the best safeguards against electrical fires. Furthermore, since electrical cords, like the wiring in the walls, may short-circuit and produce sparks when their insulation is worn, the homeowner should avoid practices which could damage a cord's insulation, such as tacking a cord to a baseboard or running a cord under a rug or carpet. However, if the cord does become frayed, the person should replace it immediately.

Another source of fire hazards in the home is the use of flammable liquids in poorly-ventilated areas. Since vapors are permitted to accumulate, even the slightest spark can cause an explosion and a fire. To avoid this hazard, the individual should always use flammable liquids in well-ventilated areas. Better still, since safer products are available and will serve the same function, he should use these rather than the highly flammable liquids.

Resource Materials

The National Fire Protection Association
470 Atlantic Avenue
Boston, Massachusetts 02210

National Safety Council
444 North Michigan Avenue
Chicago, Illinois 60611

National Smoke, Fire and Burn Institute
53 State Street
Suite 833
Boston, Massachusetts 02109

U.S. Consumer Product Safety Commission
5401 Westbard Avenue
Washington, D.C. 20207
Toll-free: 800-638-2666 in the continental United States
800-492-2937 for Maryland residents only

Activities

1. Keep a scrapbook of newspaper articles which report home fires that have occurred in the local area. Determine what percentage of the injuries and deaths are caused by smoke inhalation.

2. Purchase a smoke detector from a local store, and install the device in your home. Report to the class on your experiences.

3. Diagram a complete fire escape plan for your home. Be sure to include two routes from each room and a meeting place outside.

4. Obtain information from the local fire department about the procedures used to rescue incapacitated persons from burning homes. Inquire about the greatest difficulties in such rescues.

5. Write a paper on the selection of commercial extinguishers for the four classes of fires.

Questions

1. During a fire, how do smoke and flames move throughout a home?
2. What are the two types of smoke detectors, and how does each detector work?
3. What four factors should be considered by the homeowner when purchasing a smoke-alarm system?
4. What are "C" and "I" stickers?

5. What are the six steps in the fire escape procedure?
6. If a person is awakened at night by smoke or fire, why should he immediately switch on the nearest bedroom light?
7. How can an individual determine whether or not flames are on the other side of a closed door without opening it?
8. When exiting from a burning home, why should a person either crawl on his hands and knees or duck walk toward the door or window?
9. After escaping from a burning home, why should all family members assemble at a prearranged spot some distance from the home?
10. According to fire safety officials, what is the best piece of fire-fighting equipment that a family can have in the home?

Selected References

American Mutual Insurance Alliance. *Operation Exit Drills in the Home.* Chicago: The Alliance, 1965.

"Are Smoke Detectors Hazardous?," *Consumer Reports.* January, 1977, 52-54.

Carper, Jean. *Stay Alive!* Garden City, New York: Doubleday & Company, Inc., 1965.

"Did the Family Get Out Alive?," *Safety Education.* March, 1964, 23-26.

Fire Extinguishers: *The ABC's and the One, Two, Three's of Selection.* Washington, D.C.: Consumer Product Information, 1971.

"Home Fire Drills: They May Save Your Life," *Good Housekeeping.* February, 1969, 158-59.

"Home Fires, the ABC's of Dousing Them," *Better Homes and Gardens.* August, 1968, 83.

"If the House Catches Fire," *Changing Times.* February, 1969, 21-23.

National Academy of Sciences—National Research Council. *School Fires and Approach to Life Safety.* Washington, D.C.: The Council, 1960.

Schuler, Stanley. "20 Steps to a More Fire-Safe Home," *American Home.* November, 1971, 90.

"Smoke Detectors," *Consumer Reports.* October, 1976, 555-59.

"These Fire-Safety Rules Can Save Your Life," *Good Housekeeping.* September, 1972, 189.

Young, Warren R. "Is Your Home a Family Firetrap?," *Reader's Digest.* September, 1973, 181-84, 186.

Poisonings

9

Joey, a two-year-old boy from Denver, Colorado, took a swig from a bottle of liquid drain cleaner. Today, he is not a pretty sight. He has a hole in his throat so he can breathe and a tube jutting out of his stomach so he can be fed. In addition, he has angry red scars where surgeons implanted a new esophagus. In their total efforts physicians spent two years putting Joey together again. Still, Joey was lucky: he is alive!

Each year approximately forty-three hundred persons are not as fortunate as Joey, and die in poisonings by solids, liquids, and gases. Although poisoning accidents claim lives from all age groups and should be viewed as a problem affecting every member of the family, special attention must be directed at protecting young children against accidental poisoning. Unlike adults, children are unable to comprehend the full consequences of their actions.

Why Children Consume Poisons

In the past safety experts viewed the poisoning problem almost entirely in terms of the careless storage and the misuse of poisonous substances. Although behavior was recognized as a factor in the poisoning event, emphasis was placed primarily on providing a hazard-free environment and adequate supervision. In recent years, however, the behavior of the child has received greater attention. Today, supported by research in psychology, sociology, physiology, and growth and development, safety experts believe that the environment is a less important element in poisoning accidents than are the behavioral factors which encourage children to swallow poisonous or potentially poisonous substances.[1]

Birth to Age One

For children under one year of age, the hand-to-mouth stage of development presents the greatest concern for parents. During this stage, children

---

1. Potential poisons are substances which are safe when they are consumed in small amounts but are poisonous when they are consumed in large amounts.

will put anything in their mouths. Thus one can easily see why a child in this period of life will eagerly place poisonous substances in his mouth and swallow them. Realizing this danger, parents must take extra precautions to make sure all poisons are stored out of the reach of children. However, proper storage is only the first step in preventing behaviorally motivated poisoning. In addition, parents should provide suitable objects that children can safely place in their mouths during the hand-to-mouth stage. These nonswallowable-size toys will help lessen the possibility of the children placing poisonous substances or other swallowable-size objects in their mouths.

Age One to Age Three

By the time children have reached the age of one to three years, they will actively seek and experimentally taste most substances. In addition, their behavior is frequently strengthened by a basic drive, hunger. Numerous research studies have shown that peak times for poisonings are before meals while children are waiting to be fed. Aware of this fact, some safety experts have suggested that parents should give children fruit or small snacks during this potentially critical period.

Moreover, parents should avoid being lulled into a false sense of security by thinking that children will not eat or drink foul tasting substances. Believing this, many parents have been amazed to find that their child had consumed such repulsive substances as lye or gasoline. Unfortunately, children under three years of age have not developed a good sense of taste discrimination and a thorough knowledge about the meanings of the various taste sensations. For example, children are frequently forced to eat nutritious food that tastes bad to them. Therefore they often fail to realize that the foul taste of gasoline or other substances should serve as a warning. Furthermore, the appearance of the substance or its container may lead the child to believe that the poison is a food. For this reason, children should never be told that medicine is candy or food, in order to persuade them to take the drug, for they may seek it later on their own. Similarly, poisons should never be stored in soda bottles, jars, or other food containers. Even when an individual is temporarily working with poisons, he should avoid placing the substances in bowls or other food-related containers.

Age Three and Older

Characteristically, children over three years of age have developed better taste discrimination and accumulated more knowledge as to what the varying taste sensations mean. In addition, they are more mobile and can seek out the better tasting poisons. For these reasons, most research studies on poisonings have found that children *over* three years of age tend to consume mainly the good tasting potential poisons, such as baby aspirins, vitamins, and sleeping pills, while children *under* three years of age tend to swallow whatever substances they can reach, especially detergents, bleaches, cleaning fluids, and other substances which are stored in low places, such as under kitchen or bathroom sinks, where children can readily reach them. However, because a child is over three years of age does not mean he will never ingest a foul tasting poison. Actually, children over three years may and often do eat or drink such substances as detergents, lighter fluids, and gasoline. Obviously, the best practice is to always keep any poison or potentially poisonous substance out of the reach of children or behind locked cabinet doors.

Another behavioral characteristic which often leads to accidental poisoning of children three years of age and older is their strong desire to imitate the actions of others. For example, many parents are astonished that their child can reach a medicine cabinet, open it, and take medicine from it. For this reason, many safety experts recommend that parents should never take medicine in the presence of any child under five years of age. Furthermore, parents should warn older children not to give anything to young children, whether edible or nonedible.

Why Children Repeat Poisonings

Surprisingly, a child who has consumed poison once is likely to consume it again. As shown in numerous research studies, even the pain caused by the poison or the distress of having the stomach pumped-out is no deterrent to a repeat performance. While the reasons for repetitive poisoning are not entirely clear, research does begin to suggest possible explanations. However, the results of the studies are not conclusive and are often conflicting. Nevertheless, they do begin to shed light on the problem of repetitive poisoning.

One possible explanation as to why a child will seek repeated experiences with poisons is found within the child's psychological makeup. This is the starting point for studies dealing with pica, an abnormal craving to eat substances which are not intended for food. Although various explanations have been offered as to why pica develops, the most important consideration in terms of the poisoning problem is that pica originates and becomes well established early in a child's life. Therefore if poisoning occurs, the cause may be traced to pica and not to the social forces which may have caused pica itself. Upon recognizing pica in a child, parents should take every precaution to make certain that poisons are never within the youngster's reach. While most children will outgrow pica, some will not. In such cases parents should seek professional help from medical or psychological experts. Unchecked pica can easily lead to repeated accidental poisonings.

Another reason for repetitive poisoning involves the parent-child relationship. Frequently, children who repeat poisoning are the result of unplanned and unwanted pregnancies. As a result, such children are often resented by their parents and are forced to grow up in a hostile environment. Upon the first ingestion of a poison, the child observes the anxiety and trouble generated for his parents. Therefore, in an attempt to further strike back at his parents, the child consumes poison again. Although protecting the child may reduce the possibility of repetitive poisoning, such efforts do not solve the problem. Only a reevaluation of the parent-child relationship and professional help can effect a permanent solution.

Closely related to the parent-child relationship is the family atmosphere which surrounds the poison repeater. Frequently the atmosphere becomes cool and distant when an inordinate amount of time is devoted to a new baby, handicapped brother or sister, job, or other preoccupation. As a result, the child feels neglected and repeatedly poisons himself to gain attention. In such cases the child should be given extra attention and affection if the parents hope to prevent future poisonings. As an additional precaution, parents should keep all poisons out of the reach of the child.

Suspecting Everything As Poisonous

Even in families where parents believe they have stored all poisons out of the reach of children, poisonings still occur with frightening regularity. The reason is simple: many seemingly innocent substances are left in plain view of the child. However, parents should not be criticized too severely for this practice. With over 250,000 substances on the market, as estimated by the American Medical Association, even physicians cannot know the toxicity of every household product. Therefore, to prevent accidental poisoning, parents should suspect everything as being poisonous until proven otherwise.

As an aid to physicians, a study was conducted by Gosselin[2] to develop a reference list of toxicity ratings for a number of household products. Prepared from data compiled on over five thousand representative products, this list enables the physician to formulate an immediate prognosis when he knows the name and the approximate amount of a toxic product that has been ingested. However, the list can also be used by parents to determine which household products are more dangerous than others and which should never be left within the reach of children. In the list presented

---

2. Robert E. Gosselin, ''How Toxic Is It?,'' *Journal of the American Medical Association,* April 13, 1957, pp. 1333-37.

in Figure 9.1, all ratings are based on the lethal dose for a one hundred and fifty-pound man.

While the list of toxicity ratings does not contain categories for all products on the market, it emphasizes that most products can be classified as moderately toxic to very toxic. Accordingly, if an individual has no information about a particular product except that it is nonedible, the probability is very high that the toxicity of the product falls within this range.

Recognizing the Children's "Top Ten" Poisons

Although toxicity ratings are useful in determining which products are more poisonous than others, they do not show which products are most numerous in the home and which are most readily available to young children. Consequently, because they are often more accessible, less toxic products are frequently a greater poisoning threat than the more toxic products. This is supported by the following statistics on poisoning.

In a recent year, slightly less than 171,000 cases of accidental poisoning were reported to Poison Control Centers throughout the United States.[3,4] In analyzing these cases, the National Clearinghouse for Poison Control Centers categorized each poisoning accident according to the type of product which was ingested. Of these categories, ten products stand out as being most often ingested by children under five years of age. Altogether these products accounted for more than 40 percent of the reported cases of childhood poisonings. These products, in order of the percentage of the total, were:

1. Soaps, detergents, cleaners	6.2%	6. Perfume, cologne, toilet water 3.8%
2. Plants (excl. mushrooms and toadstools)	5.6%	7. Insecticides (excl. mothballs) 3.2%
3. Vitamins, minerals	4.8%	8. Household disinfectants, deodorizers 3.1%
4. Aspirin (baby brand, 3.1%)	4.7%	9. Internal medicines (miscellaneous products) 2.9%
5. Antihistamines, cold medicines	4.1%	10. Household bleach 2.7%

Of additional importance are several trends that have become apparent in the poisoning problem. In recent years aspirin has shown a steady decrease as reported substances in childhood poison ingestions. While the reasons for this continuing decline are not identified specifically, some of the con-

---

3. "Tabulations of 1975 Case Reports," *National Clearinghouse for Poison Control Centers Bulletin,* February, 1977, pp. 1-11.

4. "Top Five Categories of Products Ingested by Children Under 5 Years of Age in 1975," *National Clearinghouse for Poison Control Centers Bulletin,* April, 1977, pp. 1-7.

Class 1 (practically nontoxic)	**Class 2** (slightly toxic)	**Class 3** (moderately toxic)
Foods Candles Mucilages and pastes Cosmetics (especially baby products) Abrasives Pure soaps Lead pencils Modeling clays	Cosmetics (most) Adhesives (most) Lubricating oils Lubricants (most) Soap products and detergents Waxes (general, wood, window) Polishes (porcelain, some furniture) Inks (some) Incense	Polishes (metal, wood, shoe, stove) Cosmetics (hair dyes, tonics, permanent waves; liquid lipstick; nail polish, enamel, remover; perfumes) Cleaners (window, stain removers) Adhesives (rubber, linoleum, roofing, plastic cement) Bleaches Motor fuels Lighter fluids Repellents (insect, cat, dog) Antifreeze Brake fluids Mothballs (most) Preservatives (brush, canvas, roof) Matches Inks Agricultural chemicals (many)

Class 4
(very toxic)

Disinfectants (most, such as those for garbage cans)
Dry cleaner solvents (some)
Degreasers (metal, etc.)
Depilatories (some)
Drain cleaners (some)
Naphthalene moth repellents
Rust removers
Radiator cleaners
Leather dyes
Indelible inks
Fire extinguisher liquid
Agricultural chemicals (many)

Class 5
(extremely toxic)

Drain and sewer cleaners (caustics)
Fireplace flame colors (blues and greens)
Insecticides and fungicides (some)
Rodenticides (some)
Herbicides (some)

Class 6
(super toxic)

Insecticides
Fungicides (a few)
Rodenticides
Herbicides

Rating	**Probable Lethal Dose (Human)**
Class 1	more than 1 quart
Class 2	between 1 pint and 1 quart
Class 3	between 1 ounce and 1 pint
Class 4	between 1 teaspoon and 1 ounce
Class 5	between 7 drops and 1 teaspoon
Class 6	a taste (less than 7 drops)

Figure 9.1 Toxicity ratings for common household products. (From: Robert E. Gosselin, "How Toxic Is It?," *Journal of the American Medical Association,* vol. 163, April 13, 1957, p. 1334. Copyright 1957, American Medical Association.)

tributing factors involve the introduction of child-resistant safety caps, the limitation of the number of baby aspirin in each container, and the increased public awareness through governmental and private organizational campaigns on the hazards of aspirin. On the other hand, poisonings from soaps, detergents, cleaners, plants, perfumes, colognes, toilet waters, and insecticides have shown a nearly steady increase. In the case of plants, this increase is especially notable, since most people do not even consider plants a poisoning threat. The remaining products on the list have not shown any significant changes.

More important than any of the trends, however, is that aspirin accounted for approximately 15 percent of the deaths. Of further interest is that almost 80 percent of all the aspirin poisoning cases in which the type of aspirin was specified involved baby aspirin. This is not difficult to understand when one considers that children often mistake baby aspirin for candy, since the aspirin tastes good and is frequently called candy by parents who are eager to get children to take the medicine without a fuss.

However, aspirins are only a small part of the total poisoning problem. The analysis also revealed that medicines in general accounted for more than 40 percent of the deaths. This percentage merely reemphasizes that all substances must be suspected as being toxic, especially when they are misused.

Providing a Hazard-free Environment

Although childhood poisonings are greatly influenced by behavioral factors, researchers, through toxicity ratings and poisoning analyses, continue to stress that the environment is a significant factor in accidental poisonings. Naturally, a hazard-free environment and adequate supervision can often thwart behaviorally motivated actions aimed at poison consumption.

Since medicines are especially attractive to young children and account for such a large percentage of poisoning deaths each year, aspirins, tranquilizers, antibiotics, antihistamines, and certain other drugs should always be kept in their child-resistant containers. (See Figure 9.2.) In many cases the children are permitted an easy access to the medicines because their parents either leave the containers open or transfer the pills to other vials. However, even child-resistant containers may not effectively deter persistent children. In some cases the children are able to obtain the medicines by smashing the containers or biting off the tops. For this reason, all drugs, both internal and external, should be stored in a locked drawer or locked bathroom cabinet. However, since the trouble of using a key normally discourages parents from storing medicines behind locked doors, a special safety bathroom cabinet can be purchased. While adults can easily open the

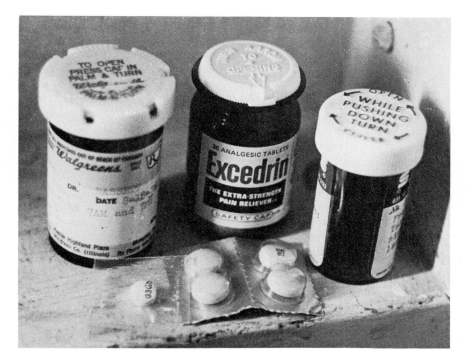

Figure 9.2   Medicines should always be stored in their original child-resistant containers.

cabinet, children are usually unable to open the receptacle even after they have been shown the method.

After making certain that children cannot obtain medicines by themselves, parents should make sure that the medicines which they give to their youngsters are indeed nontoxic when the drugs are used as directed. This means frequently examining and discarding old, illegibly labeled, and nonlabeled medicine. It also requires reading labels and directions two or three times before giving medicine to children. After a two-year-old child had become seriously ill, a young mother in Enid, Mississippi, discovered that she had given her son several teaspoons of liniment. She thought that she had given him cough syrup. Because medicinal bottles and their contents are often similar in appearance, many children are accidentally poisoned each year by their parents.

Even though medicines are always stored in a locked bathroom cabinet and then checked carefully before they are given to children, parents must always remain cautious where medicines are concerned. Only a few minutes are needed for a child to consume a fatal dose of medicine. For this reason, drug containers should always be returned immediately to a locked cabinet after their use. Also, since medicines are often found in visitors' handbags, all purses should be placed out of the reach of children. Finally, children should be supervised when they are visiting in homes where medicines are left in plain view, such as in the homes of the elderly or the incapacitated.

Other sources of poisoning which are related to medicines are vitamin tablets and mineral pills. Since vitamins and minerals are often taken at mealtime, they are usually stored with food in the kitchen. In addition, the bright colors of the tablets and pills are especially attractive to children. Consequently, youngsters identify vitamins and minerals with food or candy and frequently swallow the products in large numbers. For this reason, parents should always store vitamin tablets and mineral pills separately from food items and in a location where children cannot reach the potential poisons.

While improperly stored medicines, including vitamins and minerals, present environmental poisoning hazards, the practice of leaving household chemicals within the reach of children is just as dangerous. Yet, unfortunately, most people do just this. They store soaps, detergents, cleaners, bleaches, disinfectants, deodorizers, and other chemicals in the worst possible places, under the kitchen and bathroom sinks. Since the products are near the floor, even toddlers and crawlers can easily reach them. While parents will usually prefer the convenience of storing household chemicals in high cabinets, another solution is to install simple locks on the sink cabinets to prevent children from gaining access to the chemicals.

Other chemicals frequently incriminated in childhood poisonings and found within easy reach of children are perfumes, colognes, and toilet waters. Because they are normally left on the tops of dressing tables and bathroom sinks, the chemicals can easily be reached by young children. In addition, the sweet, unusual smells of the products may tempt youngsters into drinking the poisons. As in the case of medicines, parents should store perfumes, colognes, and toilet waters in locked bathroom cabinets.

Undoubtedly, of all the chemicals which are available for poisoning children, the insecticides, fungicides, rodenticides, and herbicides are the most treacherous. In Keokuk, Iowa, a three-year-old girl died after licking her fingers; she had merely touched the mouth of an empty insecticide container. Moreover, children do not need to swallow pesticides to become poisoned. They can inhale them or absorb them through unbroken skin. For this reason, pesticides should always be kept out of the reach of young children by locking the products inside a cabinet in an area of the home where children seldom visit. In addition, insecticides, fungicides, and similar products should always be stored in their original containers so that their identities are known to the users.

Since pesticides can be absorbed through the skin, the user should avoid spraying children's toys, cribs, and clothing. Similarly, rooms which are occupied by infants or the incapacitated should not be sprayed, since the poison can be easily inhaled. Also, before spraying a pesticide, the person should cover all food, eating utensils, and kitchen counters to prevent food contamination. Finally, empty pesticide containers should always be destroyed, or discarded where youngsters cannot reach them.

Underestimating a Child's Ability

Repeatedly, parents have been told, "Keep all poisonous and potentially poisonous substances out of the reach of children." This advice seems rather simple, but it is sometimes extremely difficult to follow.

Actually, most parents underestimate their child's ability. An enterprising young child can perform all types of stunts when he is highly motivated to reach something. In fact, children have even been known to seek hidden keys and open locked cabinets containing stored poisons. For this reason, parents should never underestimate a child's ingenuity in obtaining poisons in the home.

Identifying Dangerous Products

Naturally, parents cannot supervise their children's activities every minute. They can, however, mark all poisonous and potentially poisonous products and teach their children that the mark means danger. Ironically, the traditional mark or symbol of the "skull and crossbones" may actually encourage children to swallow poisons, since the symbol has been used in recent years in motion picture cartoons, commercial products, and amusement parks to represent pirates, adventure, and other good things. A more effective prevention symbol is the "Mr. Yuk" sticker.

Developed in 1971 by the Pittsburgh Poison Center, the Mr. Yuk symbol is a bilious, green, scowling face with a "yukky" tongue hanging out of the mouth. (See Figure 9.3.) Even without prior knowledge of the symbol, most children instantly recognize the Mr. Yuk face as meaning "bad." However, this does not mean that the symbol will automatically keep a child from swallowing a poisonous substance. Quite the opposite, for the Mr. Yuk symbol to be effective, children must be taught and must fully understand that the symbol means "DANGER." However, if a child does swallow a poison, the Mr. Yuk sticker also displays the name and the telephone number of the local Poison Center where information or help can be obtained around-the-clock from an expert medical staff.

Since only Regional and Satellite Centers of the National Poison Center Network (NPCN) may use the Mr. Yuk symbol, not all parents can obtain the stickers from their local Poison Control Center. To learn the location of

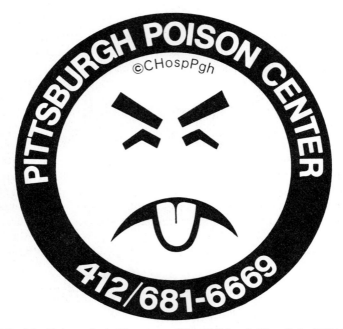

Figure 9.3   Mr. Yuk symbol. (Courtesy of the Children's Hospital of Pittsburgh)

the nearest NPCN Poison Center, parents should write to the National Poison Center Network in Pittsburgh, Pennsylvania. (See "Resource Materials" at the end of this chapter.)

Protecting Children from the Living Poisons

Unknown to many people, poisons are frequently found living in the home. Although they appear to be incapable of killing a child, certain plants are even more toxic than some of the insecticides, fungicides, rodenticides, and herbicides on the market. However, poisonous plants account for few deaths, only three or four every year. Most often, when they are ingested, the plants cause severe adverse bodily reactions, usually of a gastrointestinal nature, which may require hospitalization. Unfortunately, the incidence of plant poisoning has been steadily increasing until plants now rank as the second most frequently ingested poison by children under five years of age.

To help parents identify common poisonous plants found in and near the home, the National Safety Council has issued a list of plants and their toxic parts. (See Figure 9.4.) Published in *Family Safety Magazine,* the list

COMMON POISONOUS PLANTS

HOUSE PLANTS

Plant	Toxic Part	Symptoms and Comment
Castor bean	Seeds	Burning sensation in mouth and throat. Two to four beans may cause death. Eight usually lethal. Death has occurred in U.S.
Dieffenbachia (dumbcane), caladium, elephant's ear, some philodendrons	All parts	Intense burning and irritation of mouth, tongue, lips. Death from dieffenbachia has occurred when tissues at back of tongue swelled and blocked air passage to throat. Other plants have similar but less toxic characteristics.
Hyacinth, narcissus, daffodil	Bulbs	Digestive upset including nausea, vomiting and diarrhea when eaten even in small amounts.
Rosary pea (jequirity bean, crabs-eye, precatory bean)	Seeds	Among the most highly toxic of natural materials. Severe gastrointestinal irritation, incoordination, paralysis. Less than one seed, if thoroughly chewed, is enough to kill an adult.

FLOWER GARDEN PLANTS

Plant	Toxic Part	Symptoms and Comment
Aconite, monkshood	Roots, flowers, leaves	Restlessness, salivation, nausea, vomiting, vertigo. Although people have died after eating small amounts of garden aconite, poisoning from it is not common.
Autumn crocus	All parts, especially bulbs	Burning pain in mouth, gastrointestinal irritation. Children have been poisoned by eating flowers.
Dutchman's breeches (bleeding heart)	Foliage, roots	No human poisonings or deaths, but a record of toxicity for livestock is warning that garden species may be dangerous.
Foxglove	All parts, especially leaves, flowers, seeds	One of the sources of the drug digitalis. May cause dangerously irregular heartbeat, digestive upset and mental confusion. Convulsions and death are possible.
Iris	Underground rhizome, also developed leaves	Severe digestive upset from moderate amounts of cultivated or wild irises. However, acridity usually prevents large consumption. Boiled properly, leaf and stems may be eaten.
Larkspur, delphinium	Seeds, young plant	Livestock losses are second only to locoweed in western U.S. Therefore, garden larkspur should at least be held suspect.
Lily-of-the-valley	Leaves, flowers, fruit (red berries)	Produces glycoside like digitalis, used in medicine to strengthen the beat of a weakened heart. In moderate amounts, can cause irregular heartbeat, digestive upset and mental confusion.
Nicotiana, wild and cultivated	Leaves	Nervous symptoms. Poisonous or lethal amounts can be obtained from ingestion of cured smoking or chewing tobacco, from foliage of field-grown tobacco or from foliage of garden variety (flowering tobacco or nicotiana).

VEGETABLE GARDEN PLANTS

Plant	Toxic Part	Symptoms and Comment
Potato	Vines, sprouts (green parts), spoiled tubers	Death has occurred from eating green parts. To prevent poisoning from sunburned tubers, green spots should be removed before cooking. Discard spoiled potatoes.

Plant	Toxic Part	Symptoms and Comment
Rhubarb	Leaf blade	Several deaths from eating raw or cooked leaves. Abdominal pains, vomiting and convulsions a few hours after ingestion. Without treatment, death or permanent kidney damage may occur.

ORNAMENTAL PLANTS

Plant	Toxic Part	Symptoms and Comment
Atropa belladonna	All parts, especially black berries	Fever, rapid heartbeat, dilation of pupils, skin flushed, hot and dry. Three berries were fatal to one child.
Carolina jessamine, yellow jessamine	Flowers, leaves	Poisoned children who sucked nectar from flowers. May cause depression followed by death through respiratory failure. Honey from nectar also thought to have caused three deaths.
Common privet	Black or blue wax-coated berries, leaves	Causes gastric irritation and vomiting. Several cases in children reported in Europe.
Daphne	Berries (commonly red, but other colors in various species), bark	A few berries can cause burning or ulceration in digestive tract causing vomiting and diarrhea. Death can result. This plant considered "really dangerous," particularly for children.
English ivy	Berries, leaves	Excitement, difficult breathing and eventually coma. Although no cases reported in U.S., European children have been poisoned.
Golden chain (laburnum)	Seeds, pods, flowers	Excitement, intestinal irritation, severe nausea with convulsions and coma if large quantities are eaten. One or two pods have caused illness in children in Europe.
Heath family (laurels, rhododendron, azaleas)	All parts	Causes salivation, nausea, vomiting and depression. "Tea" made from two ounces of leaves produced human poisoning. More than a small amount can cause death. Delaware Indians used laurel for suicide.
Lantana	Unripe greenish-blue or black berries	Can be lethal to children through muscular weakness and circulatory collapse. Less severe cases experience gastrointestinal irritation.
Oleander	Leaves, branches, nectar of flowers	Extremely poisonous. Affects heart and digestive system. Has caused death even from meat roasted on its branches. A few leaves can kill a human being.
Wisteria	Seeds, pods	Pods look like pea pods. One or two seeds may cause mild to severe gastrointestinal disturbances requiring hospitalization. However, with treatment recovery occurs in 24 hours. No fatalities recorded. Flowers may be dipped in batter and fried.
Yew	Needles, bark, seeds	Ingestion of English or Japanese yew foliage may cause sudden death as alkaloid weakens and eventually stops heart. If less is eaten, may be trembling and difficulty in breathing. Red pulpy berry is little toxic, if at all, but same may not be true of small black seeds in it.

Lantana

Daphne

Oleander

Figure 9.4   Common poisonous plants found in and near the home. (From: Susan Seder, "A New Look at Poisonous Plants," Reprinted from *Family Safety Magazine,* n.d. Courtesy of the National Safety Council)

TREES AND SHRUBS

Plant	Toxic Part	Symptoms and Comment
Apple	Seeds	If eaten in large quantity, can cause death. One man died after eating a cupful.
Black locust	Bark, foliage, young twigs, seeds	Digestive upset has occurred from ingestion of the soft bark. Seeds may also be toxic to children. Flowers may be fried as fritters.
Buckeye, horsechestnut	Sprouts, nuts	Digestive upset and nervous symptoms (confusion, etc.). Have killed children but because of unpleasant taste are not usually consumed in quantity necessary to produce symptoms.
Chinaberry tree	Berries	Nausea, vomiting, excitement or depression, symptoms of suffocation if eaten in quantity. Loss of life to children has been reported.
Elderberry	Roots, stems	Children have been poisoned by eating roots or using pithy stems as blowguns. Berries are least toxic part but may cause nausea if too many are eaten raw. Proper cooking destroys toxic principle.
Jatropha (purge nut, curcas bean, peregrina, psychic nut)	Seeds, oil	Nausea, violent vomiting, abdominal pain. Three seeds caused severe symptoms in one person. However, in others as many as 50 have resulted in relatively mild symptoms.
Oaks	All parts	Eating large quantities of any raw part, including acorns, may cause slow damage to kidneys. However, a few acorns probably have little effect. Tannin may be removed by boiling or roasting, making edible.
Wild black cherry, chokecherries	Leaves, pits	Poisoning and death have occurred in children who ate large amounts of berries without removing stones. Pits or seeds, foliage and bark contain HCN (prussic acid or cyanide). Others to beware of: several wild and cultivated cherries, peach, apricot and some almonds. But pits and leaves usually not eaten in enough quantity to do serious harm.
Yellow oleander (be-still tree)	All parts, especially kernels of the fruit	In Oahu, Hawaii, still rated as most frequent source of serious or lethal poisoning in man. One or two fruits may be fatal. Symptoms similar to fatal digitalis poisoning.

PLANTS IN WOODED AREAS

Plant	Toxic Part	Symptoms and Comment
Baneberry (doll's-eyes)	Red or white berries, roots, foliage	Acute stomach cramps, headache, vomiting, dizziness, delirium. Although no loss of life in U.S., European children have died after ingesting berries.
Jack-in-the-pulpit, skunk cabbage	All parts, especially roots	Contains small needle-like crystals of calcium oxalate that cause burning and severe irritation of mouth and tongue.
Mayapple (mandrake)	Roots, foliage, unripe fruit	Large doses may cause gastroenteritis and vomiting. Ripe fruit is least toxic part and has been eaten by children—occasionally catharsis results. Cooked mayapples can be made into marmalade.

Plant	Toxic Part	Symptoms and Comment
Water hemlock (cowbane, snakeroot)	Roots, young foliage	Salivation, tremors, delirium, violent convulsions. One mouthful of root may kill a man. Many persons, especially children, have died in U.S. after eating this plant. Roots are mistaken for wild parsnip or artichoke.

PLANTS IN FIELDS

Plant	Toxic Part	Symptoms and Comment
Death camas	Bulbs	Depression, digestive upset, abdominal pain, vomiting, diarrhea. American Indians and early settlers were killed when they mistook it for edible bulbs. Occasional cases still occur. One case of poisoning from flower reported.
Jimsonweed (thornapple)	All parts, especially seeds and leaves	Thirst, hyper-irritability of nervous system, disturbed vision, delirium. Four to five grams of crude leaf or seed approximates fatal dose for a child. Poisonings have occurred from sucking nectar from tube of flower or eating fruits containing poisonous seeds.
Nightshades, European bittersweet, horse nettle	All parts, especially unripe berry	Children have been poisoned by ingesting a moderate amount of unripe berries. Digestive upset, stupefication and loss of sensation. Death due to paralysis can occur. Ripe berries, however, are much less toxic.
Poison hemlock	Root, foliage, seeds	Root resembles wild carrot. Seeds have been mistaken for anise. Causes gradual weakening of muscular power and death from paralysis of lungs. Caused Socrates' death.
Pokeweed (pigeonberry)	Roots, berries, foliage	Burning sensation in mouth and throat, digestive upset and cramps. Seeds thought to have caused one human fatality.

CHRISTMAS PLANTS

Plant	Toxic Part	Symptoms and Comment
Holly	Berries	No cases reported in North America, but thought that large quantities may cause digestive upset.
Jerusalem cherry	Unripe fruit, leaves, flowers	No cases reported, but thought to cause vomiting and diarrhea. However, when cooked, some species used for jellies and preserves.
Mistletoe	Berries	Can cause acute stomach and intestinal irritation. Cattle have been killed by eating wild mistletoe. People have died from "tea" of berries.
Poinsettia	Leaves, flower	Can be irritating to mouth and stomach, sometimes causing vomiting and nausea, but usually produces no ill effects.

Dieffenbachia   Water hemlock   Poison hemlock

Figure 9.4   Cont'd.

includes plants of varying toxicities. Some, like the wisteria, can cause a mild to severe stomach upset while others, like the yew, can produce sudden death without any symptoms appearing.

Although they are not included in the list, mushrooms should be viewed with suspicion. Contrary to popular belief, a poisonous mushroom will not always blacken a silver spoon or a silver coin. Actually, some harmless mushrooms with a high sulphur content will tarnish a spoon. On the other hand, some toxic mushrooms with a low sulphur content will leave the spoon bright and shiny. Since only experts can readily identify which mushrooms are toxic and which are not, most parents should automatically assume that all wild mushrooms are poisonous.

Since plants are ranked unusually high on the children's list of most frequently ingested poisons, toxic plants in and near the home should be replaced with nontoxic plants. Children should also be instructed to never eat plants, nibble on plant leaves, or suck on plant stocks. Parents should take every precaution to make certain that the children realize that such practices can easily lead to severe pain or death.

Checking Paint for Poison

Another unexpected source of poisoning in the home can be found on the walls, woodwork, and furniture in the form of lead-base paint. When a child eats small pieces of this paint over a period of months, chronic lead poisoning may result. The seriousness of this type of poisoning is well illustrated by the following:

> Slowly, the lead piles up in the body, especially the brain, causing a swelling that literally crushes the brain cells to death against the skull. Once this happens, there is no hope of regeneration. Lead poisoning may leave a child with a twitch, blindness, paralysis—or most cruel of all, take away his intelligence, dooming him to a life of idiocy.[5]

Since today's interior paints no longer contain high levels of lead, most modern homes are relatively safe from the hazard of lead poisoning. However, older homes, especially in slum areas, often contain the deadly lead-base paint on their walls.

To determine whether or not paint has an unsafe level of lead, a simple test has been developed at the University of Rochester School of Medicine by Dr. W. Sayre and Dr. David Wilson.[6] The test consists of placing a drop of 8 percent sodium sulfide solution, which can be obtained at a drug store

---

5. Jean Carper, *Stay Alive!* (Garden City, New York: Doubleday & Company, Inc., 1965), p. 68.
6. Maxine Lewis, "Seventy Six Ways to Save Your Life," *Family Circle,* July, 1972, p. 57.

or a chemical supply house, on a paint chip that has fallen from the wall or the ceiling. If the wetted area turns dark gray or black within a few seconds, parents can assume that the level of lead in the paint is sufficiently high to cause lead poisoning. In such cases children should never be allowed to chew on painted surfaces or to put paint chips in their mouths. In addition, when repainting walls, woodwork, or furniture, parents should always use interior paints, since they contain a safe level of lead. Exterior paints, on the other hand, often contain a high level of lead and can cause poisoning if they are used inside the home.

Recognizing the Adults' "Top Ten" Poisons

Although most people consider accidental poisoning to be a children's problem, adults account for over 95 percent of all the poisoning deaths that result from the bodily admission of solids, liquids, gases, and vapors.[7,8] Yet, adults are probably involved in only slightly more than 20 percent of all poisoning accidents.[9]

After analyzing nearly 171,000 cases of accidental poisoning in the United States, the National Clearinghouse for Poison Control Centers listed certain categories of products which were most often implicated in adult poisoning. In order of the percentage of the total, these products were:[10]

1.	Internal medicines	75.1%	6.	Petroleum products	2.2%
2.	Miscellaneous products	5.2%	7.	Gases and vapors	2.2%
3.	Cleaning and polishing agents	3.8%	8.	Plants	1.8%
4.	Pesticides	2.5%	9.	Turpentine, paints, and similar products	1.3%
5.	External medicines	2.3%	10.	Cosmetics	0.8%

All totaled, the products on the list accounted for over 97 percent of the reported cases of adult poisoning.

Respecting the Power of Medicines

In abnormal dosages all internal medicines are poisonous. "After all," as Carper notes, "drugs are nothing more than poison dished out in small

7. National Safety Council, *Accident Facts—1977 Edition* (Chicago: NSC, 1977), computed from statistics on p. 80.

8. For statistical purposes adults have been defined as persons who are fifteen years of age or older.

9. "Tabulations of 1975 Case Reports," *National Clearinghouse for Poison Control Centers Bulletin,* February, 1977, computed from statistics on p. 9.

10. "Tabulations of 1975 Case Reports," computed from statistics on p. 9.

amounts, as the similarity between the words 'poison' and 'potion' suggests."[11] Clearly, in proper doses the internal medicines, through their poisonous quality, can effectively fight infections and alleviate pain. However, in abnormal dosages the internal medicines can kill.

Many accidental deaths by poisoning are caused by the indiscriminate mixing of drugs. This is especially apparent in the flu seasons. Typically, in an effort to improve their health, individuals will consume a hodgepodge of prescription drugs and over-the-counter medicines. Still worse, some persons will foolishly wash down this medicinal mixture with several "hot (alcoholic) toddies." However, not all individuals are motivated by health reasons to consume medicines in combination. Some persons, particularly adolescents, will deliberately mix drugs in an attempt to achieve a "rush" or to "get high."

According to safety experts, all medicinal combinations are potentially lethal. However, most deaths from drug combinations are caused by alcohol-medicine mixtures. Apparently adults, who may be violently opposed to marijuana and similar drugs, feel comfortable with the use of alcohol. As a result, they, as well as their adolescent offspring, cannot fully comprehend the danger which is presented by an alcohol-medicine mixture.

As one would expect, the quantity of the consumed mixture is the most critical factor in determining the elements of danger. A person who has swallowed a large quantity of the different drugs is more likely to suffer an adverse reaction than an individual who has consumed only a small quantity. Furthermore, the combination factor will usually produce two additional risks. First, in a medicinal mixture each component drug becomes more powerful than it would be singly. This effect, as researchers say, is synergistic. Because of the wide variety of medicinal combinations, no one can predict the exact increase in potency. However, certain combinations, such as alcohol and tranquilizers or alcohol and barbiturates, may produce an effect which is four to five times greater than the simple total of their effects would indicate. Second, some persons are especially susceptible to certain medicinal combinations. As a result, one individual may not react to a particular mixture, but another person may become violently ill and even die.

In general, the depressant drugs form the most powerful mixtures within the body. The most common depressants, which slow or depress the central nervous system, include alcohol, aspirin, tranquilizers, sedatives, and narcotics. Typically, upon consuming a combination of depressants, the individual will experience increasing drowsiness. Then, if the potency of the mixture is sufficiently strong, he will lapse into unconsciousness and stop breathing.

---

11. Jean Carper, *Stay Alive!* (Garden City, New York: Doubleday & Company, Inc., 1965), p. 50.

Undoubtedly, in recent years Karen Ann Quinlan has been the most publicized victim of a drug mixture. After attending a birthday party and consuming a few alcoholic drinks, Karen, a healthy and happy twenty-one-year-old New Jersey girl, slipped into a state of unconsciousness and stopped breathing. As hospital officials discovered later, she had also consumed a small quantity of tranquilizer and aspirin, thus permitting the drugs, in combination with the alcohol, to produce a synergistic effect. In addition, since she had been on a crash diet and had not eaten at any time during the day, Karen was especially susceptible to the alcohol-medicine combination. Because of the drug-induced breathing stoppage and subsequent oxygen deprivation, she suffered irreversible brain damage. Although she survived the poisoning incident, Karen was left in a persistent vegetative state with only the most primitive parts of her brain still functioning.

As the Karen Ann Quinlan case illustrates, even a seemingly harmless mixture of drugs can easily produce permanent bodily damage or death. Consequently, all medicinal combinations should be viewed as lethal. To prevent accidental poisonings, an individual should restrict his medicinal consumption, including alcohol, to a single generic drug within each five-hour period. In addition, since many people inadvertently mix medicines, the person should avoid storing different drugs in the same container. To preserve the identity of the drugs, each medicine should be kept in its original container.

On the other hand, not all medicinal poisonings in adults are caused by the indiscriminate mixing of drugs. When they are used improperly, all internal medicines can be singly lethal. Despite living in a drug-oriented society, most people are quite ignorant about the ways in which medicines work. While the dosages for medicines are carefully planned after extensive research, many persons will double or even triple the recommended dosage. Apparently they mistakenly believe that they will receive two or three times the benefit from the drug. Actually, in an excessive quantity the medicine may become an extremely potent poison. Before consuming any medicine, an individual should read carefully the directions on the drug vial. Preferably, this should be done several times to avoid misreading. Furthermore, he should avoid exceeding the recommended dosage without his physician's approval or consuming medicines which are prescribed for another person. Either practice can easily result in poisoning and possibly death.

Another frequent cause of medicinal poisoning in adults is confusing an external medicine for an internal medicine. In many cases camphorated oil, oil of wintergreen, and other deadly liniments are mistakenly identified as castor oil or cough syrup. Apparently the most frequent victims of this type of poisoning are persons with poor eyesight. To prevent accidental poisoning by external medicines, the homeowner should insist that family members with vision problems wear their glasses when they consume their medicines. In addition, he should glue pieces of rough sandpaper on the tops of the external medicines to warn users that the substances are poisonous. Finally, the homeowner should store internal and external medicines in separate cabinets with a flashlight and magnifying glass in each cabinet.

Separating Chemicals and Foods

As mentioned earlier in this chapter, taste discrimination is primarily a function of age. Because of their immaturity, young children will drink or eat almost any substance. On the other hand, older youngsters are more selective in their tastes and, as a result, will generally prefer the good tasting products. The same is true for adults. Approximately three-fourths of all adult poisoning accidents involve internal medicines or the better tasting poisons. Yet, paradoxically, adults may consume gasoline, furniture polish, paint, and other foul tasting chemicals.

According to physiologists, the sense of smell is closely allied with the sense of taste. In fact, many of the so-called tastes of certain substances are actually odors. For example, when a person chews a piece of raw onion with his nose shut, he cannot distinguish the onion from a piece of raw potato. Since many of the foul tastes of chemicals are actually odors, the sense of smell is a significant factor in numerous cases of chemical poisoning in adults. Apparently, deprived of the sense of smell, many individuals cannot "taste" certain substances and consequently will mistakenly identify the chemicals as food.

In Memphis, Tennessee, a forty-year-old man inadvertently drank a glassful of bleach which he thought was lemonade. According to hospital officials, the man's wife, who had been washing clothes, poured the bleach into a glass, set the glass on the kitchen table, and went upstairs to gather dirty clothes. In the meantime, the man, who could not smell because of his hay fever, saw the glass, identified the bleach as lemonade, and drank the chemical. He said that he discovered his mistake when his wife complained about the disappearance of the bleach.

As a rule, most cases of accidental chemical poisoning in adults are caused by a combination of two factors: (1) the chemicals are mistaken for food, and (2) the persons are unable to smell. For this reason, the individual should never store food and household chemicals in the same location. Even when he is working temporarily with the chemicals, the person should avoid transferring the products into bowls, glasses, and other food-associated containers. In addition, because of the importance of smell, the individual should exhibit extreme caution at certain times in his life, such as during a cold or during an attack of hay fever. On the other hand, if he has lost his sense of smell for an extended period of time, the person should seek medical treatment and at all times remain cautious around household chemicals.

Handling the Killer Poisons

Pesticides are killers! They kill weeds, fungi, insects, and rodents. More important, they occasionally kill people.

As might be expected, adults will often drink or eat pesticides after mistakenly identifying them as food. A thirty-three-year-old man in Memphis, Tennessee, took a box of rat poison without looking at it from a cupboard, poured the poison into a bowl, sprinkled sugar on it, covered it with milk, and ate it. "It looked like Grape Nuts Flakes," said the man. On the other hand, adults may poison themselves by inhaling pesticides or by absorbing them through unbroken skin.

According to the Environmental Protection Agency, herbicides, fungicides, insecticides, and rodenticides are labeled with key words which indicate the relative toxicities of the pesticides. Extremely toxic pesticides are labeled with the word "DANGER." They are unsafe for use in the home. Less toxic pesticides are marked with the word "WARNING." When they are used properly, some of these pesticides are relatively safe for home use. The least toxic pesticides are labeled with the word "CAUTION." Of all the pesticides, they are the safest for use in the home. However, any pesticide can still kill if it is used carelessly or improperly.

When mixing pesticides, the homeowner should measure the amounts precisely with cups and utensils used only for this task, prepare the poisons outdoors, and mix only the needed amounts. In addition, while mixing and using pesticides, he should protect himself by wearing a buttoned-up shirt and plastic gloves and by immediately washing away with soap and water any poison that contacts the skin or clothes. While spraying pesticides, the person should avoid working downwind or remaining for a long period of time in an enclosed area. After using pesticides, he should thoroughly clean his equipment according to the label directions and then store the poisons in their original containers within a locked cabinet. As an additional precaution, the individual should wash his clothes in hot, soapy water before wearing them again.

Avoiding the Invisible Poison

Every year approximately nine hundred individuals are killed by poisonous gases in the home. Almost 90 percent of the victims are adults. Of the deaths, most can be attributed to carbon monoxide gas, a product of incomplete combustion.

Odorless and colorless, carbon monoxide cannot be detected with the senses of smell or sight. However, the gas is always found in smoke, a fact which may serve as a warning. Yet, this warning is not entirely foolproof, for a person can easily smell and see nothing, but still become poisoned by carbon monoxide. Another warning may be the signs and symptoms of impending carbon monoxide unconsciousness. The individual may experience nausea, drowsiness, mental confusion, and a throbbing and tightness across his forehead. However, again, this indication is not entirely foolproof. Often the person will not recognize the symptoms, but even if he does, he still may not be able to escape from the poisonous gas in time to save his life. Therefore the best protection against carbon monoxide is never to allow the gas to enter the home.

Unfortunately, modern, well-insulated homes are more susceptible to carbon monoxide accumulation than older, poorly-insulated homes. Consequently, all nonelectrical pieces of heating and cooling equipment can readily generate the gas in sufficient quantity to kill every member of the family. For this reason, nonelectrical equipment should be properly vented to safely carry the carbon monoxide gas to the outside of the home. In addition, since obstructed vents and defective equipment can easily lead to carbon monoxide poisoning, the homeowner should employ a qualified repairman to inspect the heating equipment at least once every year.

Although charcoal briquettes afford a convenient and pleasant method of outdoor cooking, they are not designed for use in home heating. In a confined space, such as the bedroom, the charcoal can quickly produce a lethal concentration of carbon monoxide gas. In a typical case, a Provo, Utah, husband and wife used their hibachi on a cool spring evening to warm their bedroom. During the night, the man became nauseated and vomited on the sheets and bedspread. When he started to clean up the vomitus, the man found that his wife was dead. According to the autopsy, the woman's heart blood contained a concentration of 75 percent carbon monoxide gas. By federal law, all bags of lump charcoal and charcoal briquettes must prominently display the following words: "Warning—Do not use for indoor heating or cooking unless ventilation is provided for exhausting fumes to outside. Toxic fumes may accumulate and cause death." Although some individuals will put the briquettes in the fireplace, this practice is no guarantee against carbon monoxide poisoning. Unless the fireplace has a good draft to pull the gas up the chimney, the homeowner and the members of his family may still be asphyxiated by the carbon monoxide gas.

Naturally, not all carbon monoxide is generated within the home. Often kitchen fans and air conditioners will draw automobile exhaust fumes into the home from an adjacent garage. For this reason, if the garage is attached to the house, the homeowner should block or seal any openings between the two building structures. In addition, he should avoid idling the car engine in the closed garage, since carbon monoxide gas may quickly accumulate in a lethal concentration.

Staying Away from Airborne Chemicals

Carbon monoxide, unfortunately, is not the only toxic gas which may be encountered in the home. Numerous household products can readily generate poisonous gases and vapors in sufficient concentrations to kill children and adults.

As a rule, the most dangerous gases and vapors are produced by cosmetics, polishing agents, paints, turpentine, and petroleum products, such as paint remover and paint thinner. Individuals who use these products in areas without adequate ventilation may experience nausea, headache, dizziness, and, in extreme cases, respiratory failure. In addition, if they aspirate or breathe the oil droplets, individuals may develop chemical pneumonia, an extreme inflammation of the tissues of the lungs. Sometimes the oil will work its way out of the lungs, but if it does not, the oil cannot be medically removed. Worse yet, because the inflammation is not caused by microorganisms, this type of pneumonia will not respond to the usual antibiotic treatment and can easily result in death.

When using paints, turpentine, and similar products, the person should follow the directions on the label and work only in well-ventilated locations in the home. Even outdoors, by positioning himself upwind from the products, he should avoid breathing the gases and vapors.

Oddly enough, toxic gases can also be created by simply mixing several common household products. In Portland, Maine, two elderly women were killed by poisonous fumes emanating from a mixture of household bleach and ammonia which they had used to clean away splattered eggs from the house windows on the day after Halloween. According to the medical examiner, the women's cleaning mixture produced toxic nitrogen trichloride fumes. As a rule, the individual should never mix bleach with either ammonia or strong acids, since either mixture will release a potentially lethal gas. On the other hand, to obtain a better cleaning action, the person can safely mix bleach with soaps, detergents, or sodium hydroxide products.

Resource Materials

American Medical Association
535 North Dearborn Street
Chicago, Illinois 60610

Lever Brothers Company
390 Park Avenue
New York City, New York 10022

Medical and Pharmaceutical Information Bureau
210 East 86th Street
New York City, New York 10028

National Coordinating Council on Drug Education
1211 Connecticut Avenue, N.W.
Suite 211
Washington, D.C. 20036

National Poison Center Network
125 DeSoto Street
Pittsburgh, Pennsylvania 15213

National Safety Council
444 North Michigan Avenue
Chicago, Illinois 60611

U.S. Department of Health, Education,
    and Welfare
Food and Drug Administration
Bureau of Drugs
5401 Westbard Avenue
Bethesda, Maryland 20016

Activities

1. Using Gosselin's list of toxic products, survey your home to determine how many of the products you have accumulated. Compare your list with the lists of others in the class.

2. Keep a scrapbook of newspaper articles that report childhood poisonings in the local area. Determine what percentage of the poisons named are on the "top ten" most frequently ingested list.

3. Using the National Safety Council's list of poisonous plants, survey florists and nurseries in the local area to determine which plants are purchased most often.

4. After gathering a number of different paint chips, obtain an 8 percent sodium sulfide solution from a drug store, and prepare a demonstration before the class on testing paint for high lead content.

5. Write a short paper on the dangers of taking alcoholic beverages and medicines together.

Questions

1. Why do children consume poisons for the first time?
2. Why do children often repeat poisonings?
3. What is meant by the term "pica"?
4. Which poison is most frequently ingested by children under five years of age?
5. Where is the best place to store medicines in homes having children?
6. What are the "living poisons"?

7. What is the main source of poisoning in adults?
8. What does "synergistic" mean, and why is it an important factor in medicinal poisonings?
9. Why do adults often consume gasoline, paint, and other foul tasting chemicals?
10. What is the "invisible gas"?

Selected References

Carper, Jean. *Stay Alive!* Garden City, New York: Doubleday & Company, Inc., 1965.

Gosselin, Robert E. "How Toxic Is It?" *The Journal of the American Medical Association.* April 13, 1957, 1333-37.

Lewis, Maxine. "Seventy Six Ways to Save Your Life," *Family Circle.* July, 1972, 57-61, 118, 120.

Lourie, Reginald and others. "Why Children Eat Things That Are Not Food," *Children.* July-August, 1963, 143-46.

"Make Sure Your Child Won't Be A Poison Victim," *Consumer Bulletin.* February, 1966, 20-21.

"100 Ways to Make the Summer Safe for Your Family," *Good Housekeeping.* June, 1975, 154-55.

Scherz, Robert G. "Prevention of Childhood Poisoning: A Community Project," *Pediatric Clinics of North America.* August, 1970, 713-27.

Sobel, Raymond, and James A. Margolis. "Repetitive Poisoning in Children: A Psychosocial Study," *Pediatrics.* April, 1965, 641-51.

"Tabulations of 1975 Case Reports," *National Clearinghouse for Poison Control Centers Bulletin.* February, 1977.

"Tips for Your Home and Family; Accidental Poisoning," *Today's Health.* July, 1968, 68-70.

"Tips for Your Home and Family; Veiled Killers," *Today's Health.* August, 1971, 69.

"Top Five Categories of Products Ingested by Children Under 5 Years of Age in 1975," *National Clearinghouse for Poison Control Centers Bulletin,* April, 1977.

"Ways to Use Medicine Safely with Children," *Good Housekeeping.* January, 1968, 170.

Suffocations

10

Approximately twenty-three hundred persons die each year in home suffocation accidents involving either ingested objects or mechanical means. Of this total, almost one-third are children under four years of age. After a near tragedy in Sparta, Wisconsin, a young mother graphically reported to the National Safety Council:

> Our daughter, 20 months old, was on her back holding a musical bunny above her and winding the key. It dropped into her open mouth and lodged in her throat. She was taken to the hospital emergency room, since she was choking, turning blue and vomiting. The key finally fell from her mouth.[1]

Since suffocations claim the lives of so many children at an age when they are essentially helpless to protect themselves, parents must take special precautions to safeguard their children from suffocation hazards.

Preventing Suffocation by Ingestion

To prevent suffocation by ingested objects, parents must realize that children under four years of age are experiencing a stage of development in which everything goes from the hand into the mouth. Small toys, parts of toys, household objects, and even pieces of food should always be viewed as suffocation hazards. (See Figure 10.1.) Since such items account for approximately two-thirds of the home suffocation deaths every year, special efforts should be made to keep the items away from young children.

Providing Appropriate Toys

While toys are naturally attractive to youngsters, they are especially irresistible to young children in the hand-to-mouth stage. For this reason, great care should be taken to provide young children with safe, appropriate toys.

---

1. Jean Carper, *Stay Alive!* (Garden City, New York: Doubleday & Company, Inc., 1965), p. 184.

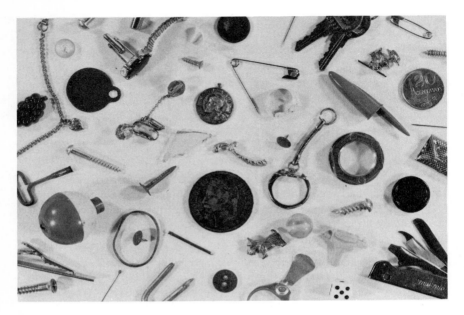

Figure 10.1   Typical objects which are ingested by young children.

For a baby who is unable to stand in his crib, a thick cord strung with beads, doughnuts, and other large, nonswallowable-size toys can be stretched across the top of the crib. Inside the crib, one-piece toys which are large, lightweight, and unbreakable may be appropriate play items. As an additional precaution, older children should be warned against giving toys to a baby without parental permission. Inappropriate toys, even those which are given with the best of intentions, can be easily ingested by a baby and can cause him to choke to death.

Although most parents believe that toys which are specially designed and manufactured for babies are safe, many toys are not. In fact, the ordinary baby rattle is often unsafe. Frequently baby rattles are small and poorly constructed, so that even brief use can cause them to break into many small pieces which can be easily ingested. For safety reasons a rattle should be large enough to prevent a baby from putting the toy into his mouth. In addition, the toy should be one piece and unbreakable.

Baby items, however, are not the only toys whose poor construction makes them dangerous. On the market are toys for young children that are composed of small swallowable-size pieces. For example, cars with hubcaps, dolls with button eyes, and other toys with decorations are easy to take apart. Before giving such toys to small children, parents should remove all ornaments that could be easily pulled off during play. Better still, they should purchase only toys with anchored or painted decorations.

While certain play items are suitable for older children, the same toys may not be appropriate for younger children. In fact, some playthings are quite hazardous. For example, foam-type toys, such as "Nerf" balls, are safe for older children. However, the toys can present choking hazards for younger children who chew off and then swallow small pieces of the foam. Because of this danger, foam-type toys are not recommended for children under four years of age. Another toy which is appropriate for older children but not suitable for the younger ones is the ordinary balloon. Often a young child, instead of blowing into the toy, will suck it into his mouth and then down into his throat, thus permitting the balloon to seal off his air passage. For this reason, children under four or five years of age should not be allowed to play with uninflated balloons. Inflated balloons are safe, if someone supervises the child's play and retrieves all the pieces when the balloons burst. As a general rule, when selecting toys for young children, parents should follow the age recommendations which are listed on the toy packaging by the manufacturers.

Keeping Small Objects Away

Every home has an array of small household objects that a baby or young child can easily ingest. Thus, needles, bobby pins, coins, buttons, beads, and other small objects should be hidden or placed where young children cannot reach them.

Normally, any small object which is lost can be quite easily found by young children. In Collinsville, Illinois, a young couple heard their nineteen-month-old baby gagging and coughing. As the parents rushed their child to the hospital, the baby started to turn blue; by the time the parents had reached the hospital, the baby was dead. To determine the cause of the baby's death, an autopsy was performed. The doctors found a poker chip lodged in the baby's windpipe. After dropping any small object, parents should search until the item is found. In addition, before putting a baby on the floor to play, they should thoroughly search the area for small objects which may have dropped unnoticed.

Making Clothes Safer

Generally, manufacturers of young children's clothing realize that pompons, bows, bells, and other tiny decorations can easily cause suffocation if they are ingested by young children. For this reason, most children's clothes are devoid of such ornaments. However, if the clothes include decorations, the objects should be removed immediately.

Fortunately, most children's clothes are equipped with zippers and snaps instead of small buttons which can be pulled off by children. When buying clothes for babies and young children, parents should select only items with zippers and snaps. For those clothes which have already been purchased, parents should replace all buttons with zippers or snaps.

Averting Mealtime Tragedy

Leaving a baby alone as he feeds from his bottle is a common but very dangerous practice in many homes. Contrary to what many people believe, a baby can easily regurgitate his milk and subsequently choke to death on the fluid. A foolproof way to prevent mealtime suffocation is always to remain with the baby until he has finished his milk.

Another precaution is to avoid giving the baby or very young child such foods as hard candy, peanuts, popcorn, raw carrots, and bacon, since these foods can easily lodge in the throat and block the air passage. Also, older children should be warned against giving food to young children. Only parents or other responsible adults should ever give food to a baby or very young child.

Displaying Proper Habits

Besides placing everything in the mouth, young children are especially impressionable and will quickly imitate the actions of other people. Consequently, parents should avoid displaying dangerous habits which children may imitate. Obviously, if a young child observes an adult holding pins, nails, or other small objects in his mouth, the youngster may attempt the same feat, but with disastrous results.

Preventing Mechanical Suffocation

Approximately one-third of the home suffocation deaths which occur each year are caused by mechanical means. Most often, the victims are babies and young children who smother in bed materials, strangle themselves with cords, clothes, and other materials, or suffocate when trapped in coolers and old refrigerators. Even a heavy object can cause suffocation if it rests on a child's chest or back, thereby preventing his breathing.

Making the Crib Safe

Tragically, every year many parents go to the cribs only to find their babies dead, needless victims of suffocation. Naturally, since a baby spends so much of his early life in his crib, parents should take every precaution to make his bed as safe as possible.

Because a baby can easily bury his face in soft material and suffocate, the mattress in a crib should be smooth and very firm. In addition, the mattress should be sufficiently large to prevent the occurrence of a gap between it and the crib into which the baby could wedge his face.

For covering the mattress, cloth material, such as muslin, is the best choice. Under no circumstances should parents improvise a mattress cover from plastic, especially from a thin plastic bag of the type obtained from dry cleaners. While it may protect the mattress, the plastic can easily adhere tightly to a baby's face. Since the plastic is extremely thin, static electricity is generated through friction. When the static electricity is combined with the suction caused by a baby's inhaling, the plastic clings to the nose and mouth, thus cutting off the baby's air supply. Furthermore, the plastic will not tear when the baby fights it, and consequently, he is unable to cry for help.

Another way in which babies frequently suffocate in their cribs is through entanglement in bed clothing. Since a baby can be kept comfortably warm in his pajamas if the room is well heated, parents should eliminate the use of blankets in the crib. Similarly, parents should eliminate the use of pillows, since a baby can readily bury his face in them and suffocate. Actually, a baby is just as comfortable without a pillow as he is with it.

Fortunately, since the spindles on modern cribs are spaced close together (three to four inches apart), the chances of a baby's sticking his head through the spindle spaces and strangling himself are slight. However, suffocation in this manner can occur if a spindle breaks, thus leaving a large space. To prevent this, parents should check frequently for loose spindles. Older-model cribs with spindles spaced widely apart (six to seven inches) should not be used.

A common practice which often results in suffocation is leaving baby clothes or diapers hanging on the sides of the crib. Such items can be easily pulled into the crib by the baby, or they may fall into the crib when it is shaken by the baby. Once they are in the crib, the clothes or diapers can become wrapped around the baby's neck and cause strangulation. To prevent this, parents should purchase a clothes rack and hang clothes, diapers, and other apparel there. Furthermore, the rack should be placed well away from the crib so the baby cannot reach any of the items hanging on it.

While toys strung on a thick cord across the top of the crib are safe for babies who cannot pull themselves up the sides of their cribs, they are very dangerous for those youngsters who can pull themselves into a standing position. Once on his feet, a baby can easily become entangled in the cord and hang himself. Obviously, such suffocations can be prevented by removing strung toys when a baby first begins to stand in his crib.

As a final note, parents should never sleep in the same bed with a baby. Often a sleeping parent will roll on top of his baby, thereby placing such pressure on the baby's chest that he cannot breathe. For this reason, even if a baby must be moved into his parents' bedroom for supervision during an illness, he should always remain in his crib.

Protecting Young Children

Since young children have considerably more strength than babies, many of the sleeping hazards associated with babies are not threats to young

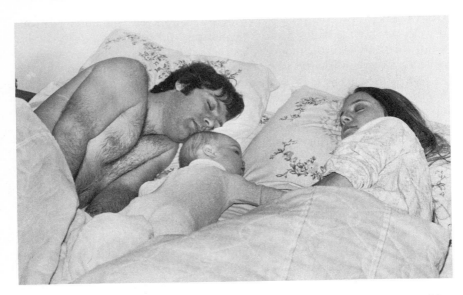

Figure 10.2   Parental companionship at night is a potential suffocation hazard for an infant.

children. Pillows and blankets, for example, are perfectly safe to use in young children's beds. However, young children have greater mobility than babies and thus face other hazards that babies do not.

Since drapery cords, belts, ropes, and similar items can become entangled around a child's neck and cause strangulation, they should be kept out of the reach of young children. Nevertheless, since youngsters can usually obtain such items without their parents' knowledge, additional precautions must be taken. Specifically, parents should warn children never to place ropes or similar items around their own necks or the necks of other children. Furthermore, parents should explain to their children that the hangings on television westerns are actually "play acting." This is extremely important, since children frequently see the "hanged" actor alive in other films and consequently they may not associate hangings with death. In fact, many children have been amazed to discover that a playmate would not come back to life after he had been playfully hanged in a game of "cowboys."

Another hazard that children should never have to face when they are playing is the plastic bag. Obviously, since the bag holds the same danger for young children as it does for babies, the best advice is to keep all plastic bags out of the reach of children.

Of all home suffocation hazards, the discarded refrigerator is perhaps the most widely publicized. Unable to open the door, many children have died playing or hiding in abandoned refrigerators. Although modern refrigerators have magnetic locks which permit the doors to be more easily opened from the inside, a frightened child can still become trapped if he makes only a feeble attempt to escape. To prevent refrigerator suffocations, old refrigerators should be destroyed; but if this cannot be accomplished immediately, the door should be removed.

Unfortunately, freezers and portable picnic chests can be just as much of a hazard as discarded refrigerators. Many children have crawled into these to hide or to play and have never come out alive. In Honolulu, Hawaii, a divorced woman returned home late at night from a date with her ex-husband. She found the babysitter asleep on the sofa, but her children were not in their beds. Thinking that the youngsters were hiding, she and the sitter searched the house. Soon, the mother heard faint crying and followed the sound to a chest-freezer in the utility room. She opened the freezer door and found her two young children. The four-year-old girl was turning blue from the cold and gasping for air, but the three-year-old boy was already dead. To prevent such tragedies, freezers should always be kept well stocked with food to eliminate large spaces into which a child could squeeze. If this is not feasible, large weighted objects can be placed in the freezer to serve the same purpose. With respect to portable picnic chests, these should always be kept in their original cardboard packing boxes and stored out of the reach of children.

Surprisingly, under certain conditions windows and furniture can easily cause suffocations. For example, if a child sticks his head through an open window, the window frame can fall on his neck and strangle him. Similarly, a piece of precariously balanced furniture can quickly fall on top of a child, trap him, and compress his chest enough to prevent his breathing. For these reasons, windows should be opened only slightly or securely fastened in place to prevent them from falling, and furniture should be properly balanced or stabilized.

Obviously, for young children backyard ditches and trenches are especially attractive play areas. However, since even the slightest cave-in can easily bury a child and cause suffocation, these below-ground playgrounds are extremely dangerous. Because of this hazard, parents should insist that ditches and trenches in the vicinity of the home always be filled as quickly as possible. Until these excavations are filled, parents should supervise the outdoor play of their children.

Averting Adult Suffocation

Although babies and children under four years of age are the most frequent victims of suffocation accidents, adults are not immune to the danger. In fact, adults account for approximately 50 percent of all home suffocations, 44 percent by ingested objects and 6 percent by mechanical means.

As mentioned earlier in this chapter, holding pins, nails, or other small objects in the mouth is an extremely dangerous habit. Besides providing young children with a poor example, the habit can easily lead to suffocation. Any sudden movement, such as a sneeze or a cough, can cause the object to be ingested, and once it has been ingested, the object can easily lodge in the airway and cause choking and suffocation. Obviously, the only way to prevent such accidents is for the individual to stop using his mouth as a storage compartment.

Another cause of adult suffocation, especially among the elderly, is the improper chewing of food. Since large pieces of food can cause an individual to choke to death, food should always be thoroughly chewed and then swallowed in small pieces. Furthermore, all bones and gristle should be removed from meat or fish before the food is eaten. When poor teeth, few teeth, or false teeth are the cause of the poor chewing habits, the individual's diet should include a large number of soft foods.

Although mechanical means account for only 6 percent of the suffocations, several precautions should be taken when appropriate. First, when working on an automobile or changing a tire, the person should secure the car so it cannot roll or fall. Second, when digging or working in trenches that are above the level of his head, the person should make sure that proper bracing procedures are followed.

Resource Materials

American Academy of Pediatrics
P.O. Box 1034
Evanston, Illinois 60204

National Safety Council
444 North Michigan Avenue
Chicago, Illinois 60611

American Toy Institute
200 Fifth Avenue
New York City, New York 10010

Toy Manufacturers of America
200 Fifth Avenue
New York City, New York 10010

U.S. Consumer Product Safety Commission
5401 Westbard Avenue
Washington, D.C. 20207
toll-free: 800-638-2666 in the continental United States
800-492-2937 for Maryland residents only

Activities

1. Obtain information from a pediatrician about the various objects that are ingested by babies and young children. Prepare a list of the items which are ingested most frequently.

2. Survey the clothing in the children's department of a local store for ingestion hazards. Write a short paper on your findings.

3. Prepare a list of dangerous habits that can cause suffocation if they are imitated by young children.

4. Obtain from a local dry-cleaning establishment the name and address of the manufacturer of its plastic bags. Then, write to the manufacturer for information on the safe use of his product.

5. Keep a scrapbook of newspaper articles that report home suffocations in the local area. Determine what percentage of the victims are adults and what percentage of the suffocations involved mechanical means.

Questions

1. Why should older children be warned against giving toys to a baby without parental permission?

2. Why are balloons dangerous for children under four or five years of age?

3. Why should babies never be left alone when feeding from their bottles?

4. Why are babies helpless to free themselves from suffocating plastic bags?

5. Why are loose spindles on baby cribs considered to be a suffocation hazard?

6. Why are strung toys dangerous for babies who can stand in their cribs?

7. Why are pillows and blankets quite safe to use in young children's beds, but not in babies' cribs?

8. Why do young children not associate the hangings on TV westerns with death?

9. Why is precariously balanced furniture considered to be a suffocation hazard?

10. In terms of ingested objects, what two practices by older children and adults can easily cause suffocation?

Selected References

"Accident-Proof Your Nursery," *Today's Health.* March, 1960, 73.

Carper, Jean. "Kids Will Swallow Anything," *Today's Health.* January, 1967, 22-25.

———. *Stay Alive!* Garden City, New York: Doubleday & Company, Inc., 1965.

Greendyke, Robert M. "Accidental Strangulation in Infancy," *Pediatrics.* August, 1965, 275-76.

Haas, Flora. "How to Keep a Creeper Safe," *Parents Magazine.* May 1961, 51, 68.

Price, Franklin S., and Melvin A. Humphreys. *Safety Practices for Home and Leisure.* Dubuque, Iowa: Wm. C. Brown Book Company, 1966.

Rakstis, L. J. "How Safe Are Your Child's Toys?," *Today's Health.* December, 1967, 20-23.

"Tips for Your Home and Family," *Today's Health.* October, 1962, 65-66.

Other Home Accidents

11

While falls, fires, poisonings, and suffocations account for over 80 percent of all home deaths, other types of accidents must still be recognized as threats to the family. Each year these accidents claim approximately forty-six hundred lives. Among the most common are firearm, glass-door, electrical, water, and lawn-mower accidents.

Unfortunately, many people consider these mishaps to be primarily freak accidents and impossible to prevent. After a Tennessee man, who had participated without injury in both World War II and the Korean War, was struck and killed by a piece of wire in his backyard, a newspaper printed the headline: LOCAL MAN KILLED IN FREAK MOWER ACCIDENT. Reinforced by the media, this erroneous attitude continues to produce many so-called "freak accidents" each year.

Firearm Accidents

More people die from firearm accidents in the home than in the field or woods, about twelve hundred every year. Tragically, over one-fourth of the victims are children under fourteen years of age.

Exposed to shoot-outs on television westerns and accustomed to playing cowboys and Indians, children often mistakenly play with real guns rather than toys and accidentally shoot themselves. Yet, a youngster with a gun is often in less danger than those around him. Many children are killed when another child playfully points a newly found "toy gun" at them and pulls the trigger. In Indianapolis, Indiana, a four-year-old boy loaded his father's pistol and fired several shots. As neighborhood children gathered to see the gun, the boy turned toward them and played "shoot-out." One child was shot in the stomach, another was hit in the face, and still another was struck in the back.

Obviously, young children are not aware of the danger presented by guns. For this reason, parents simply cannot rely on a child's judgment. To protect their children, parents should always unload the gun and immobilize the trigger with a gun lock. (See Figure 11.1.) In addition, they should store the gun in a locked drawer or cabinet separately from the ammunition. If the child should somehow obtain the weapon, the gun lock, combined with the separate storage of the gun and the ammunition, will practically eliminate the possibility of the child's shooting himself or someone else.

In addition to children, many adults accidentally kill themselves or bystanders while playing with guns. Foolishly, they perform tricks with a loaded gun, such as twirling the gun on the index finger or rapidly switching the gun from one hand to the other, or they attempt to outdraw a television gunfighter, their image in a mirror, or another person with a loaded gun. In some cases individuals even risk death by playing Russian roulette. Recently, in Memphis, Tennessee, a sixteen-year-old boy inserted a bullet into a pistol, spun the cylinder, aimed the barrel at his head, and pulled the trig-

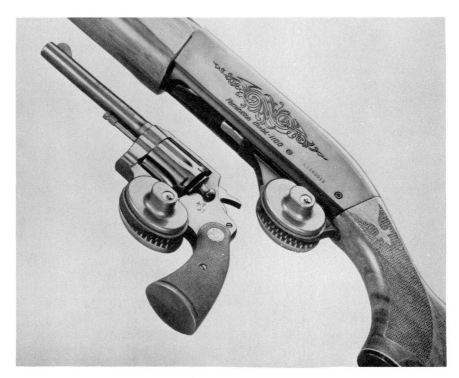

Figure 11.1   The gun lock immobilizes the trigger of the firearm, thus protecting children against accidental discharge. (Courtesy of the Master Lock Company)

ger. The gun did not discharge. Then the youth spun the cylinder again, pointed the gun at the head of a friend, and pulled the trigger again. Still, the gun did not fire! For a third time the boy spun the cylinder, aimed the gun at the head of another friend, and pulled the trigger. In this attempt the gun fired, and the thirteen-year-old girl friend was killed. Ironically, according to witnesses, each time before pulling the trigger the boy looked into the gun barrel. However, he misunderstood how the pistol worked. With a double action revolver, the act of pulling the trigger turns the cylinder one notch and places the bullet in line with the barrel as the hammer falls. Needless to say, real guns, especially loaded ones, are not designed for play. If a person must perform "gun tricks" or play "quick draw" or "Russian roulette," he should always use a toy gun. Although a toy gun may not be as masculine as a real gun, the toy is definitely safer for the modern self-styled cowboy or thrill-seeker.

On the other hand, not all firearm accidents are the result of someone's playing with a gun. Many people become involved in accidents when they mistakenly believe a gun is unloaded and fail to handle it with caution. Because guns are frequently returned to the home without being unloaded, hunting seasons are especially dangerous times of the year for a family. During these periods, many of the nonplay type of gun accidents occur as the weapons are removed from their storage cabinets for cleaning or for showing. Fortunately, preventing such accidents is simple: first, before bringing guns into the home, hunters should check to make sure the weapons are unloaded, and second, family members should at all times handle the guns as if they were loaded.

Despite the danger, many persons deliberately keep loaded guns in their homes as a means of protecting their families. Yet, according to some safety experts, for every burglar who is shot, at least eight family members are wounded or killed in home firearm accidents. In a typical case a twenty-five-year-old man in Sioux Falls, South Dakota, reached for a pistol, which he kept on a nightstand near his bed, and shot himself in the leg. According to the man, he was awakened early in the morning by a ringing telephone, and in his confusion he inadvertently grabbed the gun by the trigger. If a person feels that he must keep a loaded gun in his home for protection, he should immobilize the trigger with a gun lock and then store the weapon in a locked drawer or cabinet.

Glass-door Accidents

Modern, attractive, and functional, glass doors permit sunlight to enter the home, and provide excellent views of outdoor scenery. Unfortunately, they may also be extremely dangerous. Although they may appear to be harmless, many of these doors are actually traps which can disfigure, dismember, or kill. Constructed of ordinary glass, they can easily break into daggerlike pieces that can quickly pierce the body or into guillotinelike sheets that can slice off pieces of flesh when they drop from the metal door frame.

The reason for glass-door accidents is easy to understand: since the glass is transparent, many people mistakenly think that the door is open, and they walk or run into the glass. Because of this danger, doors are now being produced with a special glass which is many times safer than ordinary glass. This saftey glass is manufactured in three forms: wired, tempered, and laminated.

In wired glass a block-pattern of wire has been embedded in the glass. Although it is frequently seen in public buildings, for aesthetic reasons this type of safety glass is not ordinarily used in homes. Yet, because of the embedded wire, the glass is much stronger and can be seen much easier than ordinary glass.

Tempered glass is the product of a special manufacturing process which uses heat to strengthen the glass. Also found in the side and rear windows of automobiles, this type of safety glass is three to five times stronger than a comparable thickness of ordinary glass. Normally, an adult walking into the glass will not break it, but if it should break, tempered safety glass will crumble into gravellike particles which rarely cut.

Laminated glass has two layers of glass with a tough layer of plastic between them. Also found in automobile windshields, laminated glass will not shatter when it breaks, but instead, the pieces of glass will cling to the plastic. Although considerably stronger than ordinary glass, laminated safety glass can still be easily broken.

Since safety glass is more difficult to break than ordinary glass and since it does not produce the daggerlike pieces of glass that ordinary glass does, most injuries and deaths from glass-door accidents can be easily prevented by replacing ordinary-glass doors with safety-glass doors. However, installing safety glass does not necessarily render a glass door harmless. On the contrary, because the glass, except for wired safety glass, is still transparent, a person can receive a severe bump, broken nose, or black eye if he fails to see the door and walks or runs into it. Consequently, special precautions should always be taken to make glass doors more visible to members of the family.

Ideally, glass doors should be decorated at both child and adult eye level with decals, painted designs, scrolls, or other markings. Furthermore, to make certain the glass can be seen even in the dark, reflective tape or fluorescent paint should be applied in various locations. However, the homeowner should always remember that these decorations are designed to supplement safety glass, not substitute for it.

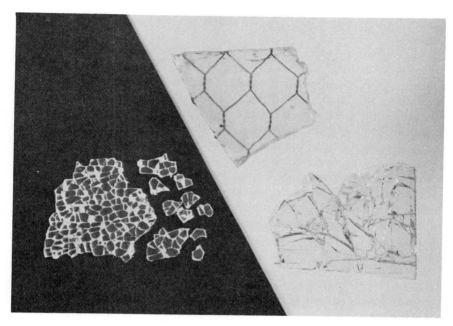

Figure 11.2   Various types of safety glass: (Top) wired, (Bottom left) tempered, and (Bottom right) laminated.

Electrical Accidents

When electricity is properly used, it is one of man's most dependable servants, but when it is misused, electricity can become a ruthless master. Despite popular belief, ordinary house current has ample voltage to electrocute a human being. However, when a person understands its behavior and appropriately respects its power, electricity can be used safely.

Continually seeking to reach the ground, electricity will always travel over the path that offers the least resistance. Since dry skin is a poor conductor, household electricity has difficulty penetrating it. Consequently, when a choice of paths is presented, electricity will invariably select wire, metal, or another good conductor rather than dry skin. However, wet skin is an entirely different matter. Water, because it is a good conductor of electricity, also makes skin a good conductor. Thus an electrical charge which would normally cause only a mild shock in a person with dry skin may produce death when the person's skin is wet. For this reason, with the exception of electric shavers and electric toothbrushes, which are so well insulated that the danger of shock is extremely small, an individual should avoid using electrical appliances near water, particularly in the bathroom. Unfortunately, every year many people ignore this advice and are electrocuted when radios, heaters, and other electrical appliances fall into bathtubs, sinks, and showers.

Although large amounts of water are involved in most electrical accidents, a small amount of moisture can still make skin extremely conductive. Even touching an appliance with sweaty hands may result in electrocution. In Biloxi, Mississippi, a thirty-two-year-old man was fatally shocked while using a portable drill on his boat. According to his wife, the man paused briefly during his work and wiped his sweaty forehead with his hand. Evidently, as the medical examiner reasoned, when the man resumed his drilling, the moisture on his hand was sufficient to conduct the electrical charge throughout his body. Naturally, in most cases defective appliances are the cause of such electrical accidents, not the small amount of moisture on the skin. To reduce the possibility of electrical accidents, the homeowner should purchase only appliances which have been tested by Underwriters' Laboratories, Inc., and found to be free of shock hazard. However, since the UL label cannot prevent subsequent wear, the person should periodically inspect all electrical appliances and have defects corrected by a qualified repairman. When appliances are in good operating condition, they are well insulated and safe to use; but when they are defective, the appliances may ''leak'' electricity and produce a severe shock or death.

Perhaps the most insidious way in which water may contribute to electrical accidents appears in the behavior of young children. Since they are ignorant of the danger associated with electricity, youngsters often stick their tongues in electrical sockets or chew on electrical cords. In many cases the moisture is more than enough to conduct electrical charges throughout their bodies, thereby producing severe facial burns or even death. To protect young children, parents should cover unused electrical sockets with safety plugs or plastic tape and place electrical cords along baseboards or elsewhere out of the reach of youngsters.

Water Accidents

While everyone is aware of the drowning danger inherent in such activities as swimming and boating, few people realize that several hundred persons die every year in their own bathtubs. Tragically, the majority of the victims are young children. Undoubtedly, many of the deaths occur because parents underestimate the danger associated with bathing and allow their children to play unattended in the bathtub.

What many parents fail to realize is that even a small amount of water in the bathtub is sufficient to cover a child's nose and mouth. Since an infant cannot rise after falling face-down into his bathwater, he is especially vulnerable to home drowning accidents. However, an older child can drown just as easily if he accidentally strikes his head on the bathtub and slips unconscious into the water. For this reason, most safety experts recommend that parents should always supervise the bathing activities of their young children, particularly those who are under six years of age.

Although a bathtub may be a deceptive hazard, there is little doubt about the dangers presented by swimming pools, water-filled ditches, wells, cisterns, and cesspools. The best way to eliminate such hazards is to construct fences around pools, fill open ditches, and cover wells, cisterns, and cesspools. However, only one foolproof solution to the problem is available: where even the slightest danger of drowning exists, parents should never leave their children unattended.

Lawn-mower Accidents

Whirling like an airplane propeller at a rate of over thirty-five hundred revolutions per minute, the blade of a power lawn mower can strike grass with over ten thousand pounds of force per square inch. For this reason, the power mower is a very efficient home tool. Yet, this machine is also extremely dangerous. Because of the tremendous force which is generated by

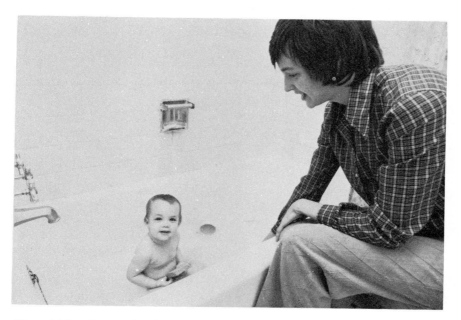

Figure 11.3   Parents should always supervise the bathtub play of young children.

the blade, the power lawn mower can cut human flesh and bones almost as easily as it can cut grass.

In a typical accident in which the operator's foot slips under the mower, the knife-sharp, whirling blade first tears through the shoe and then partially or completely amputates the toes. Unfortunately, while leather shoes offer only minimal protection, many persons fail to employ even this safeguard. Risking their toes, as well as their entire foot, individuals often foolishly mow the lawn in bare feet, sandals, open-toe shoes, or tennis shoes. Paradoxically, while safety shoes with built-in steel toes provide the best protection for the operator's feet, most people feel that they cannot justify the expense of purchasing a special pair of shoes for mowing the grass. In such cases they should at least wear thick leather shoes, preferably work shoes, for minimal protection.

Apparently, most injuries to the feet are the direct result of unsafe mowing procedures. Perhaps, of all the unsafe practices, mowing on wet grass is the most dangerous. Since the footing or traction is poor, an operator can easily slip and fall, and then while he is lying on the ground, he is helpless to prevent the mower from rolling over his feet. To prevent such accidents, the individual should avoid mowing after a brief rain or early in the morning while the grass is still covered with dew.

Another common and extremely dangerous practice is pushing a mower up and down hills. By pushing up a hill, the operator greatly increases the chances of the mower rolling back over his feet; by pushing down a hill, the operator greatly increases the chances of his feet slipping under the mower. For these reasons, the individual should always mow slopes by pushing the lawn mower sideways rather than up and down. On the other hand, if the mower is a riding model, the operator should mow slopes by driving the mower up and down rather than sideways. Because of the greater stability in this position, mowing up and down is less likely to cause the riding-type lawn mower to overturn.

As safety experts know, pulling the mower, rather than pushing it, is a frequent cause of injuries to the feet. The same is true for trying to control the direction of the mower with a foot rather than with the hands. Naturally, pulling the mower increases the chances of the person tripping and falling over objects behind him. On the other hand, using the foot to control the mower places the person's foot within inches of the blade. In either case, with one slip the entire foot can easily slide under the mower. For this reason, the person should always push, not pull, the lawn mower with his hands, not his foot.

Paradoxically, almost as many mower accidents involve the hands as the feet. One of the most frequent causes of such accidents is attempting to unclog the discharge chute of a running mower with the hands. As a result of this imprudent practice, thousands of fingers and hands are amputated every year. Before reaching under the mower, the operator should always turn off the engine and then wait for the blade to stop turning. However, since any turning of the blade by hand may start the motor again, the person should also disconnect the spark plug before working on the mower.

Naturally, not all lawn-mower accidents involve just the hands or the feet. As accident statistics verify, every part of the human body is vulnerable to serious mower injuries. Yet, oddly enough, youngsters, not adults, are most likely to sustain injuries over the entire body. In Evanston, Illinois, a four-year-old boy, riding with his father, fell from a tractor-type mower. The whirling blade of the mower passed over the left side of the boy's body, thereby necessitating the later amputation of the youngster's arm and leg by doctors. In Jacksonville, Florida, a retired businessman backed his riding-type mower over his eighteen-month-old grandson. According to a horrified neighbor, "the boy's body looked as if it had passed through a meat grinder." As these examples suggest, parents should never allow their children to ride on lawn mowers or to play in the area of mowing operations. In addition, the operator of the mower should remain alert at all times for the presence of small children.

Surprisingly, a person can receive a serious lawn-mower injury without even coming into direct contact with the blade of the mower. Because of the tremendous force which is generated by the whirling blade, a power lawn mower can easily pick up sticks, rocks, glass, and wire and then hurl the objects into human eyes, chests, and skulls. Even mower blades have been known to break after hitting certain objects, and to strike nearby persons. Although the mishap is usually referred to as a freak happening, the "mower-missile accident" is in fact quite common. Fortunately, this type of accident can be easily prevented. Before starting to mow, the individual should clear the lawn of all foreign objects. Furthermore, he should mow around, not over, fixed objects, such as boulders, tree stumps, and tree roots. Nevertheless, the person should still insist that all family members remain at least thirty-five feet away from the area being mowed, preferably inside the home.

Resource Materials

Consumer Information
Public Documents Center
Pueblo, Colorado 81009

Good Housekeeping
959 Eighth Avenue
New York City, New York 10019

Master Lock Company
2600 North 32nd Street
Milwaukee, Wisconsin 53210

National Rifle Association
1600 Rhode Island Avenue, N.W.
Washington, D.C. 20036

National Safety Council
444 North Michigan Avenue
Chicago, Illinois 60611

Underwriters' Laboratories, Inc.
207 East Ohio Street
Chicago, Illinois 60611

Activities

1. Obtain a toy "cap" gun, holster, and belt. Standing in front of a mirror, practice quick drawing while a friend records the number of times you would have shot yourself if the gun were real. Prepare a short paper on the results of your experiment.

2. Obtain small pieces of regular, wired, laminated, and tempered glass, and prepare a demonstration before the class on their breaking properties. (Be sure to cover the glass with a thick cloth before breaking.) Have the class examine the broken pieces of glass and hypothesize about the injury they would have produced if the glass had been broken by a hand or a leg.

3. Write to Underwriters' Laboratories, and request information on their testing of appliances for shock hazards. Present the information to the class in a short report.

4. Prepare and submit to a local newspaper a short article on the danger of leaving small children unattended in the bathtub.

5. Develop a checklist of unsafe lawn-mowing practices. Use this checklist to survey your neighborhood.

Questions

1. Why is the child who is playing with a gun usually in less danger than others around him?
2. What are the three most common gun games played by adults?
3. What is the primary cause of glass-door accidents?
4. What are the three types of safety glass, and how do they differ?
5. Why are electric shavers and toothbrushes relatively safe to use near water?
6. What are two practices of children which frequently result in electrical accidents?
7. Why should small children never be left unattended in the bathtub?
8. What is the only foolproof way to prevent home drownings?
9. What is the safest type of shoes to wear when mowing the lawn?
10. How can injury occur to a person who is mowing the lawn when he does not even come into contact with the mower blade?

Selected References

"Basic Rules of Gun Safety," *Good Housekeeping.* January, 1966, 139.

Carper, Jean. *Stay Alive!* Garden City, New York: Doubleday & Company, Inc., 1965.

Coopwood, Thomas B. "Missile Injuries from Power Lawn Mowers," *Texas Medicine.* April, 1976, 53-54.

Crikelair, George F. and Avtar S. Dhaliwal. "The Cause and Prevention of Electrical Burns of the Mouth in Children—A Protective Cuff," *Plastic and Reconstructive Surgery.* August, 1976, 206-09.

"Glass Doors Should Be Made of Safety Glass," *Consumer Bulletin.* May, 1964, 43, 40.

Graham III, William P. and others. "Injuries from Rotary Power Lawnmowers," *American Family Physician.* May, 1976, 75-79.

Grosfeld, Jay L. "Lawn Mower Injuries in Children," *Archives of Surgery.* May, 1970, 582-83.

"How to Avoid Glass-Door Dangers," *Good Housekeeping.* March, 1963, 142.

Knapp Jr., L. W. and others. "Power-Mower Injuries," *The Journal of the Iowa Medical Society.* June, 1969, 500-01.

"100 Ways to Make the Summer Safe for Your Family," *Good Housekeeping.* June, 1975, 154-55.

"Power Mowers: Danger in the Yard," *Changing Times.* May, 1966, 31-32.

Ross, Paul M., Edwards P. Schwentker, and Hugh Bryan. "Mutilating Lawn Mower Injuries in Children," *The Journal of the American Medical Association.* August 2, 1976, 480-81.

Sachatello, Charles and John Sawyers. "The Invisible Glass Door: Another Hazard of Modern Living," *The Journal of the Tennessee Medical Association.* April, 1968, 395-96.

"Safe Power Mowing," *Today's Health.* July, 1966, 5.

Solomon, Goody L. "Safeguarding Your Home—II. Help for House Hazards," *Reader's Digest.* March, 1975, 177-78, 180.

"Tips for Your Home and Family," *Today's Health.* December, 1968, 77-78.

"Your Power Mower—Friend and Foe," *American Home.* March, 1967, 138.

School Accidents

12

On the morning of March 24, 1972, five youngsters from Nyack, New York, were killed when their school bus was struck by a Penn Central freight train. The townspeople of Nyack in their grief erected a large stone monument in a local children's park. The monument bears these words:

The Children's Memorial

In memory of our town's most precious possession—five of our youth. Their promise, as a result of tragedy, was unfulfilled. May all who pause to share this land realize each generation carries all our hopes and our heritage.

According to the National Safety Council, more than six thousand school-age children are killed in accidents every year in the United States. However, probably fewer than one-tenth of the deaths are the result of school-related activities. As the Nyack memorial suggests, the accidental death of any school-age child, regardless of the reason, is a tragic loss, not only for friends and parents but also for society.

Going to and from School

Apparently most school-related injuries are sustained during normal activity in the classrooms or on the school grounds. However, school-related deaths are caused most often by accidents while the children travel to and from school, whether by school bus, automobile, bicycle, or foot.

Riding the School Bus

In this country school buses transport more than twenty-two million pupils and travel nearly ten million miles every school day. Despite their tremendous exposure to traffic hazards, buses are involved annually in only fifty-one thousand accidents. Fortunately, only one out of every ten school-bus accidents results in personal injury. For these reasons most people, both safety experts and parents, believe that school buses represent the safest possible transportation to and from school for their children.

Providing Safe Vehicles

The safe transportation of pupils begins with the selection and use of safe vehicles. Unfortunately, as most school safety officials realize, today's school buses are not as safe as they could be.

Over the past few years, numerous changes have been made in automotive design in an effort to protect more adequately the passengers. However, bus designers and manufacturers have neglected to show the same concern for schoolchildren. As shown in numerous experimental tests, school-bus seats are often improperly anchored. As a result, during an accident, they tend to rip out of the floor and become deadly flying projectiles. In addition, because seat backs are not of adequate height, they often cause whiplash injuries when the bus is struck from the rear. Similarly, since the backs of the seats are not padded, the exposed metal frequently produces

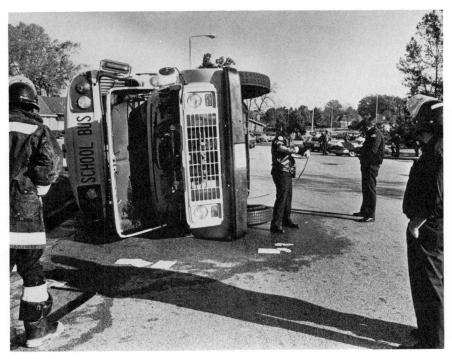

Figure 12.1   Twenty-six children were treated for minor injuries, primarily of the head and chest, when their school bus overturned after being struck by a car. (Courtesy of the *Memphis Press-Scimitar;* Photographed by James R. Reid)

severe head and chest injuries when the schoolchildren are thrown forward during a front-end collision. Undoubtedly, many of the structural deficiencies in school buses can be explained by the fact that manufacturers must contend with budget-conscious administrators and school boards.

While school buses are not as safe as they could be, the school administrator should nevertheless insist that all buses under his jurisdiction meet or preferably exceed state and federal safety standards. In addition, he should establish a stringent maintenance program to provide for the periodic inspection and repair of all school buses within his district. In situations where a school district must contract with a private company for pupil transportation, the school administrator should verify before signing a contract that the company is meeting the safety guidelines and will continue to meet them in the future.

Selecting Qualified Drivers

Regardless of the problems in school-bus design, the bus driver remains the most important factor in school-bus safety. According to some safety experts, at least one-half of all school-bus accidents could be prevented by appropriate driver action.

In an effort to improve school-bus safety, all states have established minimum guidelines and regulations for the selection, training, and supervision of school-bus drivers. Yet, despite this concern at the state level, many communities still do not devote enough attention to the process of driver selection. In certain areas men and women as old as seventy years, sometimes with heart problems, impaired coordination, partial deafness, or reduced vision, drive school buses. Even youngsters of sixteen years, statistically a dangerous age for drivers, are hired to transport pupils to and from schools on buses. Undoubtedly, part of the problem is created by an inadequate labor pool.

In most communities the school-bus driver's job is only a part-time working arrangement. In addition, except in the more affluent school districts, the job does not pay well. As a result, only certain individuals can afford to become school-bus drivers. Most often, these individuals work full-time at other jobs, such as policemen, firemen, ministers, or farmers, and then moonlight as school-bus drivers during their off-hours. However, they also may be retired persons who perform the jobs as a means of supplementing their pensions or social security benefits, or housewives who drive the buses in an effort to increase their family's income.

Because of the responsibilities of the job, the school administrator should select his bus drivers with almost as much care as he selects his teachers. As a rule, each candidate for the school-bus driver's job should meet the following standards:

1. *Age.* The person should be over twenty-one but under sixty-five years of age.
2. *Physical health.* He should present evidence that he is free from any incapacitating physical condition, such as impaired hearing, reduced vision, poor coordination, or circulatory problems, which might interfere with his safely driving a school bus. Preferably, the physical examination should be conducted by a licensed physician who has been approved by the school administrator.
3. *Mental health and emotional stability.* The individual should be congenial, self-reliant, dependable, honest, morally acceptable, emotionally stable, patient, and even tempered. In addition, when he is under stress, the driver candidate should be calm, knowledgeable, and decisive in action.
4. *Knowledge.* He should possess a thorough knowledge of the safety rules and traffic laws which govern pupil transportation and be able to successfully demonstrate this knowledge in a written examination.
5. *Physical capability.* The person should be able to demonstrate his skills, such as starting, stopping, backing, and turning, in operating a school bus safely. Also, his driving record for the three-year period immediately preceding his employment application should be free of any moving traffic violations.

Once the drivers have been employed, they should be enrolled in a short training program which provides additional instruction and practical experience in school-bus operation and pupil discipline. In addition, the school administrator should require his school-bus drivers to complete similar refresher courses prior to the beginning of each new school year.

Directing Pupil Behavior

Students who are transported to and from school on buses should always be instructed in the guidelines and rules which help promote school-bus safety. In many communities this responsibility for educating the pupils is given to the school-bus driver. However, because of the complexity of the task and for practical reasons, students, parents, teachers, the administrator, and the school-bus driver should all assume the responsibility for the safety of school-bus passengers.

Undoubtedly, one of the most dangerous times for students is the period when they are waiting for the school bus to arrive. In Pittsburgh, Pennsylvania, a seven-year-old boy was struck and dragged fifty feet along the street by a delivery truck. Despite the resuscitation efforts by a passing motorist, the youngster was later pronounced dead at the scene of the accident. According to witnesses, the boy, who was one of several children waiting for the school bus, was playing when he suddenly darted into the street and into the front of the truck. Obviously, in order to reduce the temptation of playing on the roadway, pupils should be taught to leave home at an appropriate time. However, this is only a partial solution to the problem. Because young children are often unpredictable, whenever possible, parents should supervise their youngsters until the school bus arrives. On the other hand, when a parent is not present for supervision, older students should accept the responsibility for the safety of the younger pupils.

Once the school bus has been boarded, the driver has complete jurisdiction over his passengers. However, since he must devote most of his time and attention to the task of driving, the school-bus driver, unlike the classroom teacher, cannot afford to become distracted by the conduct of his students. In general, student behavior on the school bus should equal the quality of behavior which is normally exhibited by the students in their classrooms. To permit the school-bus driver to hear the sounds of traffic, such as horns, emergency sirens, and train whistles, students should, as much as possible, talk and laugh at a reasonable level. Furthermore, they should refrain from scuffling and other forms of horseplay which might distract the driver. Unfortunately, because pupils are often unruly and difficult to control, some school administrators have been forced in recent years to organize school-bus patrols as a means of helping the driver maintain discipline. Most often, one or two teenage students are chosen to accompany each bus driver. Besides maintaining order on the bus, the student-patrol members may assist younger children in boarding or leaving the bus and in crossing streets or highways. In some communities the administrators have also trained their student-patrol members in the proper methods of stopping the school bus in an emergency, such as when the driver has been stricken by a heart attack or incapacitated in some other way.

For safety reasons, most schools provide loading and unloading zones on the school grounds or a curb area which is adjacent to the school. Consequently, students are often subjected to the greatest danger at the end of the school day, for at that time many must cross busy streets or highways in order to reach home. Preferably, before crossing a street or highway, the pupils should stand approximately ten feet in front of the school bus and wait until the driver signals them to proceed across the street. However, whenever possible, the bus driver should load and unload his passengers at locations where they will not have to cross any streets or highways. Although some children may be forced to remain on the bus until its return trip, this plan will provide for maximum pupil safety.

Preparing for Emergencies

In the event of an emergency, such as a traffic accident or a fire, the school-bus passengers' lives may be endangered if they remain inside the bus. For this reason, the bus driver, in cooperation with student school-bus patrol members and the school administrator, should periodically conduct drills which closely simulate emergency evacuations of the bus. As a part of these drills, pupils should be taught how to open the rear emergency door, as well as how to remove the side "kickout" windows. Furthermore, they should be instructed in the methods of operating the emergency brake, turning off the ignition switch, and using the fire extinguishers.

Supervising Special Bus Trips

Besides carrying pupils to and from school, buses are often used to transport athletes, cheer leaders, band members, and students on field trips. When the school bus is used for one of these purposes, the faculty member in charge of the activity should supervise the passengers and assume complete responsibility for their behavior on the bus. In addition, since the activity may be located in an area which is unfamiliar to the bus driver, thus increasing the danger of an accident, the faculty sponsor should discuss beforehand with the driver any unusual situations or problems which might be encountered on the trip.

Riding to School in a Car

Despite the increasing use of the school bus in this country, the automobile is still a favorite means of transporting students to and from school. Naturally, when they ride to school in cars, students are exposed to the same hazards as all automobile passengers. However, school-automobile transportation does present several special problems for parents, other pupils, and the school administrator.

Organizing Community Car Pools

In recent years, for financial and convenience reasons, many parents have formed community car pools for transporting their children to and from school. In spite of the responsibility which is involved, most parents do not devote enough attention to the selection of their fellow car-pool drivers. In some instances this lack of concern has resulted in tragic situations.

In Madison, Wisconsin, a car-pool driver and her three young passengers drowned when the car in which they were riding ran off the highway and plunged into a swiftly flowing river. An autopsy performed on the driver later revealed that she had enough alcohol in her blood to be considered legally drunk. Shockingly, according to her husband, all of the other car-pool parents knew that the woman had a drinking problem. In fact, one parent knew that the woman kept an opened bottle of cherry vodka under the driver's seat in her car.

Because of the importance of the driver, parents should select their fellow car-poolers with extreme care. Only persons who are emotionally stable and in excellent physical and mental health should be allowed to participate in the car pool.

Protecting Automobile Passengers

Like the school-bus operator, the car-pool driver must maintain complete control over his student passengers. By requiring the use of safety belts, the car-pool driver, besides protecting his passengers, is usually able to minimize the amount of scuffling and other forms of horseplay by the children. However, in any case of loud talking, excessive laughing, or other unruly behavior, the driver should stop the car as soon as possible and restore order among the children.

Walking or Bicycling to School

With school buses and private automobiles transporting students, the area around the school is often heavily congested. For pupils on foot or on bicycles, this congestion is especially hazardous. Often the installation of flashing 15-mph signals on the streets adjacent to the school grounds will significantly slow vehicular traffic and thus increase safety. However, in most communities additional precautions are usually necessary.

Organizing Safety Patrols

The most commonly used method of protection at school crossings is the student safety patrol. Fundamentally, school safety patrol members serve two functions: (1) they assist teachers and parents in the instruction of schoolchildren in pedestrian and bicycle safety, and (2) they direct and control other schoolchildren in crossing streets and highways. However, because they are physically, mentally, and emotionally immature, patrol members should not be allowed to direct vehicular traffic or to accompany student pedestrians across streets or highways.

Although they work in close cooperation with the local police, student safety patrol members remain under the supervision of the school board. For operational purposes the school administrator is usually given the responsibility for selecting and organizing the student members into an effective school safety patrol. To accomplish this task, he may, in turn, place the patrol members under the close direction of a competent and interested teacher. Normally, the teacher-supervisor is the most important person in the organization, since his enthusiasm will stimulate the patrol members to perform eagerly and well.

As a rule, school safety patrol members should be selected on a volunteer basis from the upper elementary grade levels and from the junior high school. During the selection process, the school administrator should give preference to volunteers who exhibit courtesy, punctuality, reliability, leadership, and a thorough knowledge of pedestrian and bicycle safety rules.

Utilizing Adult Crossing Guards

Although school safety patrol members may be properly trained and closely supervised, they cannot function effectively at congested intersections without adult assistance. For this reason, in most communities adult crossing guards are used in conjunction with student patrol members.

Basically, adult crossing guards perform two essential tasks: (1) they escort students across streets and highways, and (2) they direct vehicular traffic whenever necessary to protect the students. Because of their traffic control functions, crossing guards are often placed under the supervision and direction of both the local police department and the community schools.

Like other school personnel, crossing guards should be selected with extreme care. The school administrator should personally interview each applicant and examine his credentials carefully to assure that he possesses the physical, mental, emotional, and moral qualifications which are needed for the crossing-guard position. Once the crossing guards have been employed, they should be enrolled in a training program to provide instruction in traffic control, pedestrian safety, first aid methods, and community relations. In many communities this training program is jointly sponsored by the schools, the police department, and the local chapter of the American Red Cross.

Planning Routes to and from School

Whether children ride their bicycles or walk, getting to and from school safely is a serious responsibility and requires considerable planning. For this reason, most schools place great emphasis, particularly in the lower grade levels, on traffic safety instruction.

In the classroom the teacher should construct a large bulletin-board map of the area surrounding the school and discuss with the students the various hazards which they may encounter in traveling to and from school. In addition, the teacher should give the students folding maps of the community and ask them to draw the safest routes for school travel. With the assistance of the teacher, the students should select routes which provide minimum vehicular traffic, sidewalks, traffic control devices, marked crosswalks, school safety patrols, and adult crossing guards.

After they have chosen the best routes, the students should take the maps to their homes and ask their parents to carefully study the routes. Furthermore, whenever possible, the parents should walk with the students to and from school and verify the safety of the routes.

Safeguarding Students at School

Primarily, a safe school environment is the responsibility of the school administrator and his nonteaching staff members. However, since unsafe behavior may result in accidents in even the safest environment, teachers must always accept the major responsibility for their students' safety.

Programming for Physical Education Safety

Physical education is an integral part of the school curriculum. Consequently, like all school programs, physical education is concerned with the mental, social, and physical growth and development of the students. However, unlike other subjects, the physical education program is designed to achieve its objectives through the guided instruction and participation of the students in sports, rhythms, gymnastics, and related physical activities. Since many of these activities involve speed, agility, and bodily contact, more accidents and injuries occur in physical education classes than in ordinary classrooms.

Recognizing Activity Hazards

Every activity in the physical education curriculum has certain inherent hazards. To recognize these potential dangers the teacher must carefully analyze the nature of the activity, the environment in which it will occur, the equipment which will be used, and the level of performance which is required by the participants in the activity. By ascertaining the various hazards the teacher can then determine whether or not each hazard can be eliminated or at least controlled to some degree.

Eliminating Unnecessary Hazards

Whenever possible, unnecessary hazards should always be removed immediately. For example, each day the physical education teacher, with help from members of the school maintenance staff, should clear the activity area of all sticks, rocks, metal cans, broken glass, water, and other hazards. Similarly, with student assistance, the teacher should periodically inspect all physical education equipment and repair or replace defective items.

On the other hand, whenever unnecessary risks cannot be eliminated, the students should be removed from possible contact with the hazards. For example, the physical education teacher should not permit his students to participate in activities under lightning skies, on slippery surfaces, or in conditions of extreme fatigue. Likewise, the instructor should limit the participation of students with medical problems, such as poor vision or heart conditions.

Controlling Unavoidable Hazards

Obviously, not all of the hazards in a vigorous and exciting physical education activity can be or, for that matter, should be avoided. Some activities by their very nature present more risk than others. For instance, gymnastics and swimming are naturally more hazardous than dancing or volleyball. Nevertheless, with proper instruction and supervision, the teacher can largely control the hazards. Furthermore, certain peculiarities in the equipment or the environment may produce unavoidable hazards for physical education students. For example, the floor supports on the gymnastics balance beam may present a hazard for a falling student. However, to prevent injuries, the teacher can control this hazard by covering the supports with thick, flexible mats.

Planning for Safety in Sports

With increasing public support, participation in intramural, extramural, and interscholastic sports has grown impressively in recent years. However, because of the "all-out" effort which is required, the many situations which involve bodily contact, and the hazards which are created by throwing or striking objects, injuries are common occurrences in sports. Apparently the greatest number of injuries is sustained during the athletes' participation in football, basketball, wrestling, and gymnastics programs.

According to safety experts, inadequate conditioning is a contributing factor in many athletic injuries. In general, the first month of the season is the most hazardous period in any sport, since the athletes are usually in poor physical condition and still somewhat awkward in their movements. To reduce the possibility of athletic injuries, the coach should develop and direct off-season programs which are devoted entirely to the various aspects of physical conditioning. Furthermore, in the pre-season he should conduct conditioning sessions for his athletes during the first two or three weeks of the period and thus restrict bodily contact, scrimmage, and other forms of all-out activity until at least the last two weeks of the period.

During the pre-season period, as well as during the regular season, many athletic injuries can be prevented or mitigated by proper equipment. For this reason, the coach and his athletes should periodically inspect all sports equipment and repair or replace defective items. In addition, in sports which require personal protective gear, the coach should always select the best equipment and then carefully fit the gear on each athlete in accordance with his particular needs.

Promoting Playground Safety

Through careful research and planning, many modern elementary school playgrounds are designed to meet the highest safety standards. Specifically, the best pieces of playground equipment are selected for the various age groups and then located permanently in areas which limit physical conflict between the groups of children. Furthermore, when schools are located near busy streets, the playgrounds are enclosed by high fences. However, even the best designed playgrounds require constant attention if they are to remain free of hazards.

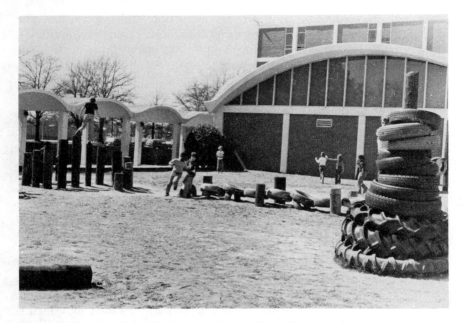

Figure 12.2   A well-designed playground will provide suitable equipment for the various age groups and through the placement of the equipment will limit physical conflict among the various groups of children.

Besides providing students with instruction in the proper use of playground equipment, the supervising teacher, with assistance from members of the school maintenance staff, should carefully inspect the play area every day and remove all sticks, rocks, broken glass, metal cans, and other hazards. In addition, the teacher should provide constant supervision for the students and stop all dangerous activities on the playground. During recess and lunch periods, the teacher can be assisted by members of the student playground patrol. Assigned a specific section of the playground, each patrol member should encourage safe pupil behavior and report any defective play equipment to the supervising teacher.

Emphasizing Safety in Shops and Laboratories

In most high schools student enrollment in shop and laboratory courses has increased substantially in recent years. Fortunately, with this increased enrollment, shop teachers have become more safety conscious than they were in past years. According to the National Safety Council, this change in teacher attitude has occurred for several reasons:

For one thing, they are increasingly aware that they may be held legally liable for injuries resulting from a shop accident. In addition, expanding enrollments in shop courses have resulted in a wider range of students than ever before. The more pronounced variations in age, mental ability and mechanical aptitude among students have caused more emphasis to be placed on teaching them to work safely.[1]

Nevertheless, with the possible exception of the gymnasium, more students are injured in shops and laboratories than in any other location in the school building.

Complicating the problem is that conditions in shops and labs are constantly changing. Materials are moved, storage boxes are emptied, waste materials are produced, and equipment, such as handtools and machines, are altered by student use, misuse, or wear. To maintain an acceptable standard of safety for the shop or laboratory, the teacher and his students should always practice "good housekeeping" principles. As the National Safety Council notes,

> Good housekeeping in school shops and laboratories certainly means "a place for everything and everything in its place." The term, however, describes other important practices such as providing for the daily removal of all sawdust shavings, metal cuttings, and other waste materials; providing a toe board and railing around all balconies used for overhead storage of supplies, equipment or shop projects; providing properly marked boxes or bins for various kinds of scrap stock; employing a standard procedure to keep floors free of oil, water and foreign materials; providing brushes for the cleaning of equipment after each use; providing for the sweeping of the shop floors at least once each day depending on the rate of scrap accumulation; locating machines and equipment in such a way as to provide easy cleaning and maintenance.[2]

In addition, with the assistance of several students, the teacher should conduct daily inspections of the shop or lab to make certain that all equipment and machines remain guarded and in good working condition and that the general work environment remains clear of any hazards.

Although students may have passed an examination on shop techniques and safety procedures and may have demonstrated their ability to operate the various shop tools and machines safely, the teacher should still remain alert at all times for dangerous work habits. Because of their inexperience, students often overestimate their abilities and become careless in their work. Whenever a dangerous practice is observed, the teacher should stop all activity in the shop or laboratory and remind all of the students about the correct method. Furthermore, to impress others, students sometimes attempt to work without personal safety equipment. When students are seen with in-

1. National Safety Council, "Safety in the Drafting Room," *Safety Education Data Sheet No. 95* (Chicago: NSC, n.d.), p. 1.
2. National Safety Council, "Coordinating Accident Prevention in Industrial and Vocational Education Programs," *Safety Education Data Sheet No. 79 Revised* (Chicago: NSC, n.d.), p. 4.

appropriate clothing or without safety goggles, the teacher should reprimand the offenders and note the violation on their class records. If they
commit the same safety violation again, the teacher should prohibit the
students from working in the shop or lab for an appropriate period of time.

Maintaining a Safe School Environment

Despite rising construction costs, most communities support the belief
that maximum safety is a prime requisite in the design of school buildings.
As a rule, new school facilities should be designed so that shops,
laboratories, supply rooms, boiler rooms, and other potentially dangerous
areas are separated from principal classroom locations. In addition, safety
innovations, such as abrasive steps, safety-glass doors, automatic fire detection systems, and automatic sprinklers, should be incorporated into
school-building design.

Naturally, all school buildings, new or old, require constant attention if
they are to remain relatively hazard-free. As Florio notes,

> Special attention should be given to the condition of corridors and stairways;
> they should be free of obstacles and sharp projections, and firm handrails should
> be located on both sides of all stairways. Although the stairways in most new
> school buildings have been constructed with rough surfaces, old stairways have
> often been worn smooth and slippery and may have to be equipped with safety
> treads. Floor surfaces should also be tested to see that they provide a sure
> footing; nonslip waxes and preservatives should be used to keep them in good
> condition.[3]

In addition, periodic inspections of the school premises should be made. As
a rule, the school administrator, along with members of the custodial staff,
should inspect the building on a daily schedule. On the other hand, a
"search team" composed of custodians, teachers, administrators, and interested community officials should inspect the school premises on a
monthly basis. While some of the problems will be minor and can be placed
on the building repair list, certain hazards, such as broken handrails and
sticking panic bars, should be corrected immediately.

Although the school building may have been carefully inspected and
made as safe as possible, the school administrator should still plan for
possible emergencies. Thus every school should develop a program of
emergency preparedness that will enable the students to seek protection
within the building, such as in a tornado or a hurricane, or to evacuate the
building, such as in a bomb threat or a fire. To be effective, however, the

---

3. A. E. Florio and G. T. Stafford, *Safety Education* (3rd ed.; McGraw-Hill Book Company,
1969), p. 122.

program must be known and thoroughly understood by students, teachers, custodial personnel, and administrators. As a means of making certain that everyone in the school knows the proper steps to take in a crisis situation, the school administrator should conduct periodic emergency drills. Besides reinforcing the correct pattern of action for any future emergencies, the drills prepare the participants to face potential panic-producing situations as calmly as possible. For information on emergency preparedness, the administrator should write to the National Safety Council. (See "Resource Materials" at the end of this chapter.)

Resource Materials

American Association for Health, Physical Education, and Recreation
1201 16th Street, N.W.
Washington, D.C. 20036

American Automobile Association
1712 G Street, N.W.
Washington, D.C. 20006

The National Fire Protection Association
470 Atlantic Avenue
Boston, Massachusetts 02210

National Safety Council
444 North Michigan Avenue
Chicago, Illinois 60611

National Smoke, Fire and Burn Institute
53 State Street
Suite 833
Boston, Massachusetts 02109

Activities

1. Prepare a slide presentation for the class on the inherent structural hazards of the modern school bus.

2. Invite several school safety patrol members to discuss with the class their responsibilities in the school safety program.

3. Write a short paper on "safety in physical education and sports."

4. Prepare a list of general safety rules and regulations for use in school shops and labs.

5. Write to the National Smoke, Fire and Burn Institute, and request information on "introducing smoke drills into school fire drills." Present a short, oral report on your findings to the class.

Questions

1. When do most school-related deaths occur?
2. What are some of the inherent hazards in school-bus design?
3. What are some of the standards which should be used to evaluate a candidate for the school-bus driver's job?
4. What are the functions of the school safety patrol?
5. What tasks are performed by adult crossing guards?
6. Why do more accidents and injuries occur in physical education classes than in ordinary classrooms?
7. What is the most hazardous period in any sport?
8. Why are shop teachers more safety conscious today than they were in past years?
9. What are some of the safety innovations that should be incorporated into school-building design?
10. What functions do emergency drills serve?

Selected References

American Association for Health, Physical Education, and Recreation. *School Safety Policies with Emphasis on Physical Education, Athletics and Recreation.* Washington, D.C.: National Education Association, 1968.

American Automobile Association. *How to Organize a School Safety Patrol.* Washington, D.C.: AAA, 1960.

Clarke, K. S. "Accident Prevention Research in Sports—an Exploration of Reform," *Journal of Health, Physical Education, and Recreation.* February, 1969, 45-48.

Florio, A. E. and G. T. Stafford. *Safety Education.* 3rd ed.; New York: McGraw-Hill Book Company, 1969.

National Safety Council. "Safety in the Drafting Room," *Safety Education Data Sheet No. 95.* Chicago: NSC, n.d.

———. "Coordinating Accident Prevention in Industrial and Vocational Education Programs," *Safety Education Data Sheet No. 79 Revised.* Chicago: NSC, n.d.

Owen, Mickey. "Play It Safe." *School Safety.* March-April, 1967, 2, 4-6.

Legal Responsibility and School Accidents

13

On January 15, 1962, in Chatham, New Jersey, a fourteen-year-old boy attempted a mid-air gymnastics stunt during a physical education class and suffered a severely crippling injury. In subsequent legal action, the court awarded the student and his parents the astonishing sum of $1,215,140.00. The award, which was reported at the time to be the largest negligence recovery in history, stunned and terrified school personnel everywhere and stimulated a renewed interest in student safety in most states. Today, the case stands as a landmark in the history of student-teacher liability suits.

Recognizing Legal Responsibilities

Teachers must always assume moral responsibility for the safety of their students. Fortunately, nearly all faculty members recognize this, and as a result, few teachers are deliberately negligent in their duties. However, many instructors are unaware of all the steps that they can and should take to prevent school accidents. Furthermore, when students are injured at school, teachers are sometimes unjustly accused of negligence. For these reasons, every faculty member should familiarize himself with his state's liability laws and his legal responsibilities for student safety.

Nature of Liability

Enforceable by court action, liability is a legal obligation or responsibility of a person, business, company, or institution. Although liability may exist in many forms, tort liability is involved in the relationship between the teacher or school, and the students. In this form of liability, the instructor and the school must accept legal responsibility for torts or wrongful acts which result in injuries to students, their property, or their reputations.

According to the courts, torts may be acts of commission or acts of omission. In addition, torts may be intentional or unintentional. Apparently, in most cases of torts which involve the schools, the wrongful part of the act is performed by omission and without intent. In general, torts include acts of malfeasance, misfeasance, and nonfeasance.

In an act of malfeasance, an illegal deed is performed. For example, in states where corporal punishment is forbidden by law, a teacher would be guilty of malfeasance if he struck a student. Because the act is against the law, the teacher would be subject to legal action regardless of whether or not the student received an injury during the performance of the deed.

In misfeasance a legal act is performed improperly, thereby causing personal injury. For example, in states which permit corporal punishment, a teacher would be guilty of misfeasance if he had injured a student by administering an excessive and unreasonable beating.

Unlike misfeasance, the act of nonfeasance is the failure to perform a legal obligation or duty. For example, if a gymnastics teacher did not station "spotters" around a trampoline and a student was injured after being thrown from the piece of equipment, the teacher may be charged with nonfeasance. Similarly, if a student were left unsupervised during a chemistry experiment and if he were severely injured by exploding glassware, the laboratory teacher may be subject to a charge of nonfeasance and legal action.

School and Teacher Liability

Traditionally, school districts, as agents of state governments, have been exempt from tort liability under the "doctrine of government immunity." This exemption is applicable for all injuries and property damage which may result from defective equipment, improperly maintained facilities, and wrongfully performed acts by employees.

The doctrine of government immunity originated in medieval England and later became incorporated into American law. Apparently, two premises form the basis for the doctrine: first, the king can do no wrong; second, the state is the king's representative and therefore can do no wrong. In theory, because states are infallible, they cannot be subjected to legal action without their consent.

Although the doctrine has substantial precedence in American legal history, many state legislatures and courts now believe that tort immunity for school districts is unjust and has no rightful place in modern society. As a result, some states have either completely or partially abolished the doctrine of government immunity. In states where the doctrine has been partially abolished, the school districts are usually liable for only a maximum amount which has been previously specified by the state legislature.

Manifestly, whether or not a school district is exempt from tort liability under the doctrine of government immunity has a direct effect on the teachers. In states where this doctrine has been completely or partially abolished, the school districts may accept all or part of the responsibility for the action of their teachers. In such cases the school districts will usually purchase insurance to cover costs which may arise from school-related student injuries. On the other hand, in states where the school districts are still protected by government immunity and thus not legally responsible for the acts of their employees, the teachers must accept the financial accountability for their actions or omissions.

Meaning of Negligence

Before a judgment can be made against a teacher or a school district for personal injury or property damage resulting from a school-related activity, the person who is bringing suit must prove that negligence was involved on the part of the teacher or the district. According to Shapiro,

> Negligence is any conduct which falls below the standard established by law for the protection of others against unreasonable risk of harm. The standard of conduct the law demands is measured against what a reasonable man of ordinary prudence would have done in the same or similar circumstances.[1]

Thus, in determining whether or not negligence existed, the court asks one important question: did the person who is being sued act as a reasonably prudent individual would have acted under the same circumstances?

In answering this question, the court must first determine what would have been the action of a reasonably prudent individual. This is referred to as the "test of foreseeability." In general, when a person could not have foreseen the results of his acts, he is not negligent and therefore not liable for his actions. On the other hand, if a person could have foreseen the results of his commission or omission of an act but did not take precautionary measures against any injurious or damaging consequences, he is considered to be negligent and legally liable for his behavior.

Besides personal injuries and property damage which resulted directly from his negligent behavior, the teacher may be judged liable for the following:

1. For physical harm resulting from fright or shock or other similar or immediate emotional disturbances caused by the injury or the negligent conduct causing it.

2. For additional bodily harm resulting from acts done by a third person in rendering aid irrespective of whether such acts are done in a proper or negligent manner.

3. For any disease which is contracted because of lowered vitality resulting from the injury caused by his negligent conduct.

4. For harm sustained in a subsequent accident which would not have occurred had the pupil's bodily efficiency not been impaired by the original negligence.[2]

---

1. Freida S. Shapiro, "Your Liability for Student Accidents," *NEA Journal*, March, 1965, p. 47.

2. National Education Association, *Who Is Liable for Pupil Injuries?* (Washington, D.C.: NEA, 1963), p. 15.

In all judgments of negligence and liability, the plaintiff, the person who had brought suit, will be directed to collect an amount of money, usually specified by the court, from the defendant, the person who had been sued. However, in many cases of obvious tort liability, the parties who are involved in the suit will settle the financial arrangements out of court by mutual agreement.

Defenses Against Negligence

In determining whether or not a teacher, or other person being sued, is guilty of negligent conduct, judges and jury members must carefully evaluate all the facts surrounding the specific incident. Since liability laws are designed to protect, not persecute, the innocent, the courts have provided numerous defenses for persons charged with negligence.

Proximate Cause

For a person to be held liable for an injury suffered by a student, the plaintiff must prove that a substantial connection existed between the wrongful act and the student's injury. In other words, proximate cause, the direct or immediate causation of the resultant student's injury, must be proven by the plaintiff. Through this line of defense, a teacher can actually be negligent and still not be held liable for damages.

In Binghamton, New York, an eight-year-old boy was struck in the eye during the noon-hour recess by a rock that had been batted by another student. At the time of the accident, the school principal who had been supervising the playground was away from the area attending to a telephone call. The court ruled that the school board's failure to provide additional help for answering the telephone was not the proximate cause of the injury. Since supervisors cannot be expected to observe all the movements of their pupils, the court reasoned that the accident could have occurred even if several teachers had been present.[3]

In another case, a student in San Francisco, California, was injured in a fight with another boy during the noon hour. Apparently, the student was pushed from the base of a flagpole, and when he refused to stay off the base, the other boy twisted his leg until it was broken. At the time of the fight, over one hundred children were on the playground under the supervision of the assistant principal. Although she was in close proximity to the spot where the student was injured, the assistant principal was not aware of the fight until it was finished. The court ruled that she failed to use

---

3. Herb Appenzeller, *From the Gym to the Jury* (Charlottesville, Virginia: The Michie Company, 1970). pp. 12-13.

reasonable care or diligence to observe the conduct of the fighting students, and thus her lack of supervision was the proximate cause of the student's injury.[4]

Contributory Negligence

If a student was injured because he failed to act with reasonable prudence to safeguard himself, he is guilty of contributory negligence. Thus, in contributory negligence the student's own negligent action contributed to his injury. When both the student and the teacher are guilty of negligent conduct, neither can recover damages from the other for the resultant injury.

In New York State, an elementary school pupil was injured when he slipped while walking on a fence near the school playground. At the time of the accident, the playground was unsupervised. In addition, a teacher had given the boy permission to play outside during the noon-hour recess. However, the boy freely admitted that he had received several warnings about the dangers of the fence but that he had deliberately ignored the warnings. As a result, the court ruled that the boy was guilty of contributory negligence and dismissed the liability charge against the principal of the school.[5]

In school liability cases the law recognizes that children do not use the same degree of self-protection as adults. Thus, in determining or assigning the responsibility for contributory negligence, courts do not employ adult standards but will consider the student's age and particular conduct in relationship with the degree of reasonable care which is characteristically shown by other children of the same age. Often, when a minor is involved, a charge of contributory negligence is not a practical or useful defense for a teacher.

In Oakland, California, a high-school girl was injured when she was struck by a garbage truck as she ran from the gymnasium to the playground. According to the girl's testimony, the members of her physical education class would meet in the gymnasium, and after the roll had been taken, they would cross the road to the school playground. Although the principal knew that students had been running across the road to the playground for the past seven years and that trucks traveled on the road between the gymnasium and the playground during the entire school day, he had not established rules or regulations to protect the students. In response to the girl's charges, the principal argued that the student was guilty of contributory negligence because she had failed to use discretion in crossing the road. In ruling in favor of the student, the court denied the principal's charge of contributory negligence by stating:

---

4. Herb Appenzeller, pp. 56-57.
5. Herb Appenzeller, p. 20.

To hold that the plaintiff was guilty of contributory negligence as a matter of law is to hold that the majority of school children in like situations have been acting in a negligent manner, a result which contradicts the very standard utilized in determining the existence of negligence.[6]

In a similar case, also in California, a seventeen-year-old boy was struck and injured by an automobile as he ran from the gymnasium to the play area. Since the principal had not established rules for the safety of his students, he was accused of negligence and sued by the boy. In response to the principal's charge of contributory negligence, the court commented:

We should not close our eyes to the fact that even boys of seventeen and eighteen years of age, particularly in groups where the herd instinct and competitive spirit tend naturally to relax vigilance, are not accustomed to exercise the same amount of care for their own safety as persons of more mature years.[7]

Comparative Negligence

In recent years some states have adopted the principle of comparative negligence. In the application of this principle, the court assigns a degree of negligence to both the teacher and the student. Thus, when the teacher's negligence is greater than the student's negligence, the court will apportion the amount of recovery for the student.

In Beloit, Wisconsin, an adult student, who was enrolled in a night vocational class, was injured in a grinding-wheel accident. According to the student, after he had activated the multiple-speed grinder, the grinding wheel fragmented, thereby causing him to suffer a serious injury. After examining the facts in the case, the court ruled that the student was 25 percent negligent and the city and school district were 75 percent negligent. As a result, the student was awarded $15,000.00 of a $20,000.00 claim for damages.[8]

Since recovery is diminished in proportion to the student's degree of negligence, the principle of comparative negligence is generally viewed as equitable for both the student and the teacher. However, the principle has not completely escaped criticism. As Kigin notes,

An argument that has been brought out against the adoption of comparative negligence is that juries are not capable of weighing relative negligence or of determining accurately the proportions of negligence of the litigants. Another objection is the fact that insurance premiums would rise, since insurance companies would be forced to pay damages in many instances where they now pay nothing under the rule of contributory negligence.[9]

---

6. Herb Appenzeller, pp. 16-17.
7. Herb Appenzeller, p. 17.
8. Denis J. Kigin, *Teacher Liability in School-Shop Accidents* (Ann Arbor, Michigan: Prakken Publications, Inc., 1973), pp. 43-44.

Despite these criticisms, in recent years the principle of comparative negligence has been gaining substantial support in this country.

Assumption of Risk

If a person voluntarily participates in an activity while thoroughly recognizing the dangers which are involved, he cannot ordinarily collect damages for any resultant injury. Consequently, when the defendant had accepted a reasonable risk and failed to exercise proper care for his own safety, the principle of assumption of risk may provide a defense for the plaintiff.

Although this principle may apply in some school tort-liability suits, courts are often reluctant to permit an assumption-of-risk defense by teachers. As Kigin explains,

> When an adult willingly participates in an activity involving certain risks of which he is aware, he cannot claim damages for any resulting injury. School pupils, however, are generally classified as minors and are not expected to possess the same degree of reasoning power that enables adults to determine possible danger of certain activities. Historically, courts have ruled that their immaturity and resultant inability to understand completely the consequences of their acts and their lack of complete responsibility for their own behavior make them incapable of assuming a given risk.[10]

Apparently, as trial records verify, the courts are inclined to allow the defense of assumption of risk only in special situations, such as interscholastic athletics, where student participation is largely voluntary.

In the State of Oregon, a high school student sustained a broken neck when he was tackled by two opposing players during an interscholastic football game. In his suit the boy charged that he had not been properly instructed by his coach. In addition, the boy claimed that because of his small size, awkwardness, and inexperience, the football coach used poor judgment in playing him against a powerful team with outstanding players. The State Supreme Court disagreed with the boy's charges on several points. First, the court declared that the boy, as well as all members of the team, had been provided with adequate and extensive training by the coach. Second, while the boy was small in stature, weighing only one hundred and forty pounds, the court asserted that many other players on his team were approximately equal to him in size. In fact, according to trial testimony, the two players who had tackled the boy weighed less than he did. Third, the court reasoned that the boy was not inexperienced in the game of football,

---

9. Denis J. Kigin, pp. 16-17.
10. Denis J. Kigin, p. 22.

since he had previously played the sport for two years. In dismissing the suit against the football coach and the school district, the court ruled that the boy had assumed the risk of injury when he voluntarily tried out for the football team.[11]

Except in interscholastic athletics, safety-patrol work, and similar functions, students are not permitted much freedom in choosing their school activities. Furthermore, because of the teacher's authority, students are often required to perform certain acts, regardless of the risks. Under these circumstances the defense of assumption of risk is rarely successful in legal actions brought by an injured student against a teacher or a school district.

Act of God

When a student is injured by an inevitable and unforeseeable consequence of some force of nature, he cannot recover damages for any resultant injury. According to Florio,

> If, for example, a student is cut by fragments from a glass transom that shattered when it was slammed shut by a sudden gust of wind, the teacher is not to blame, for such an accident could not have been anticipated and avoided by a reasonably careful, skilled, and experienced person.[12]

Unfortunately, the distinction between an injury caused by an act of God and an injury caused by teacher negligence is often obscured by other factors. As a result, when a student is injured by a force of nature, the teacher may still be liable if he could have anticipated the undesirable consequences of the force and guarded against them.

Obtaining Insurance Protection

Today, more than in any other period of history, teachers and school districts are especially vulnerable to liability suits. Because of this increased vulnerability, school personnel have shown a marked interest in insurance protection. Besides providing monetary assistance for injured students, liability insurance plans are designed to protect teachers and school districts against financial ruin.

In many states the school districts are still exempt from tort liability under the doctrine of government immunity. According to the courts, the schools cannot spend public funds for liability insurance without statutory authorization. Consequently, in these states the teachers, who are usually unable financially to withstand the burden of lawsuits, are left with the

---

11. Herb Appenzeller, *From the Gym to the Jury,* pp. 128-29.
12. A. E. Florio and G. T. Stafford, *Safety Education* (3rd ed.; New York: McGraw-Hill Book Company, 1969), p. 146.

responsibility of purchasing liability insurance for their own protection. In other states where the doctrine of government immunity has been completely or partially abolished by legislative action, the school districts are usually inclined to purchase liability insurance for their teachers and other personnel.

Often, in addition to purchasing liability insurance for the teachers, the school districts will require or make available at a nominal rate accident insurance plans for the students. As Strasser notes,

> The purchase of this insurance indirectly aids the school district in meeting its liability responsibilities. Many law suits have been initiated because this was the only method whereby the injured could collect for his medical expenses for treatment of his injury. Payment of these expenses by an insurance policy relieves the district of potential suits.[13]

Although the plans vary in the type and extent of coverage, they usually provide medical payments for all school and school-related accidents.

Even in school districts that provide for the payment of accident liability claims, teachers should make certain that they are fully covered for any eventualities. Many professional organizations now offer group liability insurance plans to all of their members. In many cases, when a teacher pays the normal yearly dues to the organization, he is automatically covered by the liability plan. Furthermore, personal or individual liability plans are available from insurance agents. These plans may be independent policies or "business-pursuits" endorsements on existing homeowner's policies.

Resource Materials

Aetna Life and Casualty Company
151 Farmington
Hartford, Connecticut 06115

Liberty Mutual Insurance Company
175 Berkeley Square
Boston, Massachusetts 02117

American Bar Association
1155 East 60th Street
Chicago, Illinois 60637

National Education Association
1201 16th Street, N.W.
Washington, D.C. 20036

Kemper Insurance Companies
4750 Sheridan Road
Chicago, Illinois 60640

Nationwide Insurance Company
246 North High Street
Columbus, Ohio 43215

Traveler's Insurance Company
One Tower Square
Hartford, Connecticut 06115

---

13. Marland K. Strasser and others, *Fundamentals of Safety Education* (2d ed.; New York: The Macmillan Company, 1973), p. 263.

Activities

1. Prepare a twenty-five question, multiple choice test over the material in this chapter. Distribute a copy of the test to each member of the class.

2. Invite a lawyer to speak to the class about the legal responsibilities of teachers.

3. Using the details from one of the negligence suits that was presented in this chapter, conduct a mock trial in the classroom.

4. Write to three insurance companies, and request information on their personal liability policies. In a short paper, discuss the benefits and costs of these various policies.

5. Write to the National Education Association, and request information on teacher liability insurance. Present a short report to the class on this information.

Questions

1. What is tort liability?
2. What is nonfeasance? (Also, misfeasance and malfeasance)
3. What is the doctrine of government immunity, and how are teachers affected by the doctrine?
4. What is negligence?
5. What important question is asked by the court in determining whether or not negligence existed in a liability case?
6. What is the "test of foreseeability"?
7. For a person to be held liable for an injury suffered by a student, the plaintiff must prove that a substantial connection existed between the wrongful act and the student's injury. What is another name for this substantial connection?
8. Unlike contributory negligence, the principle of comparative negligence is viewed as equitable for both the student and the teacher. Why is this statement generally considered to be correct?
9. Why are courts often reluctant to permit an assumption-of-risk defense by teachers in liability cases?
10. What types of liability insurance plans are available to teachers?

Selected References

Appenzeller, Herb. *From the Gym to the Jury.* Charlottesville, Virginia: The Michie Company, 1970.

Florio, A. E. and G. T. Stafford. *Safety Education.* 3rd ed.; New York: McGraw-Hill Book Company, 1969.

Kigin, Denis J. *Teacher Liability in School-Shop Accidents.* Ann Arbor, Michigan: Prakken Publications, Inc., 1973.

Mohler, J. David and Edward C. Bolmeier. *Law of Extracurricular Activities in Secondary Schools.* Cincinnati, Ohio: The W. H. Anderson Company, 1968.

National Education Association. *Who Is Liable for Pupil Injuries?,* Washington, D.C.: NEA, 1963.

Shapiro, Frieda S. "Your Liability for Student Accidents," *NEA Journal,* March, 1965, 46-47.

Strasser, Marland K. and others. *Fundamentals of Safety Education.* 2nd ed.; New York: The Macmillan Company, 1973.

Accidents and School Safety Education

14

In Milwaukee, Wisconsin, three young children died in a raging fire they had started while their mother had gone to a corner store to purchase ingredients for the baby's formula. She had been away for only fifteen minutes. In Cornwall, New York, a small girl fell into a creek, and her three young brothers, none of whom could swim, jumped into the water, one after the other, to save her. All four children drowned!

In these two accidents alone, seven youngsters lost their lives. According to the National Safety Council, every year in this country, more than six thousand school-age children are killed in accidents. What these youngsters might have accomplished as adults will never be known. Perhaps one might have been a Nobel prize winner or another might have been President of the United States. Moreover, all of them would have been precious and integral parts of the lives of their friends, relatives, and parents.

Definition of Safety Education

In today's society, children, as well as persons of all ages, do not have to die suddenly and unexpectedly with their potential unfulfilled. Accidents can be prevented, and lives can be saved. This belief was succinctly expressed in Chapter 1 by the following definition: safety is the prevention of accidents and the mitigation of personal injury or property damage which may result from accidents.

The instrument by which safety can be accomplished is safety education. Although numerous and diverse definitions for safety education are available, the following is suggested for use in this textbook: **Safety education is the entire range of events experienced by a person during his lifetime that effectively and favorably influence in him the development of certain emotions, attitudes, personality traits, habits, knowledge, and physical skills which are necessary for his safe behavior in specific environments.**

According to this definition, safety education has at least five distinct components. *First*, any of the events which are experienced by a person during his lifetime may contribute to his safety. Thus, safety education, which begins at birth and continues throughout the person's life, may originate from any number of different sources. *Second*, not all of the apparent safety-producing events experienced by a person are effective in developing safety. Consequently, while a person may have been exposed to certain safety information, he has not received safety education if this information failed to affect his subsequent behavior. *Third*, not all of the apparent safety-producing events experienced by a person in his lifetime will favorably affect his behavior. Often, a person is exposed to outdated or even erroneous safety information. In such cases he has not received safety education, and in fact, he may have received information which is actually an effective deterrent to safety education. *Fourth*, certain emotions, attitudes, personality traits, habits, knowledge, and physical skills are necessary for safe behavior. Thus, safety education is concerned with the total—emotional, mental, and physical—development of the person. *Fifth*, the safety-producing events experienced by a person in his lifetime are quite limited, and as a result, they will influence only certain developmental characteristics which are necessary for safe behavior in specific environments. Consequently, safety education is directed at specific situations, such as bicycling, operating an industrial machine, boating, or other activities.

As defined in this book, safety education has one basic goal: the integration of safety into the person's philosophy of life. When this goal has been accomplished, the individual will exhibit safety as an active part in every aspect of his daily life.

The School's Role in Safety Education

At the instant a baby is born, he is exposed to certain safety hazards. For the first part of his life, the infant, who has few self-protective resources, must be completely safeguarded by his parents. By the age of one or two years, however, the child can be taught to protect himself in limited ways. Thus, through necessity, safety education, must begin in the home under the direction of the child's parents.

Although many parents do provide excellent safety training for their children, most home safety education efforts by parents are quite inadequate, as evidenced every year by the large number of home accidents involving children. Apparently one reason for this weakness is that most parents have not received adequate safety education themselves and, as a result, they cannot provide their children with adequate safety education. In fact, in many cases, parents actually encourage accidents by their imprudent safety education efforts. Most notably, in warning their youngster not to repeat a certain accident-producing act, parents will often over-sympathize with the minor injuries of the child and give him excessive affection or cookies to make him feel better. Consequently, the child will usually forget the safety lesson and remember only that his performance of the act resulted in a reward. Another reason for the inadequacy of the home safety education efforts is that most parents have not integrated safety into their philosophy of life and, as a result, they do not exhibit safety in their everyday activities. In such cases the children will usually model their behavior after their parents' conduct, a practice which functions as a deterrent to safety education.

In addition to the home, children may receive safety education from various community organizations, such as the Girl Scouts, Boy Scouts, YMCA, YWCA, Civil Defense, Red Cross, and Coast Guard Auxiliary. However, most of these programs are directed at safety in recreational activities. Furthermore, the programs are limited in participation, since the organizations lack the personnel and facilities which are necessary for handling large numbers of children in comprehensive safety education efforts.

In an attempt to reach more people, a few national organizations, such as the National Safety Council and the National Fire Protection Association, have prepared short public service announcements on numerous safety topics. Just how effective these messages are in changing behavior, however, is still the subject of much debate among safety experts. In one instance a television campaign, which would have cost approximately seven million dollars if it had been presented throughout the entire country, was tested in a community with dual television cables. The viewers on one cable were exposed to a variety of high-quality, professionally prepared messages that encouraged people to wear safety belts; the viewers on the other cable were exposed to only normal television programming. At the end of the test, the researchers discovered that the television messages, although shown many times, did not significantly increase the use of safety belts by the viewers. In general, safety education through the use of television and other forms of mass media is still quite limited in its effectiveness.

Considering the many possible sources of safety information and training in the community, the school is certainly in the best position to provide a comprehensive safety education program for children. Besides possessing the necessary personnel and facilities for a large-scale program, the school has the distinct advantage of having direct access to millions of youngsters in a semi-captive situation. For this reason, the school must accept the major share of the responsibility for providing children with safety education.

As a rule, the educational process should be well planned, carefully organized, and adequately budgeted; and children should receive safety instruction throughout their school careers, not just in certain grades. Furthermore, the safety education efforts of the school should be carefully coordinated with those of the home and the various community organizations. Unless the safety training of the students is strongly reinforced by their out-of-school experiences, the youngsters will usually demonstrate safe behavior only when they are subjected to close supervision.

Organizing the Instructional Program

Among various schools, safety education programs will differ considerably in organization. Some programs will offer safety instruction as a separate course or as a separate unit within an existing course; other programs will correlate safety instruction with other school subjects or will integrate safety instruction into study units which involve several different school subjects. In practice, the organization of the safety education program will depend largely upon the educational philosophy of the school district and the nature of the school curriculum.

Realistically, as technological changes alter living conditions, safety hazards are invariably created along with the improvements. For this reason, the school safety education program must remain flexible in its organization. For the greatest success the instructional program should include the following elements: (1) developing a policy of safety education; (2) assigning responsibility; (3) promoting faculty cooperation; (4) determining the nature and scope of the program; (5) developing program objectives; (6) selecting the course content and the teaching methods; (7) coordinating community safety efforts; (8) evaluating the program; and (9) adjusting the program elements.

Developing a Policy of Safety Education

The superintendent of schools is primarily responsible for the inclusion of safety education in the school curriculum. As a part of his responsibility, the superintendent should develop and publish a policy of safety education which clearly expresses the school district's philosophical position on safety and its views concerning the role of safety instruction in the educational curriculum. This statement of policy should include such items as: (1) the relationship between safety and safety education; (2) the school district's desire to provide a sound, up-to-date safety education program; (3) the requirements for faculty cooperation; and (4) the organizational structure of the safety education program.

Assigning Responsibility

For the actual implementation of the safety education program, the superintendent should assign the responsibility of guidance and leadership to a specific individual. Ordinarily this person is designated as the safety coordinator or the safety supervisor. In most school districts the job of safety coordinator is an additional duty for someone, such as the assistant superintendent of schools or the district supervisor for health and physical education. Ideally, however, the safety coordinator should possess substantial formal training in safety education and devote all of his working time to the safety program of the school district.

In general, the safety coordinator serves as a connecting link between the superintendent of schools, who develops the policy of safety education, and the school teacher, who directly provides safety education to the students. Some of the safety coordinator's responsibilities include: (1) familiarizing teachers with the school district's safety education policy; (2) securing faculty cooperation in the safety program; and (3) preparing periodic reports on the safety program for the superintendent of schools and the school board. In addition, the safety coordinator should organize a curriculum committee for safety education. This committee should be comprised of representatives from the various school disciplines, as well as delegates from the superintendent's office, Parent-Teacher Association, student body, and appropriate community organizations. In each instance the exact composition of the committee will be determined by the nature of the community and the type of school for which the safety curriculum is designed.

Promoting Faculty Cooperation

Despite his training and experience in safety education, the coordinator cannot guarantee that the instructional safety program will be successful. Actually, program success is primarily dependent upon the cooperation of the faculty members. However, since most teachers have received little formal instruction in safety education, the coordinator can effectively promote faculty cooperation and thus enhance the likelihood of program success by organizing safety workshops, distributing safety education information, and preparing lists of companies and organizations which offer resource materials on the various areas of safety.

Determining the Nature and Scope of the Program

As a part of his job, the safety coordinator, with the assistance of the curriculum committee, will determine the nature and scope of the safety education program. Because the school program must be designed to fulfill the particular needs of the students, the coordinator should carefully analyze the activities of the youngsters and the environment of the community.

In his analysis the safety coordinator should answer certain questions. First, what types of activities are most frequently performed by the students in the community? Second, what types of accidents are most often experienced by the students? Third, in terms of human failures, environmental hazards, and defective agents, what are the likely causative factors in each type of accident? Fourth, in terms of the person, the environment, and the agent, what feasible countermeasures can be applied to each accident factor? In summary, the safety coordinator in his analysis of the community situation should utilize the epidemiological accident prevention/mitigation model, which was discussed in Chapter 2.

In using this model, the coordinator must rely on a multitude of sources for accident and safety information. As the foundation for his analysis, he should carefully examine accident reports from local and state safety organizations and accident records of the school district, the police department, the fire department, and local insurance agencies. Then, for a deeper insight into the needs of the students and the community, he should conduct surveys and interviews with youngsters, parents, nurses, doctors, and community leaders. As an additional source of information, the coordinator should examine published articles and accident research studies by experts in the field of safety and safety education.

Developing Program Objectives

Once the nature and scope of the safety education program has been determined by the coordinator, the curriculum committee can develop the desired objectives for a successful program. In determining these objectives the committee should describe clearly the planned accomplishments of the safety education course, including the unique contributions of the course to the overall education of the student. In addition, the committee should provide in the objectives a justification for including the course in the school district's instructional program.

Although planned accomplishments will vary greatly among different schools, certain course objectives should always form the core for the school's instructional safety program. Specifically, upon the completion of the safety education course, the student should be able to:

1. Identify the characteristics and scope of the total accident problem of the community, state, and nation.
2. Identify the meaning of accidents and the relationship between accidents and safety.
3. Identify the role of safety in everyday living and the role of the school in safety education.

4. Identify the causative factors in accidents, and implement possible countermeasures for each accident factor.
5. Demonstrate behavioral patterns which illustrate an integration of safety into the student's philosophy of life.

Since program content, teaching methods, and evaluation techniques will be selected in terms of the planned course results, the careful development of course objectives by the curriculum committee is essential for the success of the safety education program.

After the objectives for the course have been established by the committee, the classroom teacher has the responsibility of developing specific objectives for each unit of safety instruction. These instructional objectives must contribute in some manner to the fulfillment of the course objectives. In developing the instructional objectives, the teacher should explain clearly what the student will be able to do, under what conditions he will be able to do it, and to what degree he will be able to do it. The following planned accomplishments are examples of instructional (behavioral) objectives for specific units in the safety education program.

1. By oral or written means, the student will name the two types of motorcycle helmets and describe one advantage and one disadvantage of each type of helmet.
2. Given a rifle and a gun lock, the student will demonstrate the proper technique for immobilizing the trigger of the firearm.

In the classroom setting, instructional objectives provide the means by which the teacher can identify desired behavioral changes in his students and evaluate his teaching methods to determine their effectiveness in producing these desired behavioral changes.

Selecting the Course Content and the Teaching Methods

As mentioned earlier in this chapter, safety education has one basic goal: the integration of safety into the student's philosophy of life. When this goal has been accomplished, the student will exhibit safety as an active part in every aspect of his daily life. For this reason, the teacher in the instructional safety program must provide the student with practical information on a wide array of safety topics.

In general, the safety program should thoroughly survey the following topics: nature of the accident problem; causes of accidents; conceptual models of accident prevention/mitigation; automobile safety, including driver education; motorcycle safety; pedestrian safety; bicycle safety; home safety, including instruction on falls, fires, poisonings, suffocations, and firearm accidents; school safety, including safety in and around the school, as well as on the way to and from the school; work safety; recreational safety; and disaster safety. In the course of the program, the teacher will encounter numerous questions from his students. Many of these questions will originate in group discussions or from new interests which arise as the students learn more about safety and its relationship to life. For this reason, specific sub-topics or units in the safety education program will vary greatly among different schools and among different teachers within the same school.

Once the content of the course has been chosen, the classroom teacher must then select appropriate methods for presenting the safety material to the students. The teaching methods most commonly employed are lecture, discussion, demonstration, and student practice sessions. In most cases the safety education teacher will use a combination of these methods in his presentations. In addition, he may periodically select one of the following methods: guest speakers; conferences; activity simulation; programmed instruction; audio-visual instruction; individualized study; group projects; field trips; panel discussion; question and answer; problem solving; role playing; and dramatization.

Ideally, the teacher should select methods which are best suited to his personality and the collective personality of his students. However, in recent years numerous research studies have indicated that learning is significantly enhanced when the students actively participate in the instructional process. For this reason, whenever possible, the teacher should utilize methods which are predominantly child-centered, not teacher-centered.

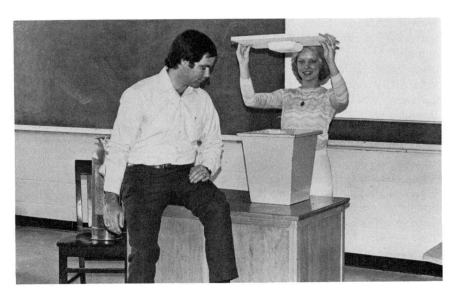

Figure 14.1   Using a demonstration teaching method, a safety education teacher explains the purpose and the value of home smoke detection units.

Coordinating Community Safety Efforts

As a rule, children tend to learn most effectively when they are able to relate their in-school training to their out-of-school experiences. Thus, for maximum success the safety education program of the school must be coordinated with the safety efforts of the community.

In every community, large or small, various agencies and organizations are available to assist the school district in its safety education efforts. Some of these groups, such as the police department and the American Red Cross, are regular sponsors of projects and programs which help citizens in the community to understand the accident problem and become more safety-minded. On the other hand, certain groups, such as the automobile club and the chamber of commerce, will occasionally sponsor safety projects as a part of their community-involvement programs. Actually, many of these safety efforts by community agencies and organizations are duplications of the safety instruction received by the youngsters in the school.

In recent years, in an attempt to avoid program duplications, some communities have established local safety councils. Generally, a safety council has the responsibility of developing and coordinating all of the safety education efforts in the community. Included in this council are representatives from the various agencies and organizations in the community, such as the school district, police department, fire department, health department, chamber of commerce, American Legion, Veterans of Foreign Wars, Coast Guard Auxiliary, Girl Scouts, Boy Scouts, YMCA, YWCA, Civil Defense, American Red Cross, and commercial and industrial enterprises.

Because of the school district's role in the safety education efforts of the community, the safety coordinator will often be asked to initiate the organization of the safety council. To assure a successful organization, he should first conduct a study of the community's accident experiences to determine whether or not a safety council is needed. At the same time he should consult the community leaders to determine whether or not they are really interested in supporting such an organization. If the coordinator ascertains that a safety council is warranted, he should invite five to ten well-known and respected persons in the community to form a steering committee. In turn, the steering committee, while working closely with officials of the National Safety Council, should develop a sound organizational plan for the safety council and then extend written invitations for admission to the various leaders in the safety community.

Evaluating the Program

Even in the best organized program, a continuous evaluation process is essential for determining and improving the quality of the safety education efforts. For this reason, the safety coordinator should periodically review the accident record of the community and carefully analyze any accident trends, both desirable and undesirable.

Although accident statistics provide the most reliable indication of program success, other sources may furnish additional, valuable information. Whenever possible, the safety coordinator should survey or consult parents to determine any significant changes in their children's safety attitudes and practices. In addition, he should carefully study the activities of the students in school and in community activities and prepare a subjective analysis of his observations.

Adjusting the Program Elements

Regardless of the success of the safety program, the evaluation process will always expose certain weaknesses. Once these weaknesses have been identified, the safety coordinator, the teachers, and the curriculum committee should reanalyze the instructional program and propose measures to correct the weaknesses. This adjustment of the program elements is a continuous process and will further improve the success of the program.

Safety Education in the Elementary Schools

As mentioned earlier in this chapter, the child's first exposure to safety education will normally occur in the home. As a rule, since young children are unable to understand and apply the knowledge underlying safe behavior, parents must rely heavily on the use of certain safety rules. For example, "Don't touch the stove; it'll burn you." or "Don't go near the street; if you do, I'll spank you." Obviously, this approach to safety education is quite simplistic. Consequently, most home safety programs are largely unplanned.

With their enrollment in the elementary school, most children will receive their first instruction in a planned safety education program. Ideally, this instruction will permit the children to develop a philosophy of safety which is consistent with their age and level of maturity. In general, elementary school children should understand that accidents, while they are unplanned, are not the result of chance but are caused by certain factors in all people and in their surroundings. In addition, they should realize that accidents can be prevented or, at least, that the consequences of accidents can be lessened. When children have successfully integrated safety into their philosophy of life, they will perform their activities correctly, and hence safely, and not avoid certain activities because of possible risks.

Without exception, the primary emphasis at the elementary school level should be on "learning by doing." Since young children possess short attention spans, brief periods of repeated practice are needed to develop the knowledge, attitudes, habits, skills, and other characteristics which are essential for safe behavior. As in the home and the community, the elementary school program should emphasize primarily the various safety activities which involve student participation. These include such activities as role playing, dramatization, student practice sessions, participation exhibits, school assemblies, field trips, bicycle inspections, playground patrols, school safety patrols, and junior safety councils.

For the most part the instructional safety program in the elementary school should stress the safe performance of everyday activities. Every child should learn the safest routes to and from school, the safest places to play, and the safest ways to use his skateboard, bicycle, and other items. Similarly, he should learn the meanings of traffic markings, signs, and signals and the various safety rules and laws for walking and bicycling in the traffic setting. In addition, with the parents' help, the child should be taught to recognize common hazards in the home and to take appropriate precautions to avoid accidents. As a part of this cooperative teaching effort, the child should acquire the knowledge and skills to protect himself during an accident, such as rolling on the ground to extinguish a clothing fire or crawling on the floor to escape a burning building.

In the elementary school the organizational pattern most commonly used for the safety education program is the correlation of safety instruction with the different school subjects. Most often, safety information is taught in subjects which are directly related to safety education, such as science, social studies, health, and physical education. However, one weakness may appear in this type of organizational pattern: teachers often do not stress safety enough to develop the mental and physical traits which are necessary for safe behavior. In many cases this weakness appears because the teachers did not receive adequate instruction in safety education during their teacher training and, as a result, they are not genuinely aware of the safety needs of their students.

Safety Education in the Junior and Senior High Schools

When children enter the elementary school, they are predominantly self-centered. Thus, for the first few years of their school life, they are most receptive to safety information which has personal significance. In other words, they are most likely to remember and utilize safety information which can help them to avoid personal accidents and injuries. Characteristically, at this stage in their development, children are not yet sufficiently concerned about the welfare of other people. However, by the time they reach the junior high school level, most children have matured considerably in their social relationships and are no longer predominantly self-centered.

As a result, they are now more responsive to safety instruction which stresses the social nature of the accident problem, and in turn they are now more likely to remember and utilize safety information which can help them to prevent accidents and injuries to other persons, as well as to themselves.

For the most part safety education in the junior and senior high schools should help students to further develop and refine their philosophy of safety. High school students should understand that they have both a moral and a social responsibility to prevent accidents and that they must cooperate closely with other persons to meet this responsibility. When they have firmly integrated this concept into their philosophy of life, youngsters will exhibit safety as an active part in every phase of their lives, both personal and social.

In the junior and senior high schools, teachers should stress both individual and group safety. Every student should learn the safest ways of driving bicycles, motorcycles, and automobiles, the safest methods for using hand tools and power tools, and the safest ways of handling household appliances and other equipment. Similarly, he should learn to recognize common hazards in his environment and to take appropriate precautions to protect himself and his family members. In addition, since most individuals seek new adventures and thrills during adolescent years, youngsters should be taught the proper information and skills relating to a variety of leisure activities, such as swimming, boating, underwater diving, hunting, fishing, and, in some regions, snowmobiling.

As in the elementary school, the organizational pattern most commonly used for the safety education program in the junior and senior high schools is the correlation of safety instruction with the various school subjects. Certain subjects, such as general science, chemistry, physics, health, physical education, agriculture, industrial arts, and home economics, are excellent means for the correlation of safety education with the other subjects. As many experts stress, the ideal place to emphasize safety is where the topic presents itself naturally during an activity.

As an exception, in the senior high school, one phase of the overall instructional safety program is almost always treated as a separate subject. This is driver and traffic safety education. As a rule, the modern driver education program is divided into two distinct parts: (1) the classroom and (2) the laboratory. The classroom phase is concerned with the knowledge components of the traffic safety program. These include traffic accidents, use of the motor vehicle, road citizenship, driver characteristics, driving skills, effects of alcohol and other drugs on the driver, traffic laws and regulations, traffic law enforcement, and traffic engineering. On the other hand, the laboratory part of the driver education program is concerned with behind-the-wheel instruction for the students. This is provided through the use of simulators, the multiple-car range, and the dual-control car.

Resource Materials

American Driver and Traffic Safety
Education Association
1201 16th Street, N.W.
Washington, D.C. 20036

American Home Economics Association
2010 Massachusetts Avenue, N.W.
Washington, D.C. 20036

The American Legion
National Headquarters
700 North Pennsylvania Street
Indianapolis, Indiana 46206

The Center for Safety
New York University
New York City, New York 10003

Employers Mutual of Wausau
Safety Engineering Department
Wausau, Wisconsin 54402

Highway Traffic Safety Center
Michigan State University
East Lansing, Michigan 48823

National Committee on Traffic Law
Enforcement
744 Broad Street
Newark, New Jersey 07100

National Committee on Traffic Training
700 Hill Building
Washington, D.C. 20006

National Committee on Uniform Laws
and Ordinances
1776 Massachusetts Avenue, N.W.
Washington, D.C. 20036

National Congress of Parents and
Teachers
700 North Rush Street
Chicago, Illinois 60611

National Education Association
1201 16th Street, N.W.
Washington, D.C. 20036

National Safety Council
444 North Michigan Avenue
Chicago, Illinois 60611

Northwestern University Traffic Institute
405 Church Street
Evanston, Illinois 60204

Safety Center
Central Missouri State University
Warrensburg, Missouri 64093

Safety Center
Southern Illinois University
Carbondale, Illinois 62901

United States Department of Health,
Education and Welfare
Division of Accident Prevention
Washington, D.C. 20036

Activities

1. Prepare and submit to a local newspaper a short article on the topic of
   "The Need for Safety Education in the School."

2. Prepare a bulletin board display which illustrates the various elements
   in the instructional safety program.

3. With the assistance of two other class members, organize and conduct
   a safety education workshop for the elementary teachers in a local
   school.

4. Select a specific unit in safety education, and develop a set of instructional (behavioral) objectives for the unit. Distribute a copy of the objectives to each member of the class.

5. Survey ten teachers to determine the extent of their safety education efforts. Present a short, oral report on your findings to the class.

Questions

1. What are the five distinct components in the definition of safety education?
2. What is the one basic goal of safety education?
3. What are two reasons for the weakness in most safety education efforts by parents?
4. Why is the school in the best position in the community to provide a comprehensive safety education program for children?
5. What are the nine fundamental elements in the instructional safety program?
6. What are the five course objectives which should always form the core for the school's instructional safety program?
7. What is the primary responsibility of the safety council in the community?
8. What should be the primary emphasis at the elementary school level?
9. What weakness may appear in the correlation type of safety education program in the elementary school?
10. What are the two distinct parts of the modern driver education program in the senior high school?

Selected References

Clark, Norma C. "Safety Education As Preventive Medicine," *The Journal of the Arkansas Medical Society,* August, 1975, 143-44

Key, Norman. "Safety Education," *Curriculum Handbook for School Executives,* ed. Wm. J. Ellena. Washington, D.C.: American Association of School Administrators, 1973.

Punke, H. A. "Safety and Early Childhood Education," *Journal of School Health,* March, 1971, 146-53.

Wilson, P. "Helping Students Develop Lifetime Safety Habits," *Forecast Home Economics,* October, 1971, 58-59.

Zirbes, Laura. "How Shall We Teach Them Safety?," *School Safety,* January-February, 1969, 4.

Industrial Accidents 15

For the American worker, the latter part of the nineteenth century and the early part of the twentieth century were periods of extreme hardship. In many cases employers were totally insensitive to the needs of their workers. As one manufacturer boldly announced to Samuel Gompers, the principal founder of the American Federation of Labor (AFL), "I regard my employees as I do a machine, to be used to my advantage, and when they are old and of no further use I cast them in the street."[1] Consequently, fostered by this attitude, work conditions were usually hazardous, and safeguards for workers on dangerous jobs were practically nonexistent. By today's standards the accident rates at the time were appalling.

Growth of the Safety Movement

Before 1910, few companies had established safety programs, much less a plan of monetary compensation for injured workers. Apparently employers did not stress accident prevention, since they believed that accidents were caused by careless workers or unavoidable circumstances. Inevitably, the accident problem grew worse over the years. By 1910, the plight of the injured worker had become a major social issue in this country.

In 1911, the State of Wisconsin passed the first effective workmen's compensation law. After the passage of this law, other states soon began to enact similar laws. Today, every state in the Union has a workmen's compensation law. Although they differ slightly in specific details, the laws all express, in effect, that regardless of who was at fault, industry must provide monetary compensation to workers who sustain on-the-job injuries.

After the passage of the early workmen's compensation laws, employers had a direct financial interest in the accident problem. To protect themselves from financial ruin, employers were forced to purchase insurance, and since insurance premiums were rated in accordance with the

---

1. Clarence L. VerSteeg and Richard Hofstadter, *A People and A Nation* (New York: Harper & Row, Publishers, Inc., 1971), p. 451.

companies' accident records, employers were predisposed to save money by preventing accidents. The first step they took was to safeguard dangerous machinery. Between 1911 and 1920, the number of disabling work injuries was reduced sharply, as employers made notable progress in safeguarding machinery. However, this was only the beginning of the modern industrial safety movement.

In 1912, in Milwaukee, Wisconsin, a cooperative Safety Council was held at the National Convention of the Association of Iron and Steel Electrical Engineers. Participating in this historic meeting were groups from industry, employee organizations, government agencies, and insurance companies. As a result of this conference, the National Safety Council was formed. Under the Council's direction and guidance, the work-accident rates in this country have been reduced considerably over the last sixty-five years.

In 1970, Congress passed the Occupational Safety and Health Act. From the viewpoint of worker safety and health, this law has the most comprehensive effects of any legislation in modern history. Basically, OSHA, as the law is called, requires every employer to comply with safety and health standards published under the act and to provide safe and healthful working conditions for his employees. To assure that employers comply with the provisions of the act, federal officers are granted the authority to inspect and investigate all OSHA-covered businesses. In addition, when a business fails to meet the standards, the employer may be subjected to rather stringent penalties. Because of these inspection and penalty provisions, the Occupational Safety and Health Act is remarkably effective in carrying out its functions.

Just how effective the modern industrial safety movement has been in this country can be seen in the accident data gathered by the National Safety Council. Between 1912 and 1976, accidental deaths per one-hundred thousand workers were reduced from twenty-one to six. In 1912, approximately eighteen thousand to twenty-one thousand workers' lives were lost. In 1976, in a work force more than double in size and producing more than seven times as much, less than thirteen thousand work deaths were recorded. The reduction in deaths and death rates since 1933 is illustrated in Figure 15.1.

Programming for Industrial Safety

Among various companies, safety programs will differ considerably in emphasis. Some programs accentuate the importance of mechanical guarding and environmental control; others stress safe work practices through strict compliance with established safety regulations; still other programs accent personal motivation in a human relations context.

For the greatest success, a personalized safety program should be

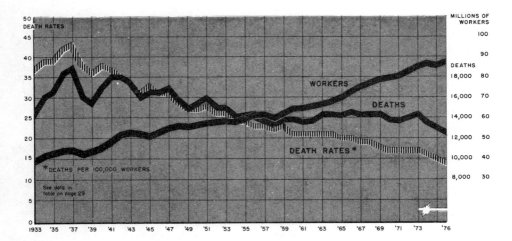

Figure 15.1   Work deaths and death rate trends. (Reproduced from *Accident Facts—1977 Edition,* p. 23, courtesy of the National Safety Council)

developed to satisfy the present and future needs of each company. However, despite this need for personalization, all industrial safety programs should include at least five basic elements: (1) providing management support, (2) assigning responsibility, (3) analyzing the situation, (4) evaluating the program, and (5) adjusting the program components.

Providing Management Support

Accident prevention/mitigation is a primary responsibility of management. In fact, the development of a safe work environment and the creation of a safety-conscious, efficient operation are economic, legal, and moral obligations of top company executives. As a part of this managerial responsibility, company executives should formulate and publish an accident prevention/mitigation policy which clearly expresses the management's philosophical position on safety and its views on the operation of the company's safety program. This statement of managerial policy should include such items as: (1) the relationship between safety and production; (2) the management's desire to provide safe working conditions; (3) the requirements for employee cooperation; and (4) the organizational structure of the safety program.

Assigning Responsibility

For the actual administration of the industrial safety program, management officials should assign the responsibility of guidance and leadership to a specific individual. Most often, this person is referred to as the safety director for the company. In large plants the safety director will normally devote all of his time to the administration of the safety program. However, in small establishments the position of safety director may be an additional duty for someone with other job responsibilities.

In general, the safety director acts as a functioning link between management executives, who formulate the accident prevention/mitigation policy of the company, and supervisors, who immediately direct the job efforts of the working groups in the company. Because of the many differences among companies, the specific duties of the safety director will vary greatly. Obviously, in large plants the safety program is more extensive, and as a result the safety director's administrative duties will be more numerous. Some of the safety director's responsibilities may include such tasks as: (1) preparing periodic progress reports for the top management executives; (2) establishing safety training programs for the supervisors; (3) studying work methods and analyzing jobs for potential accident problems; (4) inspecting the plant periodically for environmental and machinery hazards; (5) maintaining accident records and analyzing the information for accident causation; and (6) prescribing countermeasures for potential accident problems.

In spite of his importance in the industrial safety program, the safety director does not personally stop accidents. This is the primary responsibility of the first-line supervisor. For this reason, the supervisor is always the key man in every industrial safety program. As the National Safety Council explains,

> This war against accidents continues as safety is built into the regular operation and management of production. Management increasingly recognizes the important work of supervisors in preventing injuries. Many companies have set their sights on injury-free work performance. Many have succeeded. The key to this success is the supervisor.[2]

When he is supported by management and properly trained in accident prevention/mitigation, the first-line supervisor can contribute significantly to the company's safety program. Some of his responsibilities may include: (1) training new employees in proper work methods; (2) supervising and evaluating workers' performances; (3) enforcing all safety regulations established by the company; (4) constantly monitoring the working area for environmental and machinery hazards; and (5) investigating accidents involving his workers and prescribing countermeasures for similar situations in the future.

---

2. National Safety Council, *Supervisors Safety Manual* (4th ed.; Chicago: NSC, 1975), p. 10.

Analyzing the Situation

As a part of his job, the supervisor studies the plant equipment to determine the best ways for reducing breakdown-time, increasing production, and developing better product quality. In addition, he works closely with his men to help them to improve their work performances. Because of this familiarity with the industrial process, the trained supervisor will normally experience little difficulty in analyzing the work situation and in developing effective countermeasures for potential accident problems.

In his analysis of the situation, the supervisor should ask himself certain questions. First, what types of accidents could occur at this location? Second, in terms of human failures, environmental hazards, and defective agents, what are the possible causative factors for each type of accident? Third, in terms of the person, the environment, and the agent, what possible countermeasures can be assigned for each accident factor? In short, the supervisor should apply the epidemiological accident prevention/mitigation model, which was discussed in Chapter 2, to the working situation.

In applying this model, the supervisor will need information on departmental accident experience. A good accident recording system can provide this information. However, the information on accident records is only as reliable as the reports on which the records are based. For this reason, the supervisor should conduct a thorough investigation of every accident in his department. Below are listed some of the accident investigation procedures which are recommended by the National Safety Council:

1. Go to the scene of the accident promptly.

2. Talk with the injured person, if possible. Talk with witnesses. Stress getting the facts, not placing the responsibility or blame.

3. Listen for clues in the conversations about you. Unsolicited comments often have merit.

4. Encourage people to give their ideas for preventing the accident.

5. Study possible causes—both unsafe conditions and unsafe practices.

6. Confer with interested persons about possible solutions. The problem may have been solved by someone else.[3]

Once the investigation has been completed, the supervisor should write his report, using an OSHA-accepted accident form. (See Figure 15.2) This report, as well as all accident reports, should then be stored in a permanent file where the information will be readily accessible for future reference.

---

3. National Safety Council, p. 26.

MEMPHIS STATE UNIVERSITY   Case No._____
MEMPHIS, TENNESSEE 38152

SUPPLEMENTARY RECORD OF INJURY OR ILLNESS

INJURED OR ILL PERSON IS EMPLOYEE ( ); STUDENT ( ).   Check one.

1.   Name_____Social Security No._____

2.   Home Address_____City_____State_____Zip_____

3.   Age_____   Sex: Male ( )   Female ( )   Check one

4.   Occupation_____

5.   Department_____

THE ACCIDENT OR EXPOSURE TO OCCUPATIONAL ILLNESS

6.   Place of accident or exposure_____

7.   Date and time of injury or initial diagnosis of occupational illness_____

     _____

8.   Description of what happened (Be specific)_____

     _____

     _____

     _____

9.   Nature of injury or illness and body parts affected_____

     _____

10. Was injured/ill person treated at Memphis State University Health Center?

     Yes ( )   No ( ).

11. What has been done to prevent same or similar accident from recurring?   _____

     _____

12. In your opinion, was there a violation of approved safety practices/standards?

     Yes ( ) No ( ). If yes, describe violations. _____

     _____

     Date_____Signature_____Title_____

This side of report must be completed by injured student's instructor or employee's
supervisor after every accident, including those requiring first aid treatment only,
and submitted to the safety department within twenty-four (24) hours of injury/illness
occurrence.

Attachment 3
OSHA-accepted form

Figure 15.2   An OSHA-accepted accident form. (Courtesy of Safety Services,
Memphis State University)

THIS SIDE TO BE COMPLETED BY SAFETY DEPARTMENT

THE ACCIDENT OR EXPOSURE TO OCCUPATIONAL ILLNESS

13.   Was place of accident or exposure on employer's premises?_____

14.   What was the employee doing when injured?_____
       _____

15.   How did the accident occur?_____
       _____

16.   What caused this injury or illness?_____
       _____

17.   What action was taken to prevent same or similar accident from recurring?   _____
       _____

18.   Was there a violation of approved safety practices/standards? Yes ( ) No ( )
       If yes, what?_____

OCCUPATIONAL INJURY OR OCCUPATIONAL ILLNESS

19.   Describe the injury or illness in detail and indicate the part of body affected
       _____

20.   Name the object or substance which directly injured the employee_____
       _____

21.   Did employee die?_____

22.   Date and time injured/ill person reported back to work_____

23.   Lost work days_____

24.   Name and address of physician _____
       _____

25.   If hospitalized, name and address of hospital _____
       _____

       Date _____ Prepared by (Signature) _____

                                          Title _____

This side of report to be completed by safety department in all occupational injury or
illness cases, except those requiring first aid treatment only, within six (6) days of
accident.

Figure 15.2   Cont'd.

Evaluating the Program

Even in the most effective safety program a continuous evaluation process is essential for maintaining improvement. Without evaluation, the supervisor, as well as the safety director and the management executives, cannot assess the program's progress or develop additional counter-measures for alleviating the work-accident problem.

One of the most useful methods of evaluation employs the concepts of frequency rate and severity rate. The frequency rate is defined as the number of disabling injuries per one million man-hours of work. The number of man-hours is simply the total number of hours worked by all employees in the department or the company during a specified length of time. The method for computing the frequency rate is shown in the following equation.

$$\text{Frequency rate} = \frac{\text{total number of disabling injuries} \times 1{,}000{,}000}{\text{total number of man-hours worked during period}}$$

On the other hand, the severity rate is defined as the number of days charged for disabling injuries per one million man-hours of work. The number of days charged varies according to the type of disability. For temporary total-disabling injuries, the days charged is the actual number of calender days of disability. In cases of permanent partial-disabling injuries, a proportionally higher number of days is charged. For permanent disability or death, a fixed rate of six thousand days is charged. The method for computing the severity rate is given in the following equation.

$$\text{Severity rate} = \frac{\text{total number of days charged} \times 1{,}000{,}000}{\text{total number of man-hours worked during period}}$$

Because both equations use the standard index of one million man-hours of work, the concepts of frequency rate and severity rate are remarkably effective in eliminating the problem of variations in exposure time of workers to potential accident situations.

By comparing these rates with the injury experience in past years or with the injury experience in similar companies, the supervisor, safety director, and management executives can accurately evaluate the overall accident situation in a department or in the company. However, for a more detailed indicator of the effectiveness of a safety program, some companies also employ other indexes, such as accident costs, critical incidence, and measures of near-misses. Information on these indexes can be found in many industrial safety manuals.

Adjusting the Program Components

Regardless of the effectiveness of a safety program, the evaluation process will always reveal certain accident problem areas. Once these areas have been identified, the supervisor, with assistance from the safety director, should reanalyze the situation and assign new or additional countermeasures. This adjustment of the components in the safety program is a continuous process and will further improve the effectiveness of the program.

Protecting the Workers

Normally, workers possess the ability to perform their jobs well and safely. In contrast, serious accidents have a devastating effect on worker morale. Often workers lose interest in their jobs, and as a result they are involved in even more accidents. On the other hand, an outstanding safety record has a positive effect on morale. Reassured by the company's concern for their safety, workers usually develop a strong sense of job security and company loyalty, and consequently they are usually involved in fewer accidents.

Providing On-the-job Training

Accidents and injuries, as well as interrupted production and damaged equipment, are almost certain to result when workers have been inadequately trained. For this reason, most companies employ some form of on-the-job training for employees. In general, no single method of on-the-job training is suitable for all industrial situations. Consequently, numerous methods of on-the-job training have been developed. One method is job safety analysis; another is job instruction training; and still another is over-the-shoulder coaching. Depending upon the complexity of the job and the element of time, an on-the-job training method may be used separately or in combination with other methods.

Job Safety Analysis

As the term implies, job safety analysis is a method of on-the-job training in which the employee, under the direction of a supervisor, learns to perform his duties properly through a systematic analysis of the various components of the job. The steps in job safety analysis include the following: (1) selecting the job; (2) breaking down the job; (3) identifying hazards and potential accident situations; and (4) developing solutions.

Job Instruction Training

Since the instructing task is broken into four parts, the job instruction training method is often referred to as the four-point method. The four parts of the task are described as: (1) preparing the worker for the job;

(2) demonstrating the job for the worker; (3) allowing the worker to perform the job under supervision; and (4) testing the worker on his job performance. After the phases of the job instruction training method have been satisfactorily completed, the supervisor will then permit the worker to perform the job without constant guidance. Nevertheless, to assure that the employee is not "slipping up" on any necessary steps in the job, especially safe practices, the supervisor will periodically check the progress of the worker.

Over-the-shoulder Coaching

Of the three on-the-job training methods, over-the-shoulder coaching is perhaps the most flexible and direct. In this method the worker is expected to learn his job by actually performing the tasks in a typical work situation under the guidance of a qualified individual. Even more than in the other methods, over-the-shoulder coaching permits the worker to contribute to production while he is still being trained.

Requiring Protective Equipment

Where hazards cannot be eliminated or controlled at their source and where regular work clothes cannot provide sufficient protection, the employer should require his workers to wear personal protective equipment. This equipment should be purchased from reputable firms and should meet current national standards.

Because of the great variety of industrial companies, personal safety equipment is available for practically every area of the body and for almost every type of industrial hazard. Below are listed a few examples:

1. Head.—safety hat
   —protects against protruding, falling, and flying objects
2. Ears.—earplugs and earmuffs
   —protect against noise-induced hearing impairment
3. Eyes.—cover goggles, cup goggles, dust goggles, melters' goggles, welders' goggles, chemical goggles, miners' goggles, spectacles with side shields, and protective spectacles

   —protect against flying objects, molten metals, dust, radiation, and corrosive solids, liquids, and vapors
4. Face.—face shield, babbitting helmet, welding helmet, hand-held shield, acid-proof hood, and air-supplying hood

   —protect against light impact, chemicals, hot metals, and heat radiation
5. Lungs.—air purifier and air supplier
   —protect against contaminated air
6. Abdomen, trunk, and arms.—leather apron, fabric apron, asbestos apron, and coveralls

   —protect against light impact, sharp objects, and hot metals

7. Hands and fingers.—asbestos gloves, metal mesh gloves, leather gloves, rubber gloves, fabric gloves, treated fabric gloves, neoprene gloves, and vinyl gloves

—protect against sharp objects, light impact, and hot substances

8. Legs.—leggings and knee pads
—protect against light impact and hot metals

9. Feet.—metal-free shoes, gaiter-type shoes, reinforced-soled shoes, wood-soled shoes, and safety shoes with metatarsal guards

—protect against electricity, hot metals, protruding objects, wet surfaces and heavy impact

In many companies the departmental supervisor is responsible for the "personal protective equipment phase" of the overall plant safety program. In such cases, according to the National Safety Council, the supervisor should assume the following duties:

1. Be familiar with required standards and the Occupational Safety and Health Act requirements.

2. Be able to recognize hazards.

3. Be familiar with the best safety equipment available to protect against these hazards.

4. Know the procedures for supplying the equipment.

5. Know how to maintain and clean the equipment.

6. Develop an effective method for persuading all employees to dress safely and to wear the proper protective equipment when they should.[4]

To fulfill his responsibility, the supervisor should learn as much as possible about the various types of personal safety equipment. Good sources of information include local safety meetings, the National Safety Congress and Exposition (held every fall in Chicago, Illinois), manufacturers' catalogs, and the "equipment issue" of the *National Safety News* (published each March by the National Safety Council).

Maintaining Interest in Safety

In the industrial safety program, the supervisor continually seeks to develop good attitudes in his workers. He trains them in safe workmanship, supervises their progress, and repeatedly emphasizes that he expects safe behavior. However, for the safety program to function at its maximum efficiency, the supervisor must instill in the workers a sincere interest in plant safety.

Safety Committees

One of the most effective ways to develop and maintain an interest in safety is to involve workers in the operation of the safety program. This is

---

4. National Safety Council, *Supervisors Safety Manual,* p. 152.

the function of an employee safety committee. Supported by top management, the members of the committee, who are rotated periodically to permit all of the employees to participate, perform such safety tasks as inspecting plant conditions, observing workers' activities, investigating accidents, and recommending effective countermeasures.

Safety Stickers and Posters

When they are placed in prominent positions of high visibility, safety stickers and posters will alert employees to safe working practices. For best results, the material should be changed frequently by the safety director. Old posters should be rotated to new locations, and new posters should be added to the collection.

Promotional Stunts

For creating attention, safety promotional stunts are excellent change-of-pace devices. For example, to dramatize the effectiveness of personal protective equipment, an array of safety glasses, safety shoes, safety hats, and other safety gear which have actually prevented or mitigated injuries to their wearers during accidents can be conspicuously displayed in an area of the plant. (See Figure 15.3.) Similarly, to demonstrate how much work accidents cost, a guessing contest about the average cost of an injured worker being off from the job can be conducted in each department.

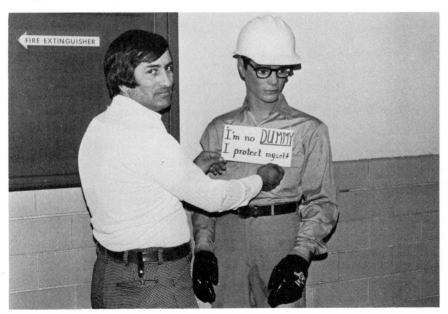

Figure 15.3   In this promotional stunt a safety director has dressed a department store mannequin with various items of personal protective equipment.

Safety Contests

Whether they are sponsored by the National Safety Council, local safety councils, trade associations, companies, or departments, safety contests are one of the most effective means devised for developing and maintaining the workers' interest in safety. As a rule, the contests are based on accident experience and are conducted over a period of six months or a year. Winners are determined by relative standings, improved performances, or other predetermined standards, and are presented with cash, merchandise, trophies, plaques, or similar awards.

Recognition Organizations

Many organizations offer awards to persons who have prevented or mitigated serious injuries by using certain types of personal protective equipment. These awards are excellent devices for rewarding safe practices and for publicizing the importance of wearing personal safety equipment.

The Wise Owl Club is the oldest of the organizations and has awards for workers who have saved their vision by wearing eye protection. For people who have survived serious automobile accidents because of the assistance of airbags, the Cocoon Club has certain awards. The Scarab Club, Ole Safety Sam Club, and Golden Shoe Club are among the organizations that provide awards to employees who have avoided serious injuries by wearing safety shoes. For workers who have been saved from serious injuries or death by falling into safety nets at the job site, the Half-Way to Hell Club will present recognition awards. The Kangaroo Club has awards for persons who have avoided serious injuries or death by wearing vehicular safety belts, whether on or off the job. (For organizational addresses see Resource Materials at the end of this chapter.)

Safety Suggestions

Because of their familiarity with the production process, workers are sometimes able to suggest methods for improving the efficiency and safety of the system. To stimulate interest in thinking about safety and in submitting suggestions, many companies have developed a plan for providing financial rewards to workers with usable proposals.

Designing and Maintaining a Safe Environment

As mentioned earlier in this chapter, the Occupational Safety and Health Act (OSHA) requires every employer to provide safe and healthful working conditions for their employees. In meeting the requirements of this law, many companies have found that increased production is a conspicuous by-product of their efforts. Apparently employees enjoy working in a clean, orderly, and well-protected environment, and as a result they perform their duties more willingly, safely, and efficiently.

Designing a Safe Plant

Safety and efficiency within the industrial plant is largely dependent upon the layout of the working facilities. For this reason, the plant should be designed in a manner that will permit raw materials and finished products to move through the various departments with a minimum of delay and rerouting. As a part of this design, the location of fixed equipment should provide workers with ample space for handling materials easily and safely. In addition, the plant should be designed to allow sufficient light and ventilation and to permit adequate operating space for maintenance work.

Promoting Good Housekeeping Practices

As a rule, if good housekeeping practices are ignored in a company, plant operations can never be really safe for the workers. As the National Safety Council describes the problem,

> There always will be some dirt and disorder when you are making a product or providing a service, but if it is allowed to accumulate, sooner or later you will have production problems, higher employee turnover, and increased accident rates. People do not enjoy working in areas that are dirty, disorderly, crowded and booby-trapped with hazards. Good housekeeping is good business.[5]

Because of the numerous problems which are presented by poor housekeeping, many companies have included good housekeeping statements within their general accident prevention/mitigation policies.

Basically, each worker should be held responsible for maintaining orderly conditions within his own working area. Before serious hazards can develop, the worker should dispose of litter, trash, dirt, scrap, waste substances, and other accumulated junk. As part of the company's responsibility, the management should provide suitable containers for these items and contract for the disposal of such materials at frequent and regular intervals. For raw materials and finished products, the management should provide spacious and readily available storage areas. In turn, the worker should maintain these areas in a safe condition by utilizing correct storage methods, such as stacking, blocking, interlocking, and height-limiting, and by preventing the accumulation of materials which could produce tripping, falling, burning, or exploding hazards. To insure that good housekeeping practices are being employed within the department, the supervisor should conduct weekly, bi-monthly, or monthly inspections of the work areas.

---

5. National Safety Council, *Supervisors Safety Manual,* p. 201.

Controlling Health Hazards

Safety professionals have always been interested in preventing or mitigating bodily injuries caused by accidents. Now, however, they are also very much concerned about controlling environmental hazards which are conducive to the development of slow, insidious diseases of various organs of the body, such as the skin, lungs, liver, kidneys and brain. Today, this deep concern for controlling health hazards within the work environment is embodied within the science of industrial hygiene. By definition,

> Industrial hygiene is that science and art devoted to the recognition, evaluation and control of those environmental factors or stresses [chemical, physical, ergonomic, and biological], arising in or from the workplace, which may cause sickness, impaired health and well-being, or significant discomfort and inefficiency among workers or among the citizens of the community.[6]

Furthermore,

> An industrial hygienist is a person having a college or university degree or degrees in engineering, chemistry, physics, or medicine or related biological sciences who, by virtue of special studies and training, has acquired competence in industrial hygiene.[7]

In modern industry the hygienist works closely with the safety professional to maintain a healthful working environment.

In most large companies the industrial hygienist inspects the plant and prepares recommendations for controlling environmental hazards. In turn, the safety professional examines these recommendations and then implements the necessary control measures. Nevertheless, in emergency situations or in small companies, in the absence of the industrial hygienist, the safety professional must be prepared for the responsibility of recognizing environmental health hazards and implementing practical, effective control measures within the plant environment.

Chemical Hazards

In the majority of industrial operations, toxic chemicals—in the form of liquids, gases, mists, dusts, fumes, and vapors—are the most common environmental health hazards. For the chemical agents to exert their toxic effects, however, they must directly contact and react with the cells of the body. This can be easily accomplished through inhalation, ingestion, or skin absorption.

Of the three methods of entry into the body, inhalation is the most

---

6. Julian B. Olishifski and Frank E. McElroy (eds.), *Fundamentals of Industrial Hygiene* (Chicago: National Safety Council, 1975), p. 3.
7. Julian B. Olishifski and Frank E. McElroy (eds.), p. 3.

dangerous because of the swiftness with which toxic chemicals can be absorbed in the lungs, transferred into the bloodstream, and carried to the brain. However, during an evaluation of the work environment, all possible methods of entry should be carefully studied.

Physical Hazards

The types of physical hazards which may be encountered in the industrial process are quite numerous. However, in general, most physical health hazards can be classified into such groups as noise, radiation, temperature extremes, and extremes in pressure.

As a rule, these hazards produce either immediate or long-term effects on the health of the workers. For this reason, during an environmental evaluation of the plant, the safety professional, as well as the industrial hygienist, should not overlook the physical health hazards.

Ergonomic Hazards

According to the National Safety Council, "the term 'ergonomics' literally means the customs, habits, and laws of work."[8] By this definition, ergonomic hazards are those that involve worker reaction to monotony, fatigue, mechanical vibration, and repeated shock.

In studying the ergonomic health hazards, the safety professional and industrial hygienist are actually looking beyond the goals of productivity, health, and safety. In essence, they are considering the total psychological and physiological demands of the job upon the workers.

Biological Hazards

Environmental hazards of the biological type are most often related to problems with viruses, bacteria, molds, fungi, rickettsiae, and grain dusts. Often, the effects of these biological hazards appear in the form of some disease, such as tuberculosis, fungus infections, anthrax, Q-fever, byssinosis, brucellosis, erysipelas, and upper respiratory tract infections. Since the biological hazards for most industrial operations are well known, the safety professional, as well as the industrial hygienist, will ordinarily encounter less difficulty in recognizing and controlling these hazards than in dealing with the chemical, physical, and ergonomic health hazards.

Control of Hazards

To maintain a healthy working environment for employees, the safety professional and the industrial hygienist must familiarize themselves with the various methods which are available for controlling environmental

---

8. Julian B. Olishifski and Frank E. McElroy (eds.), p. 37.

health hazards. The following general methods of control are listed by the National Safety Council:

1. Substitution of a less harmful material for one which is dangerous to health.

2. Change or alteration of a process to minimize worker contact.

3. Isolation or enclosure of a process or work operation to reduce the number of persons exposed.

4. Wet methods to reduce generation of dust in operations such as mining and quarrying.

5. Local exhaust at the point of generation and dispersion of contaminants.

6. General or dilution ventilation with clean air to provide a safe atmosphere.

7. Personal protective devices, such as special clothing, eye, and respiratory protection.

8. Good housekeeping, including cleanliness of the workplace, waste disposal, adequate washing and eating facilities, healthful drinking water, and control of insects and rodents.

9. Special control methods for specific hazards, such as reduction of exposure time, film badges and similar monitoring devices, continuous sampling with preset alarms, and medical programs to detect intake of toxic materials.

10. Training and education to supplement engineering controls.[9]

The exact type and extent of these controls will depend upon the chemical and physical properties of the hazard, the intensity and the duration of the exposure of the workers, and the operational mechanics of the control method.

Safeguarding Power Tools and Machinery

Even the most skilled worker is never one hundred percent alert during his job. As the National Safety Council notes, "There is no method yet devised that will keep a person's mind on his work every minute of the working day."[10] Thus no matter how much training and experience a worker may possess, he can be injured by hazardous power tools and machinery. However, the probability of worker injury, because of human error, poor equipment design, or mechanical failure, is greatly reduced by proper safeguarding methods.

Enclosing Dangerous Parts

Injury-producing accidents are inevitable where workers operate tools and machines without proper guards. According to the National Safety

9. Julian B. Olishifski and Frank E. McElroy (eds.), p. 44.
10. National Safety Council, *Supervisors Safety Manual,* p. 282.

Council, guards can protect against, and prevent injuries from, the following sources:

1. Direct contact with exposed moving parts of a machine—either points of operation on production machines (such as power presses, machine tools, or woodworking equipment), or power-transmitting parts of mechanisms (such as gears, pulleys and sheaves, slides, or couplings).

2. Work in process, such as pieces of wood that kick back from a power ripsaw, or metal chips that fly from tools or from abrasive wheels.

3. Machine failure, which usually results from lack of preventive maintenance, overloading, metal fatigue, or abuse.

4. Electrical failure, which may cause malfunctioning of the machine, or cause electrical shock or burn.

5. Operator error or human failure caused by distraction, worry, zeal, anxiety, misunderstanding, indolence, deliberate chance-taking, anger, illness, fatigue, and so on.[11]

Despite the many types of industrial tools and machines, guards can be classified into such groups as the fixed guard or starters, the interlocking guard or barriers, and the automatic protection device. In addition, semiautomatic or automatic feeding and ejection methods are typical means of safeguarding machine operations.

Regardless of the types, the best guards are the ones provided by the equipment manufacturer. Yet, far too often industrial companies buy stripped-down equipment in an effort to save money and then build guards after the machinery has been installed. Frequently such makeshift guards are flimsy, ineffective, and even hazardous in themselves. For these reasons, top management executives should always support the purchasing of equipment with all of the built-in guards offered by the manufacturer.

Utilizing Preventive Maintenance

Through repeated operation, even the safest tools and machinery will eventually show wear and deterioration. While it cannot be prevented, wear can be reduced to a minimum by the utilization of a good preventive maintenance program.

As a part of his responsibility, the maintenance worker should establish a regular schedule for the lubrication of the equipment. In addition, he should periodically inspect the most important parts of the equipment and replace worn parts before they can malfunction. By keeping the equipment in good operating condition, the maintenance worker not only prevents many accidents, but he also promotes in the employees a sense of security which, in turn, results in improved production.

---

11. National Safety Council, pp. 283-84.

Resource Materials

Cocoon Club
51 Weaver Street
Greenwich, Connecticut 06380

Factory Mutual Engineering Corporation of the Factory Mutual System
1151 Boston-Providence Turnpike
Norwood, Massachusetts 02062

Golden Shoe Club
1509 Washington Avenue
St. Louis, Missouri 63166

Half-Way to Hell Club
533 Second Street
San Francisco, California 94107

Kangaroo Club International
P.O. Box 950
Coatesville, Pennsylvania 19320

National Institute of Occupational
Safety and Health
U.S. Department of Health, Education,
and Welfare
5600 Fishers Lane
Rockville, Maryland 20852

National Safety Council
444 North Michigan Avenue
Chicago, Illinois 60611

Occupational Safety and Health Administration
U.S. Department of Labor
1726 M Street, N.W.
Washington, D.C. 20210

Ole Safety Sam Club
9th and Greenleaf Streets
Allentown, Pennsylvania 18105

Scarab Club
Emmaus, Pennsylvania 18049

Wise Owl Club
Director of Industrial Service
National Society for the Prevention of
Blindness, Inc.
79 Madison Avenue
New York, New York 10016

Activities

1. Secure the November 24, 1975, copy of *U.S. News & World Report,* and read the article titled "Protecting People on the Job: ABC's of A Controversial Law." Present a short, oral report to the class on the negative aspects of the Occupational Safety and Health Act.

2. Contact the management of a local company, and secure a copy of their accident prevention/mitigation policy. Discuss this policy statement with the other members of the class.

3. Prepare a class exhibit of the various types of personal protective devices which are commonly used by workers in industry.

4. Design several industrial safety posters, and display them in the classroom.

5. Invite an industrial hygienist to speak to the class about his professional training and his experiences in recognizing, evaluating, and controlling environmental hazards in the work situation.

Questions

1. Why were the early workmen's compensation laws important in accelerating the industrial safety movement in this country?
2. What are two general requirements of the Occupational Safety and Health Act?
3. What are the five basic elements of all industrial safety programs?
4. What are some of the accident investigation procedures which are recommended by the National Safety Council?
5. What three methods of on-the-job training are commonly used in industry?
6. What are the six methods by which the supervisor can develop and maintain in his workers an interest in plant safety?
7. What is industrial hygiene?
8. What are the four classes of environmental health hazards?
9. According to the National Safety Council, what are some of the general methods that may be used to control environmental hazards?
10. Why is preventive maintenance important in industry?

Selected References

Mazor, John. "How Accurate Are Employers' Illness and Injury Reports?" *Monthly Labor Review,* September, 1976, 26-31.

National Safety Council. *Supervisors Safety Manual.* 4th ed.; Chicago: NSC, 1975.

Olishifski, Julian B. and Frank E. McElroy (eds.). *Fundamentals of Industrial Hygiene.* Chicago: National Safety Council, 1975.

"Protecting People on the Job," *U.S. News & World Report,* November 24, 1975, 69-71.

Tillery, Winston. "Safety and Health Provisions Before and After OSHA," *Monthly Labor Review,* September, 1975, 40-43.

VerSteeg, Clarence L. and Richard Hofstadter. *A People and A Nation.* New York: Harper & Row, Publishers, Inc., 1971.

Agricultural Accidents

16

For many years agricultural work has ranked as the third most hazardous occupation in this country. Only mining, including quarrying and petroleum drilling, and construction have higher death rates. (See Figure 16.1.) Fortunately, however, the death rate for agricultural accidents, conforming to national work trends, has decreased steadily since the early part of the twentieth century. Yet, despite this decrease, the agricultural death rate is still almost four times greater than the national average for all occupations.

Today, with the exception of construction, agricultural accidents claim more lives each year, approximately nineteen hundred, than any other type of work accident. Apparently, part of the agricultural-accident problem can be attributed to the multi-occupational nature of the work. Unlike other workers, the farmer must perform the tasks of numerous craftsmen, such as

Industry Group	Workers* (000)	Deaths		Death Rates**			Disabling Injuries‡ 1976
		1976	Change from 1975	1976	1966	% Change	
ALL INDUSTRIES	**87,800**	**12,500**	**−500**	**14**	**20**	**−30%**	**2,200,000†**
Trade	**20,300**	**1,300**	**0**	**6**	**8**	**−25%**	**400,000**
Manufacturing	**19,000**	**1,700**	**+100**	**9**	**10**	**−10%**	**470,000**
Service	**20,800**	**1,800**	**−100**	**9**	**13**	**−31%**	**400,000**
Government	**14,900**	**1,700**	**0**	**11**	**13**	**−15%**	**320,000**
Transportation and public utilities	**4,800**	**1,500**	**−100**	**31**	**40**	**−23%**	**180,000**
Agriculture††	**3,500**	**1,900**	**−200**	**54**	**69**	**−22%**	**190,000**
Construction	**3,700**	**2,100**	**−200**	**57**	**74**	**−23%**	**200,000**
Mining, quarrying	**800**	**500**	**0**	**63**	**108**	**−42%**	**40,000**

Source: NSC estimates (rounded) based on data from the National Center for Health Statistics, state departments of health, and state industrial commissions; numbers of workers are based on Bureau of Labor Statistics data. **Deaths per 100,000 workers in each group.
*Workers are all persons gainfully employed, including owners, managers, other paid employees, the self-employed, and unpaid family workers, but excluding domestic servants.
‡Disabling beyond the day of the accident. Totals include deaths.
†About 4,000 of the deaths and 100,000 of the injuries involved motor vehicles.

Figure 16.1 Death rates for the various occupations. (Reproduced from *Accident Facts—1977 Edition*, p. 23, courtesy of the National Safety Council)

mechanics, electricians, and carpenters. In addition, much of the agricultural work is performed away from direct observation and supervision; as a result the mistakes of the farmer, unlike those of other workers, are not noticed and corrected immediately. In fact, many mistakes are not detected until they cause accidents.

Operating Machinery in Safety

Powered by electrical and internal combustion motors which range in size from a fraction of a horsepower to hundreds of horsepower, machines are a dominant element in modern agriculture. At almost every point, from soil preparing to harvesting to storing and to marketing, machines have brought increased efficiency to the farm. However, they have also brought increased danger to their users. Machines, which account for approximately 28 percent of all agricultural accidents, are responsible for producing the greatest number of severe and fatal injuries to agricultural workers.

Protecting Against Tractor Upset

Of the various types of accidents involving farm machinery, tractor overturns are the most serious. According to the National Safety Council, between four hundred and five hundred persons die in tractor overturns each year. More important, over one-half of all deaths in tractor accidents are caused by overturns.

In a typical overturn accident the operator is not thrown off the machine by its rolling motion, but instead he is trapped in a near-normal position on the tractor. As a result, when the tractor comes to rest in an inverted position, the operator is pinned underneath the machine. However, the operator can be spared serious injury if he is on a tractor equipped with roll-over protective equipment and is belted into his seat.

At present, roll-over protection is available in two forms: (1) a protective frame and (2) a crush-resistant cab. Both types of roll-over devices are equipped with safety belts. Basically, the protective frame surrounds the operator and prevents his being crushed by the tractor during an overturn accident. In addition, the safety belt provided with the frame prevents his being thrown off the tractor and holds him securely within the zone of protection afforded by the frame. On the other hand, the crush-resistant cab encloses the operator in a reinforced box and, like the protective frame, prevents his being crushed during an overturn. Furthermore, the safety belt provided with the cab prevents the operator from being thrown around inside his protective box.

Through testing and field analyses, agricultural equipment engineers have discovered that roll-over protective devices on tractors will in many cases significantly alter the nature of the accident. As a rule, a tractor will overturn with minimal inertia. Consequently, a roll-over device is often able to limit the roll to a 90° angle, thus permitting the machine to come to rest on its side with very little damage. By comparison, a tractor without a roll-over device will roll through a 180° angle and come to rest on its top. Because of the overhead protection and the alteration of the accident pattern, some safety experts estimate that almost 90 percent of all deaths from tractor overturns could be prevented by the use of tractors with roll-over protective equipment and safety belts.

Obviously, as additional information concerning tractor accidents becomes available, manufacturers of farm machinery will continue to modify and improve the various types of roll-over protective devices on their various makes and models of tractors. However, at the present time, when purchasing a new tractor, the farmer should probably select a model with a crush-resistant cab. Because it encloses the operator, the cab provides a more pleasant, healthier working environment than a protective frame. Besides shielding the operator from insects, low branches, and obstructions, such as flying parts and ruptured hydraulic lines, the crush-resistant cab reduces noise, controls temperature, maintains relatively dust-free air, and protects against rain and intense sunlight. For an older model machine without overhead protection, the farmer may be able to purchase a cab or, at least, a protective frame that can be specially fitted to the tractor.

Although they can prevent many deaths, protective frames and crush-resistant cabs cannot prevent tractor upsets. This remains the responsibility of the operator. In most tractor overturns, excessive speed is a significant factor. While a hidden log, stump, or stone can cause an upset in the field, many speed-related overturns occur while the tractor is being driven to or from the work site. Obviously, to prevent such overturns, the operator must remain alert at all times and maintain a speed which is appropriate for the ground conditions. Another common circumstance in many overturns is the use of the tractor on steep slopes or near ditches and banks. On steep slopes, because of the reduction in the machine's base of support, even the slightest shift in weight may cause the tractor to upset. When crossing slopes or moving down or up hills, the operator should drive slowly and remain alert for dips, rises, rocks, and gullies. In addition, on extremely steep hills he should shift into a lower gear when driving downhill and shift into reverse and back the tractor when driving uphill. Near ditches and banks, because of the sudden loss of support, a cave-in or a slippage of a wheel is a constant threat. As a rule, the tractor operator should remain at least five feet away from ditches, banks, and similar hazards.

While they are perhaps the most common elements in overturn accidents, excessive speed and the use of the tractor on steep slopes or near ditches and banks are not the only factors which may be involved in such accidents. In

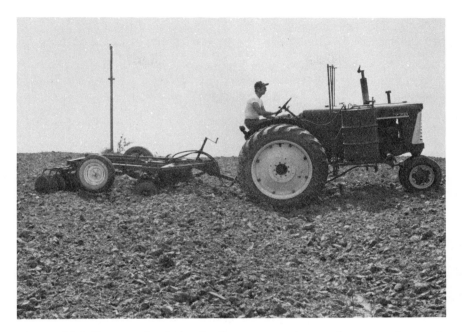

Figure 16.2   Slopes and a lack of roll-over protection are important factors in tractor overturns and operator deaths.

many cases the attachment of a mired vehicle or a tree stump to the axle or the seat bracket of the tractor can produce a backward rotational effect and cause the machine to overturn. To prevent such backward overturns, the operator should hitch only to the drawbar or to regular hitch points recommended by the manufacturer. In other cases the presence of excessive weight on a front-end loader or a two-wheeled implement, such as a manure spreader, can produce a similar rotational effect and cause a frontward, backward, or sideward overturn. To lessen the rotational effect and thus reduce the possibility of such accidents, the tractor operator should add either rear wheel weights or front end weights, depending upon the position of the load. In addition, he should avoid abrupt turns, jerky starts, and sudden stops.

Staying on Machinery

According to numerous accident surveys, falls are responsible for approximately one out of every four farm-work injuries. Naturally, many falls occur while persons are loading and unloading vehicles, climbing ladders, working in and around buildings, and tending livestock. However, most of the falls are connected with the use of farm machinery. Of the various types of machines, tractors are involved in the largest number of falls, followed by wagons and combines.[1]

Generally, falls involving machinery are almost always more serious than other types of falls. In many cases the victims fall beneath or in the path of moving equipment, into machines, onto sharp objects or hard surfaces, or between machines and stationary objects, where they are crushed. As a result, if they survive, the victims of such falls often will be handicapped by their injuries for the rest of their lives.

Naturally, many falls involving machinery result in the operators' being seriously injured or killed by their own equipment. However, the victims are often extra passengers on the machines. While a person standing on a side platform or a drawbar may easily slip off moving equipment, riders are usually thrown by a sudden jolt, as when the machines hit an obstacle, deep rut, or bump, or when they make an abrupt start, stop, or turn. Because of the danger presented by farm machinery, the operator should never permit extra riders, especially youngsters, on a tractor, wagon, combine, or other piece of equipment unless the machine has special seating provisions for passengers.

In the machinery falls involving operators, slippery surfaces are probably the most common causative factors. Mud, water, snow, ice, manure, and slop are common hazards on almost all farms. To assure better footing and thus lessen the possibility of slippage, the farmer should always wear shoes or boots with slip-resistant soles and heels. In addition, before mounting or dismounting machines, he should clean the footwear as well as possible. Unfortunately, until quite recently, manufacturers did not equip tractors and similar machines with handrails and steps or ladders to assist the operators in safe mounting and dismounting, particularly under slippery conditions. Consequently, a farmer with an older tractor or piece of machinery should always mount and dismount with extreme caution.

Unlike the industrial worker, the farmer is not limited by a daily or weekly work regimen. As a result, in busy seasons he may work twelve to eighteen hours per day in a seven-day work week. Because of the physical stress the farmer is susceptible to skill-inhibiting fatigue and accidents, particularly falls. In addition, he may aggravate the situation by consuming alcoholic drinks or certain medications shortly before or while operating farm equipment. For continued alertness and good workmanship, the farmer should, whenever possible, take short coffee or snack breaks in the mid-morning and the mid-afternoon. Furthermore, he should avoid taking alcohol or medications which, besides altering his physical skills, may cause

---

1. National Safety Council, "Falls Prevention Agricultural Work," *Rural Accident Prevention Bulletin* (Chicago: NSC, n.d.), p. 1.

him to exercise poor judgment, such as jumping from one piece of moving machinery to another.

Avoiding Mechanical Entanglement

While many different kinds of farm machinery exist, they all possess similar characteristics and hazards. Equipped with cutting edges, gears, chains, revolving shafts, rotating blades, levers, and other devices, agricultural machinery is designed to cut, pull, turn, pound, grind, and shake farm products in such a manner as to render them usable by the farmer. If fingers, hands, and feet become entangled in their mechanisms, the machines are not selective in their functions. They will cut, pull, crush, and tear human flesh just as easily as farm products. Obviously, farm machines respond only to controls, regardless of the intent of the worker.

Unfortunately, far too often farmers become entangled in machinery because they wear loose-fitting clothing when they are around moving parts, or because they fail to shut off the equipment before servicing it. Apparently, one of the most dangerous entanglements involves the power take-off (PTO) on tractors. Near Waterloo, Illinois, a forty-nine-year-old farmer was killed when he became caught in the PTO while spreading anhydrous

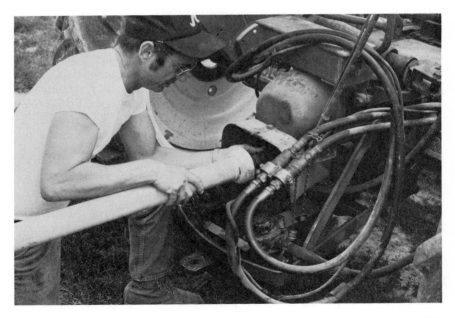

Figure 16.3 When working around machinery, the farmer should wear clothing that reduces the possibility of his becoming entangled in the equipment.

ammonia. According to authorities, while he was off the tractor, the man brushed his clothing against the PTO and became entangled in the equipment. All his clothing was torn off in the accident. Because of the tremendous horsepower which is attached to the revolving shaft, the PTO can easily dismember and kill a person if his clothing becomes entangled in it. Since even a single thread can become entangled and cause injury, the farmer should avoid wearing loose-fitting or torn clothing when working around machinery. Furthermore, before adjusting, oiling, or unclogging machine parts, he should always shut off the engine and wait until all motion has stopped.

Despite such precautions, a farmer will never be completely alert and safety conscious at all times during his work. Consequently, modern pieces of farm equipment are manufactured with guards to protect the worker. However, many parts of farm machinery cannot be completely shielded and still perform their tasks. For example, a cutting blade cannot be totally enclosed, since it would not be able to cut the product. Yet, guards are still the farmer's best protection against rapidly-moving machine parts, such as power take-offs (PTO's) on tractors, PTO shafts on implements, and augers on grain conveyors. For this reason, when selecting new equipment, the farmer should always exhibit caution and make sure that the machine parts are properly equipped with approved guards.

Naturally, through repeated operation, farm machinery will eventually show wear and deterioration. When this happens, the farmer may be forced to remove certain guards before making the necessary repairs. Then, if he is in a hurry, he may neglect to replace the guards. On the other hand, if the guarding is defective, the farmer may remove the guards with the intent of replacing them at a later date. Apparently, many persons are injured or killed each year as a result of these actions. Always, before operating equipment, the farmer should replace any guards that he removed during his maintenance work.

Clearing the Work Area

Because of the unique home-work environment, many youngsters are injured or killed each year on the farm. In numerous cases the children become entangled in machines; in other instances they are run over by heavy equipment. As a general rule, unless they are accompanied by a responsible adult who will provide them with constant supervision, small children should not be allowed in the work area. However, youngsters, as well as other farm workers, may inadvertently wander into the work area. In addition, with large field machines, such as cotton pickers, potato harvesters, pea viners, vegetable harvesters, sugar beet harvesters, hay cubers, and grain or corn combines, the operator's view is usually limited by the size of the machine. For these reasons, the farmer should carefully check to make

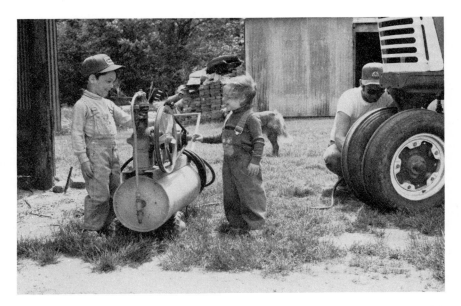

Figure 16.4 Small children, unless they are provided with constant adult supervision, should not be allowed in the work area.

sure that everyone is safely away from the machine before starting forward or backward in the barnyard or field.

Transporting Equipment on Public Roads

Over the years agricultural machinery has been greatly modified and improved. Because of these changes modern machinery now enables relatively few farmers and ranchers to produce sufficient food for a growing population. However, as farms increase in size, more and more farmers are forced to utilize public roads and highways in order to reach isolated sections of their property. Inevitably, this practice increases the probability of road collisions between automobiles and slow-moving vehicles.

As a result of studies on the many aspects of the problem of slow-moving vehicles on rural roads and highways, a unique emblem, which can be attached to the rear of farm vehicles as a warning to other motorists, was developed in 1963 at Ohio State University. The slow-moving vehicle (SMV) emblem is a fourteen-inch-high, fluorescent-orange triangle with a dark red reflective border. Because of its flourescent and reflective materials, the SMV emblem is highly visible in the daytime and at night.

By federal law the SMV emblem must be displayed on any vehicle operated by hired employees and designed to travel less than twenty-five miles per hour. Moreover, many states now require the emblem on vehicles operated by owners. Yet, regardless of the law, the farmer should still use the emblem for safety reasons. The emblem can be purchased at most implement dealers and farm supply stores.

For greatest visibility the SMV emblem should be placed in a center position on the rear of the vehicle and approximately three to five feet from the ground. At this level the emblem will provide the quickest eye contact and at night is within the normal headlight pattern of approaching vehicles. However, since the emblem will gradually lose its fluorescence, thus making it difficult to spot at night, the farmer should replace the SMV emblem every three to five years.

According to safety officials, the emblem is designed for use in conjunction with lawfully-required safety lighting and markings. Consequently, for night transportation at least one or two red taillights are required on the rear of slow-moving farm vehicles. At a great distance the red taillights will alert fast-moving motorists to the vehicle's presence. Then as the motorists approach even closer, their headlights will illuminate the SMV emblem, thereby identifying the farm machinery as a slow-moving vehicle. In short, the red taillights alert; the SMV emblem identifies.

Handling Animals Safely

Among the various types of agricultural accidents, conflict with animals is one of the most common. Approximately 10 percent of all agricultural accidents are caused by farm animals. However, animals also present an additional threat in the form of disease. Of the 209 diseases which affect humans, more than 100 are transmitted by animals.[2]

Working with Livestock

Many farm animals can cause serious and even fatal injuries if they are not handled properly. According to accident reports, milk cows are involved in more accidents than any other animals. If they are inadvertently startled or physically irritated by the farmer during the milking process, cows may kick, butt, hook, and trample. Next to cows in farm accident involvement are horses. Since they are easily frightened by sudden noises, horses will often kick without looking. Together, cows and horses are involved in nearly one-half of all farm-animal accidents.

As a rule, unless they are handled properly, cows and horses, as well as many other animals, will harbor a natural suspicion of humans. For this

---

2. "Animal Disease and Human Health," *Farm Safety Review,* March-April, 1965, p. 12.

reason, the farmer should always treat animals with kindness and patience. Before entering their stalls he should speak to the animals. Then if they are not too nervous, the farmer may want to stroke their backs or necks as he approaches. When they are handled gently and firmly, cows, horses, and other animals are more likely to trust the farmer and thus behave more calmly and predictably.

Unfortunately, even apparently gentle animals may become vicious when they are trying to protect their young. Besides cows and horses, sows are well-known for displaying their "maternal instinct." Many persons, often youngsters, have been attacked and savagely bitten when they thoughtlessly petted or attempted to move a sow's young. Because of the danger presented by animals with their young, small children should be forbidden to play in or around barns, pens, and feedlots. In addition, when he is working in their quarters, the farmer should avoid, whenever possible, any actions which the animals might interpret as a threat to their young.

As would be expected, many animals are always dangerous, since they may suddenly attack without any provocation or warning. Goats and rams will often butt; boars will often bite; and bulls will often butt, hook, gore, and trample. When he is working with these animals or in their quarters, the farmer should always remain especially cautious and watch them at all times. Furthermore, whenever possible, he should keep such animals isolated in their own areas with sturdy corrals, stalls, or pens.

Managing Animal-related Diseases

Despite the fact that this country has one of the best health quarantine systems in the world, animal-related diseases are still problems on many farms. Among the animal-related diseases which present hazards for the farmer and his family are:

1. brucellosis (called undulant or Malta fever in man), which is transmitted by drinking raw milk from infected animals, through contact of a wound with the aborted fetus or afterbirth structures of infected animals, or by inhaling the infectious organisms at the time of slaughter,
2. leptospirosis, which is spread through contact with infected urine or with soil, feed, water, or other materials contaminated with infected urine,
3. anthrax, which is transmitted through contact with infected animals or infected hair, hides, wool, or other products,
4. bovine tuberculosis, which is spread by drinking raw milk from infected animals, by inhaling discharges from the respiratory tract of infected animals, or through contact of a wound with the vagina, penis, semen, urine, or feces of infected animals,

5. Newcastle disease, which is transmitted through contact with infected fowl or with used egg crates or unsterilized feed bags from farms with infected fowl,
6. swine erysipelas, which is spread through contact of a wound with infected animals,
7. trichinosis, which is transmitted by eating uncooked or partially cooked pork infested with parasites,
8. tularemia, which is spread through contact with infected animals or by bites and stings from infected ticks and insects,
9. tetanus, which is transmitted through contact of a wound with soil or animal feces containing the infectious organisms, and
10. rabies, which is spread by bites of infected animals or through contact of a wound with the saliva of infected animals.

Unfortunately, effective treatment is not yet available for many of the diseases contracted from animals. Thus prevention is of prime importance.

In employing preventive and control measures, the farmer should remain alert at all times for any sign of disease in his animals. Yet, even in the absence of disease signs, he should still avoid certain practices, such as drinking raw milk, exposing open wounds to animals or animal-related items, and eating undercooked pork. If he suspects illness in his animals, the farmer should immediately seek a diagnosis from his veterinarian. When a disease is confirmed, he should apply every precaution recommended by the veterinarian in the quarantine and treatment of sick animals and in the disposal of dead animals. Whenever possible, he should restrict his contact with the animals, but if handling diseased animals or their carcasses is unavoidable, the farmer should wear full-body clothing and rubber gloves and later dispose of the items by burning or burying.

Tetanus

Commonly found in the soil and in animal feces, tetanus bacilli, rod-shaped bacteria, are the causative agents in tetanus. Since the bacilli are anaerobic, which means they grow and multiply best in the absence of oxygen, deep puncture wounds present the greatest danger. However, tetanus can result from even the most minor open wound.

Upon multiplying within the wound, tetanus bacilli produce a potent toxin which travels by way of the bloodstream to the spinal cord and the brain stem. At these sites the toxin acts upon the nerves which supply the voluntary muscles, thereby causing generalized rigidity, spasms, and convulsions. Because of the rigidity, the victim will experience difficulty in opening his jaws; thus, tetanus is often referred to as "lockjaw." If the rigidity and spasms are severe enough to interfere with respiration, the victim may die from asphyxiation.

In general, of every five persons who develop tetanus, three will die. However, through immunization, tetanus can be easily prevented. Because of their greater exposure to soil and animal feces, the farmer and his family members should always be vaccinated and revaccinated at recommended intervals against tetanus. Then, if they are injured, they will be protected. However, if the wound is deep, extremely contaminated, difficult to clean, or contaminated with soil from areas frequented by animals, they should still seek medical help. Besides receiving a thorough cleaning of the wound to prevent other types of infection, the farmer or his family member may require a tetanus booster to assure adequate protection.

Rabies

Found in the saliva of rabid animals, a virus is the causative agent in rabies infection. Although the virus ordinarily enters the body through a wound caused by the bite of a rabid animal, the organism can also enter if the animal's saliva comes into contact with an open wound or an intact mucous membrane. In addition, the rabies virus can also be transmitted by means of dust, specifically in bat-infested caves, but the exact nature of this transmission is still unknown.

Upon entering the body, the virus moves through the nerves and spinal cord to the brain, where the virus multiplies. This causes uncontrollable excitement in the victim, with excessive salivation and painful spasms of the throat muscles. Because these spasms result from the slightest irritation of the throat, the victim, although extremely thirsty, will refuse to drink water. For this reason, rabies is often referred to as hydrophobia, "the fear of water." Once the signs and symptoms of rabies develop, the victim will almost inevitably die within three to five days from exhaustion, general paralysis, or asphyxiation.

Fortunately, rabies can be prevented. Since the symptoms of rabies usually do not develop until thirty to fifty days after the virus enters the body, the suspected-rabid animal is confined and observed for a period of ten to fifteen days. If the animal dies or develops rabies during this time, treatment is started immediately. The same is true in cases where the animal cannot be observed or where it is a wild animal.

In this country the development of rabies in man is no longer common. While thirty years ago approximately twenty cases of rabies were reported annually, only one or two cases a year are now reported. Generally, this decline has occurred because the rabies vaccine is now readily available to all persons who are bitten by presumably rabid animals.

Because of an extensive animal vaccination program, the incidence of rabies in dogs and other domestic animals has also declined in recent years. As a result, domestic animals are no longer the greatest source of rabies transmission. Today, wild animals, particularly skunks, foxes, and bats, account for most of the cases of rabies in animals.

Contrary to popular belief, not all rabid animals are vicious and will run around attacking persons (furious rabies). Quite the opposite, some are actually gentle and even friendly (dumb rabies). Thus whenever possible the farmer should always avoid any animal, particularly a wild animal, which exhibits uncharacteristic behavior.

If he is bitten, the farmer should capture the animal and then notify the local health department. In a situation where he was forced to kill the animal to prevent further bites, the farmer should save the carcass so the animal's brain can be analyzed for the presence of rabies. Since rabies is the most serious human affliction transmitted by animals, the farmer should always secure medical help after an animal bite.

Working Safely with Agricultural Pesticides

According to authorities, nowhere in the world is a single agricultural crop being grown without insects living on its roots, stems, leaves, seeds, or fruit. In addition, many other pests are often serious threats, such as rodents, worms, snails, slugs, fungi, and weeds. Without agricultural pesticides, as much as 90 percent of the food produced by man would be destroyed by insects and other pests.[3] Furthermore, agricultural pesticides are vitally important to animal health. As insects plague the animals, dairy cattle, without pesticide protection, will experience a drastic reduction in milk output. Under the same conditions, beef cattle will lose valuable weight. On practically every farm, pets and livestock are now protected by a wide variety of chemical products.

While they have greatly improved agricultural production, pesticides have also created new hazards. Besides killing pests, many of them are highly toxic to humans. In some cases the pesticides may gradually accumulate in the body until only a minor final exposure can be enough to produce severe illness. In other cases the pesticides may produce death rapidly. Furthermore, pesticides may enter the body in numerous ways, such as by swallowing, inhaling, or absorbing through unbroken skin.

According to the Federal Environmental Pesticide Act of 1972, pesticides are classified into two groups, general and restricted. With normal precautions pesticides in the general group can be used with relative safety. However, because of their extreme toxicity, pesticides in the restricted group must be used only by certified persons or under their supervision. By

---

3. Manufacturing Chemists' Association, Inc., *Agricultural Chemicals* (Washington, D.C.: The Association, 1963), p. 12.

demonstrating his ability to handle the chemicals properly, the farmer can obtain certification in the use of restricted pesticides.

Generally, the safest method of handling an agricultural pesticide is determined by the nature of the chemical. Thus, by federal law all pesticides must be labeled with directions for their proper use and storage. Before using a pesticide, the farmer should always read the label and follow the instructions carefully. If the label recommends protective clothing, he should then contact his local farm agency representative for information on the best type of mask and clothing for the job. (See Figure 16.5.) When dusting or spraying a pesticide, the farmer should avoid working downwind. However, despite this precaution, he will still experience some exposure to

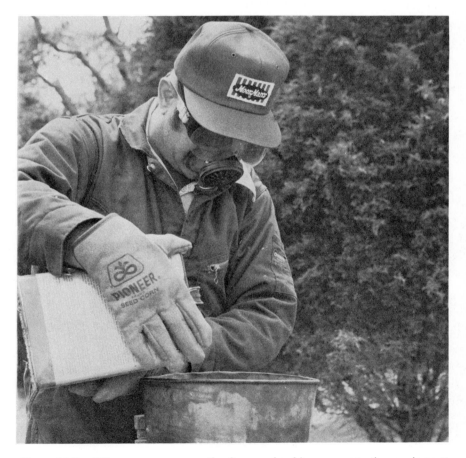

Figure 16.5 Whenever necessary, the farmer should wear protective equipment when handling pesticides.

imperceptible dust or spray particles. For this reason, the farmer should bathe or shower after dusting or spraying, and then wash his clothes in hot, soapy water before wearing them again. Furthermore, after using a pesticide he should store the poison in its original container within a locked storage room.

Because of the large quantities of poisons which are used on the farm, surplus pesticides and empty pesticide containers are a constant threat. Unless they are disposed of properly, they can cause serious illness or deaths in pets, livestock, and humans, as well as contamination of the environment. As a general rule, the farmer should dispose of surplus pesticide by burying the chemical, without its container, in a deep pit which has been dug in sandy soil. Then, since the safest method for disposing of the pesticide container is dependent upon the type of container as well as the pesticide, he should contact his chemical supplier for disposal information. Until it can be disposed of safely, the farmer should keep the empty pesticide container in a locked storage room.

Protecting the Farm Against Fire

Each year fires destroy hundreds of millions of dollars in farm property in this country. According to the National Safety Council, "When a fire occurs on farm or rural property, the damage is three to six times greater than in the average city fire."[4] Apparently, the higher losses are the result of the greater distance from fire departments and the lack of an adequate supply of fire-fighting water on most farms.

Handling Farm-machinery Fires

Farm-machinery fires are usually small and easy to handle. However, any fire, if uncontrolled, can destroy or severely damage the machinery, spread through the fields, burn farm buildings, and kill livestock as well as humans.

In most small fires involving farm machinery, the causative elements are fuel leaks, malfunctioning carburetors, electrical shorts, exhaust sparks, defective sediment bulbs, and dust or chaff accumulations. To reduce these fire hazards, the farmer should periodically inspect the machinery in detail and follow the manufacturers' servicing instructions. Besides improving the safety of the machines, periodic inspection and servicing will help to maintain the machinery's efficiency and reliability.

In explosions and large fires one of the most common causative factors is

---

4. National Safety Council, *Farm and Ranch Safety Guide* (Chicago: NSC, 1973), p. 27.

improper refueling of machinery. When sparks or hot surfaces are present, diesel fuel and gasoline can burst into flames in a matter of seconds. During the refueling of machinery, the farmer should always shut off the engine and then, if feasible, allow it to cool before filling the tank. In addition, he should refrain from smoking at all times during the refueling process. (See Figure 16.6.)

Because of the danger presented by farm-machinery fires, the farmer should equip each of his machines with a fire extinguisher. For use on most machinery, an extinguisher with a minimum 4-B:C rating is recommended. This multipurpose dry chemical extinguisher is suitable for handling the most commonly encountered sizes and classes of fires in farm machinery. However, an extinguisher with a higher rating, although it is more expensive, will provide an added margin of protection and a much greater fire-fighting capacity. Thus before purchasing a fire extinguisher, the farmer should probably consult with his local fire department or a local extinguisher distributor about the best protection for a specific piece of machinery.

Once an extinguisher has been purchased, the farmer must then determine the best position for mounting the extinguisher on the machinery. In an emergency he will need to reach the extinguisher immediately. Therefore, accessibility is the primary consideration in the mounting of an extinguisher. As a general rule, the farmer should be able to reach the mounted extinguisher both from the operator's platform and from the ground.

Storing Flammable Products

Flammable liquids and gases are commonly stored in large quantities on most modern farms. Designed to meet the demands for the refueling of machinery, refurbishing of equipment and buildings, and heating of workshops and homes, these products are essential for maximum efficiency on any farm. Yet, at the same time flammable liquids and gases are constant fire and explosive hazards. Fueled by these products, even a small fire can quickly spread out of control and eventually engulf the entire farm.

In general, the farmer should set above-ground gasoline storage tanks at least forty feet from all buildings. Tanks near a burning building will sometimes explode and spread the fire. (See Figure 16.6.) In addition, the farmer should equip the tanks with hand pumps, not faucets which might leak. On the other hand, despite a lack of a specific distance requirement for underground tanks, the farmer should probably locate the storage tanks at least twenty feet from all buildings.

On some farms large storage tanks with LP (liquefied petroleum) gas, used for cooking or heating and commonly called "bottled gas," are almost as much of a fire and explosive hazard as gasoline storage tanks. For this

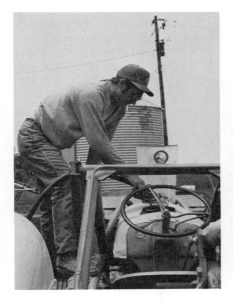 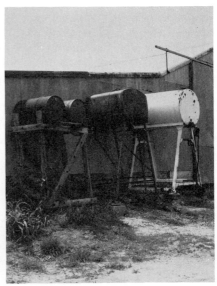

Figure 16.6   Smoking while refueling machinery and storing fuel near buildings are common fire hazards on farms.

reason, the farmer should set large LP tanks at least fifty feet from the nearest building. Furthermore, since LP gas is heavier than air and will settle in low places, he should never place small household tanks in the basement, on a low porch, or directly over a window or ventilator. As a general rule, the farmer should locate the tanks at least three feet from a window or door and at least six feet from a lightning rod cable.

Because most fires and explosions with LP gas involve leaks or system failures, improper transfer of liquid from one tank to another, or accidental line or tank ruptures, producers have odorized the gas as a warning to consumers. If he smells a strong and persistent odor of gas, the farmer should immediately turn off the tanks' valves, open windows and doors to ventilate the building, telephone the gas service dealer, and then evacuate the building.

Although gasoline and LP storage tanks present the greatest danger of fires and explosions, solvents, paints, starter fluids, and similar products are also common hazards on the farm. Because of their flammable nature, such products should always be stored by the farmer in their original containers and in a locked storage shed, thereby shielded from the sun and other sources of heat.

Preventing Electricity-related Fires

In an age of expanded mechanization, electricity is a frequent cause of farm fires. Even the slightest spark in an environment of stored products, such as grain and hay, or in wooden buildings may generate a major fire.

On the farm, as in the city, poor wiring and overloaded circuits are frequent causes of electricity-related fires. Sometimes poor wiring is the result of faulty installation or subsequent physical damage to the system. However, on older farms poor wiring may be the result of aging and deterioration by chemicals, heat, and moisture. In addition, the wiring on many older farms, although it was once adequate, may not be designed to service a large number of electrical machines and devices. Consequently, overloaded circuits are common problems.

Since overloading the circuits may cause the wires to burn their insulation, short-circuit, and give off sparks, electrical systems are protected by fuses or breakers which will "blow" or "break" when their safe carrying capacities are exceeded. Therefore the continual blowing of fuses or the breaking of circuit breakers is the most reliable warning that overloading has occurred. If he suspects overloading, the farmer should switch off all unnecessary lights and devices or connect them to other circuits. If this fails to solve the problem, he should contract with an electrician for the adding of new circuits or the rewiring of the old circuits to increase their capacity. The farmer himself should never tamper with fuses or breakers in an attempt to keep them from blowing or breaking, since they are the best safeguards against electricity-related fires.

In addition to poor wiring and overloading, electrical-device failures are common causes of farm fires. Often motors, due to excessive dirt, overloading, poor ventilation, arcing, or sparking, will ignite chaff, grease, trash, and other combustible materials on or near them. Also, shorts or internal failures will sometimes cause motors to burst into flames. Similarly, power tools, sweepers, heaters, and other electrical devices will often ignite nearby combustible materials or burst into flames as a result of internal wiring failures, faulty power cords, or malfunctioning switches.

To lessen the possibility of electrical-device failures, the farmer should clean motors periodically, provide adequate ventilation for them, and keep the areas around them free of flammable and combustible materials. In addition, he should periodically inspect all electrical devices for shorts, frayed insulation, and faulty switches and then service the devices according to the manufacturers' instructions. However, if he notices that a device fails to work or works poorly, makes unusual sounds, smokes or produces a burned smell, or pops or gives off sparks, the farmer should unplug the device and secure the services of a qualified repairman to correct the problem.

In addition, on many farms ordinary light bulbs are unexpected causes of electricity-related fires. According to tests, the surface of a clean 200-watt light bulb may reach a temperature of 437 degrees Fahrenheit. However, if it is dusty or dirty, the bulb may become even hotter, since the dust keeps the heat from escaping into the surrounding air. By comparison, dry hay or similar material will ignite when it is exposed to a temperature of about 400 degrees Fahrenheit. Chaff and cobwebs, on the other hand, will start to burn at a lower temperature.

Because of the fire hazard presented by bulbs, dust, and combustible materials, the farmer should protect light bulbs with glass globes or guards in dusty areas, such as granaries and barns. The glass fixtures will act as heat barriers. Furthermore, in areas frequented by animals, the farmer should protect the light bulbs and their glass globes or guards against breakage with heavy metal guards.

Making the Farm Lightning-proof

Sometimes referred to as "nature's electricity," lightning is an effect of electrification within a thunderstorm. According to whether or not the flow of current lasts long enough to ignite flammable materials, a lightning bolt may be classified as either "cold" or "hot." Approximately one out of every three bolts are hot.[5] Despite their relatively fewer number, hot bolts occur with sufficient frequency to establish lightning as a major cause of farm fires. Each year over 30 percent of all rural fires are caused by lightning.

In its constant effort to reach the ground, lightning will always travel over the shortest path which offers the least resistance. Thus barns, loafing sheds, livestock buildings, and other tall structures with metallic parts are especially vulnerable to bolts of lightning. In a typical strike a lightning bolt will follow a path along the metal frame of the building to the ground. At points along the metallic path, the main bolt may leap from the frame to electrical wiring or metal plumbing fixtures, or parts of the bolt may sideflash to metal livestock stalls or farm machinery. Since lightning may generate as much as 250,000 amperes of electric current and reach a temperature of 36,000 degrees Fahrenheit, the bolt will usually ignite flammable materials as it travels along the metallic path.

At present a lightning-protection system is the only means of preventing lightning-related fires on the farm. Basically the system is designed to provide a direct, low-resistance path for a lightning bolt to follow to the ground and thus to prevent damage, injury, and death as the bolt travels along its path. According to the National Safety Council, a properly designed, in-

---

5. Merrill S. Timmins, Jr., *Lightning Protection for the Farm* (Washington, D.C.: U.S. Government Printing Office, Revised January, 1968), p. 2.

stalled, and maintained lightning-protection system will provide farm buildings with almost 100 percent protection.[6]

For the surest and safest protection, the farmer should select a lightning-protection system which will be installed under the Master Label quality inspection program of Underwriters' Laboratories. Only Master Label installers, as accredited by the Laboratories, can make installations under the program. Quite simply, the Master Label indicates that the lightning-protection system has been manufactured and installed according to the Underwriters' Laboratories most exacting specifications.

Harvesting and Storing Hay

Green, uncured, or wet hay has been involved in numerous farm fires in recent years. Because they can occur at any time, day or night, such fires are often beyond control at the time of their detection.

In a process called spontaneous combustion, wet hay gives off carbon which then combines with oxygen in the air. During this chemical reaction, energy changes occur in which heat is liberated at a tremendous rate. As a result, the stored hay bursts into flames.

To reduce the possibility of spontaneous combustion, the farmer should harvest loose or chopped hay at a low enough moisture content to prevent molding, a key factor in the reaction. However, some hays, long after their leaves appear to be perfectly dry, retain moisture in their stems. Thus for further protection the farmer should equip his storage area with an approved electric fan to dry and cure the hay.

After storing the material, the farmer should check daily for at least several weeks for steaming, irritating odors, or wet spots. If he suspects heating, he should then drive a pipe deep into the hay and lower a thermometer through the pipe. After ten minutes the farmer should raise the thermometer and read the temperature. If the reading is 175 degrees Fahrenheit or greater, a fire may soon be imminent. For this reason, he should then remove the hay or divide the hay into small, shallow stacks. However, if the reading is 212 degrees or greater, a fire is imminent and may occur at any moment. In this situation the farmer should call the fire department, remove animals and machinery from the building, and then cool the hay with water.

Burning Off Fields

Because of the possibility of an uncontrolled fire, safety officials do not recommend burning as a method of clearing fields. Yet, for various reasons, many farmers feel that they must use this method. If he plans to

---

6. National Safety Council, "Fire Prevention on the Farm and Ranch," *Rural Accident Prevention Bulletin* (Chicago: NSC, n.d.), p. 4.

burn off a field, the farmer should first plow a six-foot-wide firebreak around the area to be burned and then alert the fire department. In addition, he should always burn against the direction of any breeze, never with it. Obviously, because of the danger, he should never burn during high winds.

Preparing for Fires

One of the chief problems on most farms is the lack of suitable resources for firefighting. In the absence of proper equipment, even a small fire may quickly develop into a large, uncontrolled blaze that can cause considerable damage to farm machinery, stored crops, livestock, and buildings.

In order to fight small combustible-material fires (Class A), the farmer should place buckets and water barrels in all major buildings on the farm. In addition, if he has water under pressure, he should place numerous garden hoses in locations where they can be quickly unrolled to reach the buildings during a fire. On the other hand, for fighting flammable-liquid (Class B) and electrical (Class C) fires, the farmer should mount commercial extinguishers in high-risk buildings such as machine sheds and barns. In general, for maximum utility, the extinguishers should be of the multi-purpose type, either carbon dioxide or dry chemical. Before purchasing any fire extinguishers, the farmer should always check with his local agricultural representative and his local fire department for advice on the best types and sizes of extinguishers for his particular farm.

Unfortunately, not all farm fires are small; hence the local fire department is still the best source of firefighting help. However, to function effectively the fire department must have access to large quantities of water. For this reason, the farmer should provide an emergency water supply pond within pumping distance of all buildings. Ideally, the pond should be designed to provide a year-round supply of water, as well as an easy access road for fire department pumpers. If he cannot provide a pond, he should build an emergency three-thousand-gallon or greater capacity cistern in an area centrally located near the farm buildings. For plans on building a pond or cistern, the farmer should contact his local farm representative.

Resource Materials

American Farm Bureau Research Foundation
225 Touhy
Park Ridge, Illinois 60068

American Insurance Association
85 John Street
New York City, New York 10038

4-H Program
Extension Service
U.S. Department of Agriculture
Washington, D.C. 20250

Future Farmers of America
National FFA Center
Box 15160
Alexandria, Virginia 22309

Manufacturing Chemists' Association
1825 Connecticut Avenue, N.W.
Washington, D.C. 20009

National Consumers Committee for Research and Education
1785 Massachusetts Avenue, N.W.
Washington, D.C. 20036

National Agricultural Chemicals Association
1155 15th Street, N.W.
Washington, D.C. 20005

U.S. Department of Agriculture
Agriculture Research Service
Federal Center Building
Hyattsville, Maryland 20782

Activities

1. Visit at least five local farms, and prepare a slide presentation on the safe operation of farm machinery.

2. Obtain a slow-moving vehicle (SMV) emblem, and demonstrate its unique characteristics to the class.

3. Invite a veterinarian to speak to the class about the quarantine and treatment of sick farm animals and about the disposal of dead farm animals.

4. Diagram the layout of a local farm, and suggest suitable firefighting resources for each building and the farm in general.

5. Design a poster which compares the hazards found in agricultural work to those found in industrial work.

Questions

1. What type of accident is the leading cause of tractor-operator deaths?
2. What measures can be taken by the operator to prevent tractor upsets?
3. What is the PTO, and why is it dangerous?
4. Why is the slow-moving vehicle (SMV) emblem highly visible in the daytime and at nighttime?
5. What is the relationship between "maternal instinct" and farm-animal accidents?
6. What measures should be taken by the farmer when handling diseased animals?
7. What is the proper method for disposing of surplus pesticides?
8. What is the primary consideration in the mounting of fire extinguishers on farm machinery?
9. Why are light bulbs considered to be fire hazards on many farms?
10. Why are ponds or cisterns necessary on farms?

Selected References

"Animal Disease and Human Health," *Farm Safety Review,* March-April, 1965, 12-15.

"Developing An Effective SMV Emblem Program for Your Community," *Farm Safety Review,* March-April, 1965, 3-7.

"15 State Accident Report," *Farm Safety Review,* Special Issue, 1976, 1-16.

Knapp, Jr., L. W. "Agricultural Injury Prevention," *Journal of Occupational Medicine,* November, 1965, 545-53.

Manufacturing Chemists' Association, Inc. *Agricultural Chemicals.* Washington, D.C.: The Association, 1963.

National Agricultural Chemicals Association. *Disposing of Pesticide Containers.* Washington, D.C.: nd.

National Safety Council. *Farm and Ranch Safety Guide.* Chicago: NSC, 1973.

———. "Falls Prevention Agricultural Work," *Rural Accident Prevention Bulletin.* Chicago: NSC, nd.

———. "Fire Prevention on the Farm and Ranch," *Rural Accident Prevention Bulletin.* Chicago: NSC, nd.

"Prevent . . . Protect Against Tractor Upset," *Farm Safety Review,* September-October, 1967, 7-10.

Timmins, Merrill S., Jr. *Lightning Protection for the Farm.* Washington, D.C.: U.S. Government Printing Office, Revised January, 1968.

University of Illinois at Urbana-Champaign, Cooperative Extension Service. *Safety.* Urbana-Champaign, Illinois: The Service, April, 1975.

———. *Safe Disposal of Empty Pesticide Containers and Surplus Pesticides.* Urbana-Champaign, Illinois: The Service, nd.

———. *Hazard Hunt Checklist.* Urbana-Champaign, Illinois: The Service, June, 1975.

U.S. Department of Labor, Occupational Safety and Health Administration. *Guarding of Farm Field and Farmstead Equipment & Cotton Gins.* Washington, D.C.: The Administration, 1976.

Swimming and Boating Accidents

17

Each year swimming and boating accidents claim nearly four thousand lives, most of them through drowning. As one would expect, a large majority of the accidents occur on weekends during the summer months and involve nonswimmers. In addition, most of the accidents occur in lakes, many of which are specially designed for leisure pursuits. Although the circumstances of the accidents vary greatly, the underlying cause is usually the same: the victims were unable to cope with water emergencies. As one safety expert notes, "In an emergency most victims react as if the human body were a clumsy, heavy, metal robot."

Swimming Accidents

Undoubtedly, swimming is the most popular water activity in this country. Each year an estimated one hundred million individuals participate in some form, whether wading, floating, or actually swimming. Unfortunately, however, almost one-half of the participants cannot swim or cannot swim more than a few feet. As a result, approximately twenty-seven hundred persons drown in swimming accidents every year.

Swimming to Stay Alive

Before entering the water every individual, regardless of his age, should learn to swim at least well enough to save his own life in an emergency. While even an elderly person can learn to swim if he has the physical capability and is highly motivated, the best time for an individual to learn to swim is while he is still a child. Not only are swimming skills learned more easily at an early age, but a child may find himself in a water emergency at any time. In a typical case, in Barry, Illinois, a two-year-old boy accidentally fell into a cistern. However, although he was "doing absolutely terrible" in his YMCA swimming course for babies, the boy was able to stay afloat until he was rescued. As a rule, the exact age at which a child can best learn to swim depends upon his own maturity and motivation; but most children can become proficient swimmers by the age of six years. By contacting the Red Cross, the YMCA, the community swimming pool, or other local

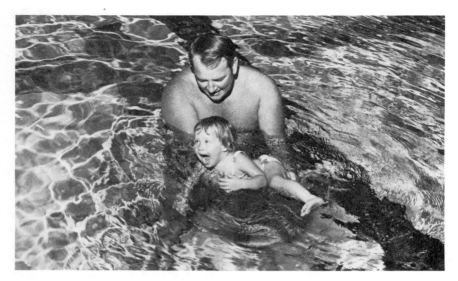

Figure 17.1   Since a child may find himself in a potential drowning situation at any time, he should be taught to swim at the earliest possible age.

groups, parents can easily arrange swimming lessons for their children, as well as for themselves.

Obviously, learning to swim is only a partial solution to the problem. Even though a person's chances of drowning decrease as his swimming skills improve, a good swimmer can still find himself in a potential drowning situation if he becomes fatigued, develops cramps, or loses consciousness. If the person is swimming in an unsupervised area, such as a pond, lake, river, or old quarry, no qualified person will be available to rescue him, and he will most likely drown. For this reason, an individual should always swim in an area which is supervised by a competent lifeguard.

However, even in a supervised situation the individual should always swim with another person who has the ability to help whenever necessary. Since the lifeguard may have several hundred people to watch, a single swimmer can easily slip below the water surface while the guard's attention is focused on another swimmer. With a swimming companion who can rescue him or alert the lifeguard, the swimmer will have a much better chance of surviving his predicament.

Since fatigue is a major factor in a large number of drowning and near-drowning situations, every swimmer should know his limitations in regard to the distance he can swim, his ability to tread water, and his ability to change directions in deep water and return to shore. Unfortunately, the feat in which most swimmers overestimate their abilities is the long distance swim. Each year many people drown while attempting to swim across large lakes or wide rivers. Before attempting a long distance swim, the swimmer should always prepare well in advance by gradually building up his distance capacity. During these training swims, as well as during the actual long distance swim itself, the individual should always swim parallel to the shore and use a back float or resting stroke whenever he is tired. Furthermore, at all times he should be accompanied by a boat with at least two occupants, one to observe and help him whenever necessary and one to steer the boat.

In addition to long distance surface swimming, many swimmers drown while attempting long distance underwater swims. Most often, the drownings are the result of hyperventilation, the common practice of taking several deep breaths before an underwater swim. While the practice will enable a swimmer to secure more oxygen, hyperventilation will also lower the carbon dioxide level in his lungs, and without a certain level of carbon dioxide in the lungs, the swimmer will not feel any need to breathe. Consequently, he will deplete his oxygen supply long before the carbon dioxide level has a chance to rise enough to signal him to breathe, and deprived of oxygen, he will suddenly, without any apparent warning, lose consciousness. Unless help is available the swimmer will quickly aspirate water and drown. Because of the danger associated with hyperventilation, the underwater swimmer should always guard against this threat. Furthermore, since hyperventilation can also result from strenuous exercise, the person should refrain from underwater swimming after vigorous surface swimming.

Regardless of the type of water activity, whether wading, floating, or swimming, children should be supervised by an adult, even when qualified lifeguards are present. In addition to supervision, small children who are playing near the water, especially if they are nonswimmers, should wear life-saving devices, preferably of the vest type, whenever the devices are available and are permitted. Under no circumstances should nonswimmers, whether children or adults, rely on water wings, inner tubes, air mattresses, or other types of free-floating artificial supports in deep water, since a loss of contact with the support or a sudden leak in it can quickly place the user in a drowning situation.

Handling Water Emergencies

Despite the observance of good safety practices, the swimmer may find himself in serious trouble if he encounters a strong current, swims into underwater plants, or develops a cramp. Yet, if the individual remains calm and takes appropriate action, these water emergencies need not result in drowning.

River Currents

Caused by flowing movements of the water, currents are always dangerous for the swimmer, since they tend to pull him away from the shore, often before he is aware of it. In rivers where the flow seldom follows the contour of the river bed, these currents are especially deceptive. Determined by back waters, islands, projecting headlands, and the windings of the stream's course, river currents tend to wander from shore to shore, even in relatively straight stretches, thus producing outward flows along both shores. Since these currents often move at four to six miles per hour, while even a good swimmer moves at less than three miles per hour, a person caught in a river current should never attempt to fight it. Instead, he should always swim downstream and diagonally toward the bank. Although swimming diagonally will bring the swimmer ashore some distance from where he entered the water, the action will at least enable him to reach safety without becoming exhausted.

Ocean Currents

Like the flow of a river, ocean currents can readily drag a swimmer away from shore. Of the several types of ocean currents, the rip current is the most dangerous, sometimes running between two and three miles per hour. Often clearly marked by the agitated water or by foam or brownish sediment on the surface of the water, a rip current is a strong outward-moving, mushroom-shaped flow of water, usually between fifty and one hundred feet wide near shore and between four and five hundred feet wide farther out. Since the current is strong enough to frustrate the swimming efforts of most individuals, the swimmer should never attempt to swim directly back to shore. Instead, he should swim parallel to the shore until he is free of the rip current. Then he can easily swim toward shore with the aid of the incoming waves.

Waterweed and Eel Grass

Commonly encountered in shallow ponds, streams, tidewater rivers, saltwater lagoons, and shallow bays, waterweed and eel grass can easily constitute a hazard for an inexperienced swimmer. Unfortunately, upon touching the weeds or grass, the person will often immediately panic and convulsively attempt to fight his way clear. However, instead of freeing the swimmer, the thrashing movements only wrap the plants tighter around his legs and arms, thereby holding him securely. Instead of fighting the waterweed or eel grass, even though they bind him tightly, the person should gently shake his limbs and slowly draw them away from the plants. At the same time he should move his entire body in the direction of the current, as the flow will help untangle and loosen the weeds or grass.

Cramps

While a cramp is ordinarily more annoying than dangerous, it can easily result in drowning for a panicky swimmer. Producing discomfort and pain, a cramp is actually a spasm or tight knot in a muscle, usually caused by cold or fatigue. Most often it will occur in the calf of the leg or the sole of the foot. However, a cramp may in infrequent cases occur in the abdomen or stomach. When it does, the cramp is extremely painful for the swimmer, typically causing him to involuntarily draw his knees and head to his chest. Fortunately, contrary to popular belief, a cramp, regardless of its location, does not incapacitate and can be easily relieved.

Upon feeling the tingling sensation which signifies the onset of a cramp, the swimmer should immediately stretch the muscles in the affected area, a procedure which will usually relieve the cramp before it can become more serious. However, if the cramp worsens, the swimmer should quickly take a deep breath, assume a facedown floating position, and, while stretching the affected muscles, massage the cramped part with both hands.

Rescuing Struggling Swimmers

Tragically, hundreds of people drown every year trying to rescue struggling swimmers. In a majority of the cases the amateur rescuers lose their lives because they panic and jump into the water after the victims, often irrespective of their ability to effect the rescue and, in some cases, regardless of whether or not they can swim. Paradoxically, while the would-be rescuers drown, the victims often are able to overcome their initial panic and swim to safety.

Without question, the worst mistake an amateur rescuer can make is to jump into the water and attempt physical contact with a struggling swimmer. Besides being unnecessary in most cases, such action can easily result in the rescuer's being drowned by the victim. Typically, in an effort to stay above the water, the struggling swimmer will seize his rescuer and climb onto him, thus forcing the rescuer's head beneath the surface of the water. Because the swimmer possesses extraordinary strength due to the adrenalin released during his panic, he can easily maintain this grip until the rescuer drowns.

Instead of immediately jumping into the water after the struggling swimmer, the rescuer, assuming he is within five to ten feet of the victim, should first try to extend some object to him. When extending a belt, shirt, towel, paddle, oar, tree branch, fishing pole, or other object, the rescuer should grip it firmly, brace himself, and slowly pull the victim to safety. According to water safety officials, even a submerged person, provided he is conscious, will instinctively grasp a firm object pressed against his chest.

When the victim is within arm's reach of the shore, pool deck, or pier and an object is not readily available, the rescuer should lie flat and extend one arm toward the victim. Upon contact, the rescuer should grasp the victim's wrist and slowly draw him to safety. However, when the rescuer cannot reach the victim from a lying position, he should then quickly slip into the water, and while firmly grasping the pool ladder, pier edge, or similar support with both hands, he should extend his feet to the victim. After the victim grabs his feet, the rescuer should either pull the victim to safety or allow the victim to pull himself to safety by means of the rescuer's extended body.

If the struggling swimmer is a great distance from shore, the rescuer should immediately toss the victim a buoyant or floatable object. Examples of such objects include beach balls, inner tubes, thermos jugs, picnic chests, wooden planks, paddles, oars, ring buoys, and cushions. Whenever any doubt exists about the buoyancy of the available objects, the rescuer should throw all of them, since at least one of the objects will most likely float. Using the object for support, the victim can then either kick his way to safety or remain afloat until a trained rescuer can be summoned.

Only as a last resort should a rescuer dive into the water and attempt to pull a struggling swimmer to safety. Yet, even then, physical contact with the victim should be avoided if possible. When swimming to a victim, the

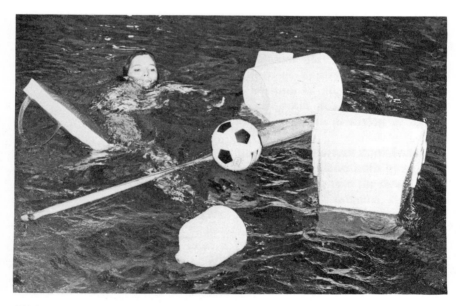

Figure 17.2   Many objects are sufficiently buoyant to support a struggling swimmer until he can kick his way to safety or until he can be rescued by another method.

rescuer should carry a towel, shirt, paddle, oar, ring buoy, or similar buoyant object and extend it to the victim upon reaching him. After the victim has grasped the object, the rescuer should slowly and carefully pull toward shore. If the victim panics and climbs across the object toward the rescuer, the person should immediately release his grip and swim away from the victim.

In the absence of any suitable rescue objects, the rescuer should swim to a position behind the victim and seize his hair. Then, using a side stroke, the rescuer should swim forcefully toward safety. If little or no progress is made or if he is in danger of being grabbed by the victim, the rescuer should release him and swim to safety.

Boating Accidents

With slightly less than one-half million boats being sold every year, boating has gradually become one of the most popular water activities in this country. Today there are an estimated eight million boats and forty million boaters in the United States. However, with this tremendous growth in boating activity, the number of boating accidents has also increased. Each year they account for almost thirteen hundred deaths and over eleven hundred injuries.

Keeping Out of Trouble

One of the most frequent types of boating accidents involves collisions with other crafts, floating objects, and persons. In a majority of the cases these accidents can be traced to the operator's inadequate knowledge and inexperience in handling and maneuvering the boat. However, they may also be caused by the operator's drinking while driving the boat or not paying enough attention to the course. Regardless of the reason, collisions rank as the leading cause of boating injuries in this country.

Although many boaters are ignorant of the fact, certain "rules of the road" regulate the movement of water traffic. The most important of these rules inform the operator which boat has the right-of-way in a crossing situation, on which side to pass another boat when meeting or over-taking it, and how to signal his intentions. When these rules are broken, collisions are likely to occur. Free copies of the boating "rules of the road," as well as instruction in all aspects of small-boat seamanship, can be obtained from the United States Coast Guard, the Coast Guard Auxiliary, the United States Power Squadron, the American National Red Cross, and other agencies. Before venturing onto the water, every boat operator, whether he has a motorboat, houseboat, sailboat, rowboat, or canoe, should thoroughly familiarize himself with these water rules.

Since many persons drink during their leisure outings, alcohol is also a significant factor in a large number of boating collisions. Typically, upon consuming three or four beers, the boat operator will demonstrate slower reflexes, poorer timing and coordination, reduced peripheral vision, decreased light and sound discrimination, and poorer judgment. To prevent alcohol-related collisions and other accidents, the boater should avoid drinking before starting onto the water, as well as while on the water. Nevertheless, if the person has been drinking, he should allow one hour of nondrinking time for each beer consumed, thus permitting the effects of the alcohol to wear off before he operates the boat.

As would be expected, numerous collisions also occur when boaters fail to see submerged or floating objects, or observe the objects too late to avoid them. Since most objects are largely underwater, even a small-looking piece of debris may actually be large enough to upset a boat or damage its hull. To spot and subsequently avoid objects in the water, the boater should be especially attentive to his course. Better still, he should avoid shallow areas where submerged objects are most readily found.

In addition to submerged or floating objects, many collisions occur when boaters inadvertently run over swimmers, skin divers, scuba divers, and water skiers. In almost all of these boat-person collisions, the individual in the water is the only injury victim, often having a limb amputated or being sliced to death by the whirling propeller. Fortunately, by paying attention to his course, the boat operator can easily avoid public beaches, coves, scuba diving flags, and ski boats, and thus prevent such accidents.

Staying Upright on the Water

Of the various types of boating accidents, capsizing-and-sinking is the leading cause of death, accounting for about one-half of all small-boat fatalities. Most often the accident is the direct result of overloading. Since overloading causes the boat to float lower than normal, a high wave or even a slight shift in weight can easily result in capsizing-and-sinking. The best way to prevent overloading is to limit the passenger weight to less than the maximum recommended by the manufacturer. By federal law each new boat must carry a capacity plate which states the maximum safe-weight load of the vessel. (See Figure 17.3.) For small, older boats which lack this information, the boater can easily estimate the number of individuals which can be safely carried by multiplying the length of the boat by its width and then dividing that product by fifteen. However, since individuals vary in weight, the number of seats in the boat is not an accurate indication of the number of persons that can be safely taken aboard. In terms of total passenger weight, a boat with every seat occupied may actually be overloaded.

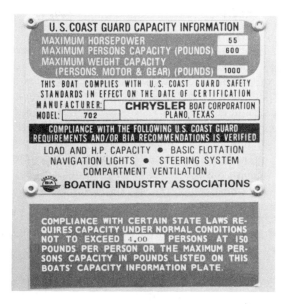

Figure 17.3 Capacity information plate.

Besides the practice of overloading a boat, capsizing-and-sinking may result from improper loading. With an excess amount of weight in a single place, the improperly loaded section of the boat will float lower than normal, thus making the boat particularly vulnerable to capsizing. Most commonly, an improperly loaded boat is the result of placing too many passengers on one side or of placing passengers in the front or the back in an effort to give the boat better trim. Generally, improper loading can be avoided by evenly distributing the passengers on both sides of the boat and by placing them in the seats provided by the boat's designer—measures which automatically give the boat its proper trim.

While most capsizing-and-sinking mishaps result from overloading and improper loading, each year a small number of the accidents involve properly loaded boats. Most often, the accidents occur when the boats are subjected to rough water. The best way to avoid such situations is to check with the nearest weather bureau or Coast Guard station for advance weather information, and to stay docked when the weather may produce rough boating conditions or when a small-craft warning has been issued. However, when the boater is already on the water, he should continually check for changes in weather conditions and immediately head for shore whenever rough weather threatens.

If for some reason the boat does swamp or capsize, the best advice is to remain calm and stay with the boat. Almost all boats, even though filled with water or upside down, will continue to float after the accident. More important, they will still support their normal passenger loads. Specifically, the occupants of a swamped boat should remain seated and, whenever possible, hand-paddle toward shore. The occupants of a capsized boat, on the other hand, should cling lightly to the outside of the boat, thus allowing most of their weight to be supported by the water. (See Figure 17.4.) Only in rare situations, such as an upcoming waterfall or a series of rapids, should the passengers abandon a swamped or capsized boat. Most swimming efforts toward shore are unsuccessful; but by staying with the boat, the occupants may be seen more easily by a search plane or rescue boat.

Remaining Afloat After Falling Overboard

Accounting for almost one-fourth of all small-boat fatalities, falling overboard ranks, behind capsizing-and-sinking, as the second-leading cause of boating deaths. Surprisingly, many of these overboard accidents occur before the boat has even left the dock, as individuals lose their balance while fueling, loading, or boarding the boat or while pulling up the anchor or pushing off. However, most of the accidents occur while the boat is underway and, as one might expect, result from unsafe practices, such as sitting on decks and gunwales, standing or walking without holding onto the boat, or suddenly turning the boat sharply at a high speed. Fortunately, most overboard accidents can be prevented by wearing proper footwear and by observing safe practices. However, since individuals may fall overboard in spite of these precautions, boaters should still insist that children, poor swimmers, and nonswimmers wear life-saving devices at all times. Furthermore, even better swimmers, if they are not wearing devices, should be instructed to don them immediately whenever the weather or other circumstances cause the slightest concern for safety.

Technically referred to as "personal flotation devices" or PFD'S, four types of life-saving devices are approved by the Coast Guard and are available to the boating public. (See Figure 17.5.) Type I and Type II PFD'S are wearable devices which turn an unconscious person from a facedown position in the water to a vertical or slightly backward position, thus keeping him from drowning. Permitting freer movement for the person who must swim some distance to safety, the Type III device is also wearable, but it is designed to keep a conscious victim in a vertical or slightly backward position. The Type IV life-saving device, unlike the others, is not wearable, but instead it is designed to be thrown to the person in the water.

According to federal law, every boat over sixteen feet in length must carry one wearable (Type I, II, or III) United States Coast Guard-approved life-saving device for every person on board. In addition, the boat must carry

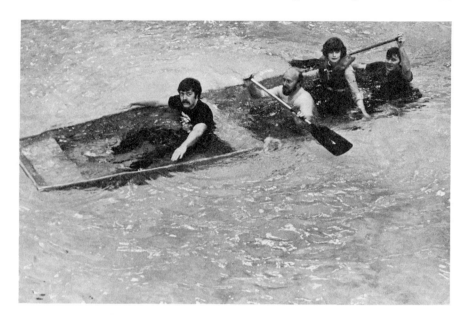

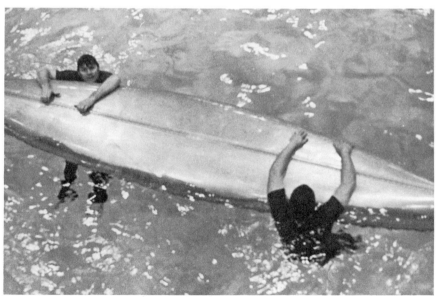

Figure 17.4 (Top) The occupants of a swamped boat should remain seated and hand-paddle for shore. (Bottom) The occupants of a capsized boat should cling lightly to the outside of the vessel and wait for help from other boaters.

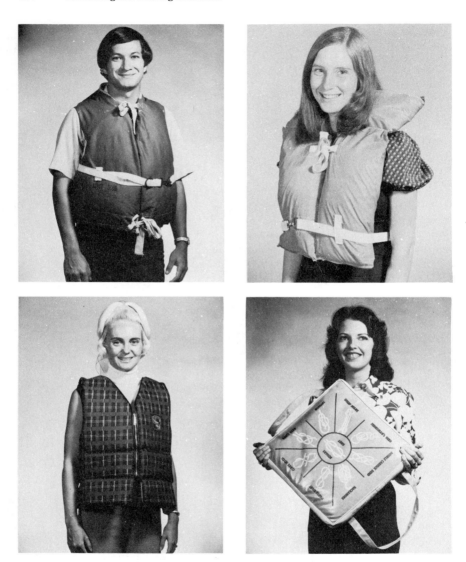

Figure 17.5 Various types of personal flotation devices: (Top left) Type I—recommended for offshore cruising, the device has more than 20 pounds of buoyancy. (Top right) Type II—recommended for closer, inshore cruising, the device has at least 15.5 pounds of buoyancy. (Bottom left) Type III—recommended for inwater sports, for close inshore operation, and on lakes or impoundments, the device has at least 15.5 pounds of buoyancy. (Bottom right) Type IV—designed to be thrown to a person in the water and not worn, the device has at least 16.5 pounds of buoyancy.

one approved throwable device (Type IV). Every boat under sixteen feet, on the other hand, must carry one approved life-saving device, either wearable or throwable (Type I, II, III, or IV), for each person on board. The same federal law provides that the devices must be in good condition and readily accessible in an emergency.

While nothing can replace an approved life-saving device, most persons who are suddenly thrown overboard can remain afloat without a device, even though fully clothed, simply by inflating a piece of their clothing and using it as a makeshift flotation device. All that is needed is an ability to tread water or at the very least an ability to float for a short period of time.

To inflate a shirt while still wearing it, either of two methods may be used. In the first method the person should tie the shirttail ends together at the waist and fasten all the buttons. Then, after taking a deep breath, he should bend his head forward into the water and blow air into the shirt between the second and third buttons. After several exhalations an air bubble will form over the person's shoulders to help support him. On the other hand, if the second method is used, the person should first fasten all the buttons and assume a floating position on his back. Then, holding the shirttails just under the surface of the water with one hand, he should cup the other hand, raise it above the surface, and quickly splash downward, thus causing air to enter the shirt. After repeating this procedure several times, the person should assume a vertical position again, thus permitting the trapped air to form a supportive bubble over the shoulders.

Unlike a shirt, slacks or trousers must be removed before they can be inflated. To accomplish this, the person should take a deep breath, bend forward, unfasten his waistband or belt, and remove the trousers one leg at a time. After the trousers have been removed, they can then be inflated by either of two methods. In the first method the person should tie the legs together at the cuffs, bend forward, and blow air into the open waistband, while keeping the trousers below the surface at all times. If the second method is used, the person should tie the legs together at the cuffs, pull up the zipper, and grasp the back of the waistband with one hand. Holding the open waist just under the surface of the water, he should then cup the free hand, raise it above the surface, and rapidly splash downward, thereby forcing air into the trousers. After inflating the trousers by either of these methods, the person should gather the waistband together and slip his head between the legs near the point where they have been tied together.

When faced with the decision of inflating either the shirt or the trousers, the person should realize that each article of clothing has its own advantages and disadvantages. For example, the shirt can be easily inflated while it is still being worn, but unfortunately, it will trap only a small amount of air. Consequently, the person must still stroke and kick to stay afloat. On the other hand, the trousers will trap a large amount of air, thus allowing the person to stay afloat without additional effort. Unfortunately, however, they must be removed before inflation, a procedure which may prove difficult for a poor swimmer.

Preventing Explosions and Fires

Even with water all around, explosions and fires are common causes of boating accidents. The reason for this is simple: being heavier than air, gasoline vapors will readily settle in the lower parts of a boat. In a confined area, such as the bilge, as little as one cupful of vaporized gasoline can produce the same explosive power as fifteen sticks of dynamite.

Most often, especially in boats with inboard motors, the source of the gasoline can be traced to a leaky carburetor or fuel line. When the gasoline is allowed to accumulate, the vapors will mix with the air, and any subsequent spark, no matter how slight, can quickly ignite the resultant explosive mixture. To prevent such an occurrence, the boater should frequently check to make sure that all the fuel connections remain tight and the bilge remains clean.

While less common, accumulated vapors may also result from careless fueling. To safely fuel outboard boats which have portable fuel tanks, the boater should remove the tanks from the vessel and fill them on the dock. Before the tanks are returned to the boat, they should be carefully wiped with a thick cloth or thoroughly flushed with water to remove any spillage. On the other hand, to safely fuel inboard boats and outboard boats with permanently installed tanks, the person should close all doors, hatches, and ports, turn off engines, fans, and motors, and extinguish galley fires, pilot lights, and cigarettes. All this should be done before he starts to fuel. During fueling, the boater should always keep the hose nozzle or the fill can in direct contact with the tank fillpipe to prevent static sparks. In addition, he should never fill the fuel tanks to full capacity, since the gasoline will expand with a rise in temperature. After fueling, he should fasten the fill cap tightly, wipe up or flush with water any spillage, and reopen the ports. In addition to these precautions, before getting underway the person should ventilate the boat for at least five minutes.

If additional gasoline must be carried aboard the boat, the boater should store the fuel in containers that have been specially designed for this purpose. Plastic bleach bottles, milk bottles, or beverage bottles are not safe storage containers for gasoline. When they are exposed to hot temperatures, such as in the bow of a boat, the plastic bottles can easily dissolve, permitting gasoline vapors to accumulate within the confined stowage compartment.

If a fire should develop aboard the boat, the operator should stop the vessel at once, thereby preventing air from fanning the flames. Then, if the burning object is small and movable and if there is no danger of burning the hands or catching the clothing on fire, he can extinguish the flames by tossing the object overboard. However, when the burning object is large or immovable or if there is danger in trying to move the object, the person should quickly put out the fire with an extinguisher. By federal law fire extinguishers must be carried in all motorboats with one or more of the following:

1. Closed compartments under thwarts and seats wherein portable fuel tanks may be stored, or
2. Double bottoms not sealed to the hull or which are not completely filled with flotation materials, or
3. Closed living spaces, or
4. Closed stowage compartments in which combustible or flammable materials are stored, or
5. Permanently installed fuel tanks.[1]

Information on the exact types and number of fire extinguishers which are required by law for the various classes of boats can be obtained by contacting the United States Coast Guard or the Coast Guard Auxiliary.

Surviving While Adrift at Sea

Being adrift at sea is perhaps the most frightening experience through which any boater can suffer. At the mercy of the elements, the person's ultimate survival is largely dependent upon his own resourcefulness. Without question, ignorance and panic in this situation is the surest route to death.

Upon finding himself adrift at sea with a dead motor, the boater should immediately tie any unneeded equipment to the anchor line and throw the anchor overboard. Even when the anchor cannot possibly reach the bottom, the vessel's drift will be slowed considerably by the dragging of the equipment through the water. Without this action, a drift of only three miles an hour will shift the boat thirty-six miles overnight, thereby increasing a rescuer's search area from a few square miles to more than three thousand square miles. Next, to make the vessel more visible to a rescuer, the person should attach a large piece of bright-colored cloth to a high mast and then drape mirrors, metal cooking utensils, and other shiny objects over various structures of the boat.

Since a rescue may take several hours, days, or even months, the boater should avoid, as much as possible, direct exposure to the elements, since this is the principal cause of death for persons stranded at sea. While a cabin will provide the best protection, adequate shelter can be obtained on boats

---

1. *New! Federal Requirements for Recreational Boats.* (Department of Transportation—Coast Guard, February, 1974), p. 5.

without a cabin by simply stretching a blanket, sheet, or sail from a mast. In hot weather the shelter will protect the individual from the glaring rays of the sun, thus preventing severe sunburn or heat stroke (sunstroke). Similarly, in cold weather the shelter will protect the person from wind, spray, and rain, thereby averting cold exposure. Without shelter, a stranded boater's chances of survival are practically null.

In addition to shelter, the boater will need a minimal supply of fresh water. Without it he can, with moderate temperatures, expect to live only eleven days at the most. When the boat is equipped with a device for desalting seawater, fresh water can usually be obtained easily. However, when a desalting device is unavailable, rain will be the only source of fresh drinking water. To catch the rain, the person should place bowls, pots, pans, skillets, and other containers around the boat. In addition, he should spread clothing, blankets, and other absorbent material on the deck. After a heavy rain the material can then be twisted and squeezed to release the water.

Since even the slightest activity requires energy, the boater will also need food. Without food he can survive at the most only twenty or thirty days in moderate weather; but in cold or hot weather he may not even survive this long, since many calories are needed each day simply to maintain an adequate body temperature. When fishing gear is available or when it can be improvised from lines and metal pins, the person's diet will consist largely of fish. Fortunately, while it may have a bad taste, fish meat, as long as it is fresh, can be eaten in its raw state. To supplement his diet, the boater should look for small crabs and shrimp which frequently attach themselves to drifting seaweed. In addition, he can scrape the barnacles from under the hull and eat the soft insides or use them for fishing bait.

Undoubtedly, despite shelter, fresh water, and food, a boater who is adrift can perish if he is unable to alert a passing boat or ship of his plight. To signal for assistance in daytime, the boater should grasp an article of bright-colored clothing in each hand, extend his arms outward at shoulder height, and raise and lower them about once every second. To signal at night, the same motion can be used effectively by simply substituting flashlights or flares for the clothing. Because the motion is slow and deliberate, it is always recognized as a distress signal and not as a friendly wave.

Resource Materials

The American National Red Cross
(Contact your local chapter for
  materials)

Boating Industry Associations
401 North Michigan Avenue
Chicago, Illinois 60611

Boat Manufacturers Association
401 North Michigan Avenue
Chicago, Illinois 60611

Council for National Cooperation in
   Aquatics
Three Hillandale Drive
New Rochelle, New York 10804

Department of Transportation
United States Coast Guard
Office of Boating Safety
Washington, D.C. 20590

National Safety Council
444 North Michigan Avenue
Chicago, Illinois 60611

Outboard Boating Club of America
401 North Michigan Avenue
Chicago, Illinois 60611

United States Power Squadrons
50 Craig Road
Montvale, New Jersey 07645

Activities

1. Contact the YMCA or the local chapter of the American Red Cross, and request permission for the entire class to observe a swimming session for babies and/or older adults.

2. Invite a lifeguard to speak to the class about the many problems that he encounters while guarding a large group of swimmers.

3. Prepare a bulletin board display depicting the various methods of rescuing a struggling swimmer without making direct contact with him.

4. Contact the nearest United States Coast Guard office, and request information on boating "rules of the road." Summarize these rules in a list, and distribute a copy to each member of the class.

5. Secure the four types of personal flotation devices, and model them, preferably in a swimming pool, for the class members.

Questions

1. When is the best time in life for a person to learn to swim?
2. Why is the practice of taking several deep breaths before an underwater swim extremely dangerous?
3. What is the most dangerous type of ocean current for the swimmer?
4. How can the swimmer relieve a cramp?
5. What is the worst mistake that an amateur rescuer can make when attempting to rescue a struggling swimmer?
6. Of the various types of boating accidents, which is the leading cause of death, and how can it be prevented?

7. On a boat which lacks a capacity information plate, how can the person estimate the number of individuals which can be safely carried aboard the vessel?
8. What are the four types of PFD'S, and how do they differ in performance characteristics?
9. Why is gasoline especially dangerous when it is allowed to accumulate around a leaky carburetor or fuel line on a boat?
10. Upon finding himself adrift at sea with a dead motor, why should the boater immediately tie any unneeded equipment to the anchor line and throw the anchor overboard?

Selected References

The American National Red Cross. *Basic Outboard Boating.* Washington, D.C.: ANRC, 1964.

———. *Lifesaving, Rescue and Water Safety.* Garden City, New York: Doubleday & Company, Inc., 1974.

———. *Basic Rescue and Water Safety.* nc: ANRC, 1974.

Capen, Edward K. and Helen B. Watson. *Swimming and Water Safety.* Dubuque, Iowa: Wm. C. Brown Company Publishers, 1968.

Carper, Jean. "Boating Safety Is No Accident," *Reader's Digest,* May, 1973, 57-60, 61.

———. *Stay Alive!* Garden City, New York: Doubleday & Company, Inc., 1965.

Department of Transportation—Coast Guard. *New! Federal Requirements for Recreational Boats.* Washington, D.C.: Department of Transportation, February, 1974.

———. *(Almost) Everything You Ever Wanted to Know About Boating . . .* *. . .But Were Ashamed to Ask.* Washington, D.C.: Department of Transportation, July, 1976.

Smith, F. D. Walton. *The Seas in Motion.* New York: Thomas Y. Crowell Company, 1973.

Sparano, Vin T. "How Safe Is Your Boat," *Outdoor Life,* February, 1974, 16-19.

Troebst, Cord-Christian. "How to Survive . . . Anywhere," *Popular Science,* August, 1966, 62-65, 172, 175.

Waters Jr., John M. "How to Avoid Getting in Trouble with Your Boat," *Popular Mechanics,* February, 1967, 161-63, 213.

Underwater Diving Accidents

18

Along the coastal regions of this country, skin- and scuba-diving accidents have presented a problem for safety officials for many years. More recently, as the sports have grown in popularity, more and more persons are dying in quarries, rivers, and lakes throughout the United States. While the exact number is unknown, an estimated two hundred persons are killed in underwater diving accidents every year.

In Miami Beach, Florida, two skin divers, while looking for underwater life, inadvertently swam too far out to sea; only the younger and stronger diver made his way back to the beach to tell the story. After a two-day search, authorities in Dayton, Ohio, were finally able to recover the body of a young scuba diver. Although the man was wearing a diving watch to tell him how much air he had left, an investigation revealed that the diver had exhausted his air supply and drowned. As these cases illustrate, the circumstances surrounding skin- and scuba-diving accidents are quite varied. Yet, as some safety experts believe, many diving accidents may result from the same underlying cause: modern equipment items make the sports too easy for overconfident, novice divers.

Skin-diving Accidents

Skin diving has become in recent years one of this country's fastest growing water sports. Today, encouraged by reports on the beauty and adventure to be found in the underwater world, more than eight million individuals engage in some aspect of the sport, such as spearfishing, rock or reef exploration, underwater photography, or treasure hunting.

Choosing the Sport

Without question, skin diving is one of the more strenuous water sports. In terms of energy expenditure, swimming underwater at only one mile per hour is equivalent to running on land at six miles per hour. For this reason, before attempting any skin diving the person should receive a complete physical examination and secure his physician's approval to participate in the sport. While the examination will usually reveal nothing out of the ordinary, the physical may in some cases disclose a problem which could lead to the death of the person if he engaged in skin diving. For example, a heart condition, respiratory ailment, circulatory problem, ear abnormality, or other serious illness would definitely rule out an individual's participation in this sport.

Besides being in good physical condition, the person must be a skilled swimmer and lifesaver. Contrary to popular opinion, the equipment worn by a skin diver is designed as an aid for the experienced swimmer, not as a substitute for swimming ability. Before an individual is qualified to learn skin diving, he must at least possess the following abilities: swim three hundred feet on the surface while using a breast stroke with the arms and a flutter kick with the legs; swim fifty feet underwater without surfacing for air; tread water for five minutes while using only the hands; and perform a swimming rescue.

Like any other sport, skin diving has certain unique skills which must be learned by the participant. Since these skills may someday mean the difference between life and death, he should seek expert instruction before attempting his first dive. By contacting the Red Cross or the YMCA, the person can arrange for skin diving lessons, as well as scuba instruction, for little or no cost.

Selecting the Equipment

The most important piece of equipment for the diver is the mask. Designed to provide an air space between the eyes and the water, thus permitting the skin diver to see as clearly as possible, diving masks can be purchased in a variety of types and designs. However, for the beginner, a sturdy, oval or circular-shaped mask with a shatterproof glass plate is generally recommended.

To assure a good fit when purchasing a mask, the person should place the mask in the normal position over his nose and eyes, and then inhale through his nose. If the mask remains in place on his face, he can assume that it fits properly, a condition which is extremely important if the strap breaks while the person is underwater.

Next in importance to the mask for the skin diver is the snorkel or breathing tube. Composed of a mouthpiece on which the skin diver bites and a tube which remains out of the water, the snorkel is designed to allow the diver to breathe at the surface or slightly under the surface while swimming facedown in the water. Since the diver expends very little energy in remaining at the surface in this position, he can easily swim for hours while submerged, thereby keeping his full attention on the underwater world. In addition, when he observes something interesting on the

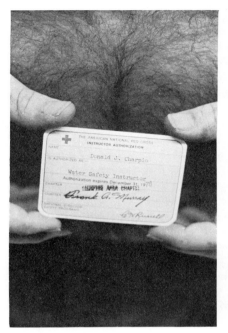 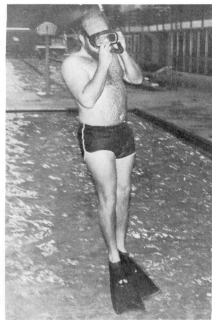

Figure 18.1   The individual must be an experienced swimmer and must learn certain unique skills to participate safely in the sport of skin diving.

bottom, the skin diver can inhale through the snorkel, hold his breath, and dive. When he surfaces again, the skin diver can quickly clear the water from the snorkel by simply blowing through his mouth.

When purchasing a snorkel, the skin diver should avoid any model with a floating valve, such as a piece of cork or a ping-pong ball, on the exposed end of the tube. Designed to automatically prevent water from entering the tube if the diver submerges or a wave breaks overhead, the valve usually allows some water to leak into the tube. More important, it often remains closed when the skin diver desperately needs air. Instead, the skin diver should select a straight-end snorkel with a smooth, comfortable mouthpiece. Besides permitting the diver to breathe easily, the straight-end snorkel will not catch on kelp, weeds, or fishing lines.

Like a mask and a snorkel, fins are essential equipment for the skin diver. Besides enabling the diver to swim about fifty percent faster than he could without them, swim fins greatly conserve his energy. Although they are available in a variety of types and designs, the beginning skin diver should select a pair of flexible fins, since they will not tire his legs as easily as a rigid pair. As his legs become accustomed to the fins, the diver can then gradually switch to the more powerful, rigid type of fins. Furthermore, if the diver plans to swim around sand, rocks, coral, or other obstructions, he should make certain that the fins have enclosed heels to protect his feet.

In fitting a pair of fins, comfort is the most important consideration. Fins which are too tight can interrupt circulation and cause cramps; fins which are too loose can lead to chafing and sores. Before purchasing a pair of fins, the skin diver should test each fin by putting it on the foot and then by moving the foot up and down several times. If the fins do not place abnormal pressure on any particular area and if they do not wobble when the feet are moved, the diver can usually assume that they fit properly.

Another valuable piece of equipment for the skin diver is a knife. However, contrary to what many people believe, this is rarely used as a weapon against sharks or other aggressive fish. Most often it is used by the skin diver as a tool to free himself from entanglement with kelp, weeds, fishing lines, ropes, or nets, or as a tool to pry loose submerged objects or to clean speared fish.

In purchasing a knife, the skin diver should select a model that has a blade made of high-tempered steel, preferably chrome steel, to prevent rusting. In addition, the blade should have two edges, one sharp edge for cutting and one serrated edge for sawing. When carrying a knife, the skin diver should make certain that the blade is enclosed within a protective sheath and that the knife can be drawn quickly without danger of causing injury.

Like the knife, an inflatable vest is a valuable part of any skin diver's equipment. Designed to inflate by cartridge or by mouth, the vest will support the diver's head in a face-up position in an accident or in a fatigue situation. Because an emergency can occur at any time, the skin diver should always wear an inflatable vest when he is diving in open-water areas.

In the selection of a vest, utility is always an important consideration. Ideally, the skin diver should choose a vest which inflates both by mouth and by a carbon dioxide cartridge. By simply blowing into the device, the diver can use the vest for support at any time he feels fatigued, thus saving the cartridge for a real emergency in which he does not have the time or the energy to inflate the vest by mouth.

Like an inflatable vest, a float is always essential when the diver is swimming in open-water areas. While a small boat is the best type of float, since it can provide transportation back to shore for a tired diver, an improvised float can be easily constructed by securing a clothes basket, a large potato sack, or some fish netting to an inflated automobile inner tube. When it is equipped with an anchor and a long sturdy line, the float will provide not only a resting place for the skin diver but also an excellent storage raft for small articles retrieved from the bottom.

Furthermore, since boaters in the area may venture dangerously close to the float, the skin diver should always attach a diver's flag to the device. A reddish-orange rectangle with a diagonal white stripe, the diver's flag is generally recognized as a warning that a skin diver is swimming within the vicinity of the float. When it is attached to the device, the flag should be at least three feet above the float to provide for good visibility. However, if the diver is nowhere near the flag, warning boats to keep their distance is meaningless. Therefore the skin diver should always restrict his activity to within one hundred feet of the flag.

Diving to Survive

Although a person's chances of drowning or seriously injuring himself decrease as his knowledge and skills improve, even an experienced skin diver may at any time find himself in trouble. For this reason, whether the skin diver is a beginner practicing in shallow water or a professional with many years of diving experience, he should always dive with another person who has the ability to help in the event of an emergency. Besides being safer, most persons find that diving with a partner is usually more fun than diving alone. In fact, some activities, such as searching for treasure or recovering items for salvage, may require the cooperative efforts of several divers.

Before diving in an unknown location the skin diver should always find out as much as possible about the area. Normally, an excellent source of information is local divers, swimmers, and fishermen who are familiar with the peculiarities of the location. By talking to these people beforehand, the diver may learn about currents, weeds, rocks, pilings, or other hidden hazards which should be avoided. As an additional advantage, the diver may discover that the community has a much better location for spearfishing, exploring, or studying underwater life than the one originally selected.

Generally, the best methods for entering the water are always the slow immersions, such as wading backward from shore, climbing down a ladder, or lowering over the side of a boat. Since rocks or other objects may lie unseen beneath the surface, the skin diver should avoid jumping into the water whenever possible. However, if he is going to swim in an area where he must jump into the water, the skin diver should hold his mask firmly in place with one hand and enter feet first so that his fins will break the force of the jump. Because the impact of the mask's striking the water can cause serious injury, the diver should never jump headfirst into the water.

When descending or swimming deeper, the skin diver will frequently experience discomfort in his ears and sinuses. Caused by increasing water pressure, this discomfort can be relieved only by equalizing the pressure between the air confined in the head and respiratory passages, and the water pressing against the eardrum. To equalize this pressure, the skin diver should stop, rise again, and swallow several times. When the pressure equalizes, he will hear a slight "popping" sound and will immediately feel normal again. However, if swallowing fails to relieve the discomfort, the diver should then hold his mask firmly against his face and exhale gently through his nose. If this method also fails, the diver should return to the surface and swim toward shore, suspending his diving activities until another day. He should never attempt to disregard the discomfort, since such action can easily result in a ruptured eardrum, even when he is diving in only ten feet of water.

When exploring the ocean, lake, or river bottom, the skin diver should always avoid swimming into tight places. This is especially important for the diver who is searching for valuables or salvage aboard a modern sunken ship. Since a weakened bulkhead can easily collapse and trap the diver within the hull, he should make certain before entering the wreck that the structure is sound and that more than one exit is available for escape in the event of an emergency. Furthermore, since many naval ships still harbor depth charges and live explosives, the skin diver should never enter this type of vessel. Even the slightest jar by the diver could easily result in a violent explosion.

When spearfishing with a spring, rubber, powder, or gas gun, the skin diver should handle the weapon as if it were a high-powered rifle. Most spearguns at close range can easily propel a spear underwater completely through a swimmer or another diver. On land the guns are even more powerful; some are even capable of driving a spear over three hundred feet. Because of the gun's greater range in air, the diver should never load the weapon until he is safely in the water. Even then he should make certain that the speargun is carried with the point down in case it should accidentally discharge. Furthermore, before firing at his prey, the skin diver should always make sure of his target, especially in water with low visibility where another diver could easily be mistaken for a fish. Naturally, after a day of spearfishing, the diver should unload the gun before leaving the water.

When ascending or returning to the surface, the skin diver should pause briefly about five feet below the surface of the water and listen in all directions for approaching boats. In addition, since a quiet inboard boat directly overhead may sometimes be mistaken for a noisy outboard boat several hundred yards away, the diver should look in all directions before surfacing. When the visibility is poor, he should extend one hand toward the surface to prevent injury to his head if he should strike a whirling propeller, an anchored boat, or a floating object. Upon reaching the surface, the diver should turn in a full circle and look carefully for approaching boats.

Dealing with Hostile Marine Life

Perhaps the greatest concern for most saltwater skin divers is the possibility of an unexpected attack by hostile marine life. Fortunately, most sea creatures are relatively harmless, and even the dangerous creatures will usually cause little difficulty for the diver if he stays away from them. However, since the skin diver may inadvertently attract or provoke many potentially hostile marine creatures, he should be able to recognize and cope with them whenever they are in his diving vicinity. Of the various forms of dangerous marine life, moray eels, barracudas, and sharks usually present the greatest threat to the diver.

Moray Eels

Found in warm waters, moray eels are long, slender, almost finless creatures with strong jaws and razor-sharp teeth. While there are several species of moray eels, the most vicious is the green moray, which sometimes reaches a length of ten feet and a girth of eighteen inches. Most often, the moray eel is found with its head protruding from a hole in a coral reef, a pile of rocks, or a shipwreck, but it can be found in almost any underwater area with a large enough hole in which to hide and a sufficient supply of fish on which to feed.

Although the moray eel is not poisonous, it is sometimes referred to as the "rattlesnake of the sea" because of its short temper, quickness to strike, and lightning-fast vicious bite. Fortunately, the creature will not attack a diver unless it is disturbed in its hiding place or antagonized in open water. Since a moray eel is difficult to spot, the diver should avoid reaching into any hole or crevice without first cautiously determining its contents. When a moray eel is sighted, the diver should always leave it alone, since trying to spear it or swimming back and forth in front of it may provoke an attack.

Barracudas

Inhabiting the warm coastal waters of the southern United States, barracudas are elongated, slender fish with fanglike, knife-sharp teeth. Except for the great barracuda which may grow eight to ten feet long, the barracuda averages about three feet in length. It is commonly found around coral reefs, buoys, wrecks, and wharves, usually resting almost motionless just beneath the surface.

When the barracuda is aroused to attack, it is the most dangerous of all the marine creatures, including the shark. Because of the barracuda's speed, which is often greater than thirty-five miles per hour, the fish can easily strike a skin diver and retreat before the diver has the chance to react. Thus the diver can never hope to repel an aggressive barracuda with a speargun, knife, camera case, or other piece of diving equipment.

Fortunately, except in self-defense, the barracuda will seldom deliberately attack a skin diver. However, it may strike by mistake, as when a part of the skin diver's body resembles the barracuda's prey. Since light-colored or shiny objects may look to the barracuda like the underbelly of a fish, the diver should avoid wearing white clothes which may flutter in the water or small metal ornaments which may catch the light. In addition, because rapid movements may be mistaken by the barracuda for the thrashing of a wounded fish, especially in murky water where the barracuda has only a partial view of the diver, the skin diver should avoid excessive splashing when he is swimming on the surface or slightly below it.

Despite the fact that the barracuda will seldom deliberately attack a diver unless it is provoked, the fish's behavior is always frightening for an inexperienced diver. Possessing a great deal of curiosity, the barracuda will often sneak up on the diver from behind. Usually when the diver discovers the presence of the fish and turns toward it, the barracuda will swim away without confronting him. However, if the barracuda begins wiggling its tail, flexing its jaws, and shaking its entire body—behavior which often precedes an attack—the skin diver should retreat in a slow, quiet, back-pedaling manner toward the boat or the shore, watching the barracuda at all times.

Sharks

A "living fossil," the shark has descended with few changes from fish that inhabited the seas millions of years ago. It has a cartilaginous skeleton, an extremely tough hide, much like coarse sandpaper, and, most important to the skin diver, powerful jaws and sharp teeth which tear rather than cut away large chunks of flesh from its prey. Ranging in size from two feet to thirty feet, depending upon the particular species, the shark is undoubtedly the most-hated, as well as the most-feared, creature in the sea. As Williams notes:

> When men catch sharks, they do not simply kill them, they mutilate them as though in the grip of an ancient rite. They hatchet fins, chop out jaws, slit open bellies. Men hate sharks. They hate them a lot. But the reality of the creature's existence cannot truly be confronted. The shark is deft and original and very ancient. Dead or alive, it inhabits impossible depths and will inhabit them forever.[1]

Contrary to popular opinion, the shark is not by nature a man-eater.

---

1. Joy Williams, "Tigers of the Sea," *Reader's Digest,* October, 1974, p. 156.

Although some old, sick, wounded, or diseased sharks, which are too slow to compete with other sharks for their normal prey, will turn to man and other slower creatures for food, the shark is usually eager to retreat when it confronts a skin diver. Nevertheless, while the shark is generally timid and cowardly, it is also unpredictable and thus very dangerous.

Obviously, the shark is always capable of deliberately striking at a diver, but most attacks seem to occur when skin divers inadvertently become involved in the shark's feeding pattern. For this reason, the skin diver should always view the shark as a perpetually hungry creature which is constantly searching for food, and he should take special precautions to avoid attracting the shark or arousing it to attack. Since the shark may view a flapping object near the surface as food, perhaps because it is accustomed to finding wounded fish and garbage from ships there, the diver should avoid wearing loose fitting clothes or splashing when he is swimming near the surface. Furthermore, because the blood and flapping of a wounded fish may attract the shark from a great distance, the spearfisherman should never carry his catch around his waist. Instead, he should either tow the fish on a minimum of twenty feet of line or, better still, immediately remove the speared fish from the water. Moreover, the skin diver should always leave the water as soon as possible if he is injured or bleeding.

Since the shark's behavior is determined by its species, its state of hunger, and its emotional state, no set of rules for dealing with the creature will apply in every encounter. In some instances the shark may be extremely curious, but in other cases he may be timid and eager to retreat. Generally, however, the shark will pursue a skin diver if he attempts to flee from it, but the creature will retreat if the diver swims toward it as if to attack. "Apparently," as Carrier notes, "the shark feels that any creature which dares attack it must be a formidable adversary indeed."[2] If a shark approaches the skin diver, he should remain submerged, face the creature, and simulate an attack by moving toward it and jabbing in its direction with a speargun, camera, or other piece of diving equipment. However, if this fails to frighten away the shark, the diver should then slowly swim backward toward the boat or the shore, facing the shark at all times until he reaches a safe location.

Scuba-diving Accidents

Sooner or later most skin divers, especially those who are intrigued by salvage work, treasure hunting, or underwater photography, become

---

2. Rich and Barbara Carrier, *The Complete Book of Skin Diving* (New York: Wilfred Funk, Inc., 1963), p. 31.

interested in scuba diving. Equipped with scuba equipment (Self-Contained Underwater Breathing Apparatus), the diver, much like the fish that swim around him, can explore the underwater world for hours with almost complete freedom. However, like skin diving, scuba diving is only as safe as the participant.

Selecting Additional Equipment

In addition to the basic equipment which is used for skin diving, the scuba diver must select and purchase a self-contained underwater breathing apparatus, a watch, a depth gauge, and a compass. Also, if he plans to dive in cold water, the person must purchase some type of exposure suit.

The self-contained breathing apparatus is composed of five parts: (1) a metal cylinder which acts as a storage tank for the compressed air; (2) an air valve which fits into the top of the cylinder and retains the compressed air until it is ready to be used; (3) a breathing regulator which reduces the pressure of the air in the cylinder to a pressure equal to that of the water around the diver, no matter what the depth; (4) a breathing tube and a mouthpiece which deliver air to the diver; and (5) a harness which attaches the entire breathing apparatus to the diver's back. For guidance, before purchasing a self-contained underwater breathing apparatus, the beginning diver should discuss his needs with a certified scuba instructor or a diving equipment representative.

Next to the breathing apparatus in importance for the scuba diver is the underwater wristwatch. While it is essential on long dives to provide a record of the time spent at a depth, thus allowing the person to avoid decompression or to make decompression stops, the wristwatch is used primarily by the diver to estimate the amount of air left in his cylinder. Before purchasing a wristwatch the scuba diver should check the manufacturer's statement concerning the maximum depth at which it will remain waterproof. If no statement is available, the diver should avoid buying that particular watch, for it may leak at greater depths because of the increased water pressure.

Like the pressure-proof wristwatch, the depth gauge is an essential piece of equipment for the scuba diver. Only by watching his depth gauge can the sport diver avoid depths which, if he remains there too long, will require decompression. When purchasing a depth gauge, the diver should generally select a model with a small depth range, since this feature permits easier, more accurate reading of the gauge.

Another piece of essential equipment for the scuba diver is the underwater compass. During searches or explorations, especially in murky water, the compass is the diver's only way of telling direction. When selecting a compass, the diver should consider the frequency with which it will be used. If he will only occasionally use the instrument, the scuba diver should probably choose the less expensive combination compass and depth gauge. However, if the diver will be doing a great deal of work with the instrument, he should select the more precise single unit compass.

For the person who plans to dive in water colder than 70 degrees Fahrenheit, an exposure suit is also a necessary piece of equipment. Designed to insulate the diver, thus conserving his energy and making him comfortable in cold water, exposure suits are available in two basic types: the dry and the wet. Constructed of thin rubber or plastic and worn over woolen underwear or other insulating garments, the dry suit is designed to exclude water, thereby maintaining an insulating layer of air between the diver's body and the suit. On the other hand, the wet suit, which is generally made from a thick, spongy material called foam neoprene, is designed to permit a small amount of water to enter and to be warmed by the diver's body heat. This water, along with the thousands of tiny air bubbles in the material itself, acts as an insulating layer. Although each type of exposure suit has its advantages and disadvantages, the wet suit is far more practical for the sport diver than the dry suit, since in the event of a sudden tear, it will not lose its overall insulating properties or its buoyancy.

Avoiding Unique Scuba Hazards

Besides the usual problems encountered by skin divers, the scuba diver must face many unique hazards created by his breathing compressed air at great depths. Of these hazards, nitrogen narcosis, decompression sickness, and air embolism claim the most lives.

Nitrogen Narcosis

When the scuba diver is swimming underwater at great depths and breathing air from his cylinder, his blood absorbs large amounts of nitrogen gas, which is the major component (79%) of the air. While nitrogen gas is normally inert, under pressure it produces a curious effect on the nervous system, similar to that of alcoholic intoxication. This condition, referred to as nitrogen narcosis or "rapture of the depths," hampers normal mental activity, produces changes in mood, inhibits coordinated body movements, and causes an overpowering feeling of drowsiness—factors which reduce the diver's ability to accomplish a task. More important, nitrogen narcosis eliminates the scuba diver's instinct for self-preservation, thus causing him to act in foolish ways. For example, even Jacques Cousteau, the famous diver and "father of scuba," reports his having experienced a case of nitrogen narcosis in which he saw a fish and wanted to give it his mouthpiece so the little thing would not drown.

While the condition occurs suddenly, individuals differ in their susceptibility to nitrogen narcosis. Some scuba divers begin to feel its effects at a depth of seventy-five feet, while others start to sense the effects at one hundred and thirty feet. Most divers, however, begin to experience some impairment at a depth of one hundred feet. As the scuba diver reaches increasingly greater depths, this impairment becomes even greater, often to the extent that he cannot escape the extreme drowsiness which eventually leads to unconsciousness and finally to drowning.

To prevent nitrogen narcosis, the scuba diver should always limit his dives to depths of less than one hundred feet. Even then, with the slightest feeling of intoxication at any depth, the diver should immediately ascend to a higher level. Similarly, if his diving companion begins to show signs of unusual behavior, the diver should promptly escort him to a higher level.

Decompression Sickness

Like nitrogen narcosis, decompression sickness, which is also referred to as "the bends" or "caisson disease," results from the effects of nitrogen gas while it is under pressure. Upon entering into solution in the blood, the nitrogen travels by way of the bloodstream to all the body tissues, where it stays in solution until the diver rises to a higher level. Then, when the diver ascends, the nitrogen, because of the decrease in water pressure, leaves the tissues, enters the blood, and moves through the bloodstream to the lungs for elimination from the body.

As long as the diver ascends slowly, thus permitting sufficient time for the removal of most of the gas, the nitrogen in his body does not cause problems. On the other hand, if he ascends too rapidly, large amounts of nitrogen remain in the blood and in the body tissues, and, in turn, readily form small bubbles which expand, thus blocking blood circulation to vital organs or causing tissue damage in different parts of the body.

Generally, the amount of nitrogen that enters into solution in the blood and the body tissues depends upon the depth of the dive and the length of time spent at the depth. When too much gas enters into solution, the scuba diver must ascend in stages to permit the nitrogen to leave his body without bubbling, a procedure referred to as decompression. Before starting his dive, the diver should check a decompression table to determine how much time he can spend at a depth before decompression becomes necessary.

Normally, the sport diver should avoid any dive that requires decompression. By staying at depths of less than thirty-three feet, the diver can remain underwater indefinitely without need for decompression. However, if he chooses to exceed this depth, he continually should watch his bottom time and take care not to exceed the maximum bottom time listed in the decompression table. During his ascent, the diver should never rise faster than his air bubbles, or one foot per second.

Lung Injury and Air Embolism

When the scuba diver breathes from his air cylinder while underwater and then ascends, the air in his lungs expands because of the decreasing water pressure. For example, if the diver were to inhale one lungful of air at thirty-three feet, it would double in volume by the time he reached the surface. Obviously, unless the diver removes part of the air on his way to the surface, the expanding air will cause his lungs to burst.

While a burst lung is always serious, it is not necessarily fatal in itself. Far more dangerous is the possibility of an air embolism. With the bursting of the lung, air will frequently pass into nearby blood vessels. Once in the bloodstream, a bubble of air can easily become lodged in one of the small blood vessels supplying a vital part of the body, particularly the brain or the heart, and cause a circulation blockage. Unless prompt recompression is obtained to reduce the size of the air bubble—now referred to as an air embolism—and eventually force it into solution, the diver will usually die, or at the very least suffer a permanent disability.

Fortunately, air embolism can be easily prevented by proper diving technique. In fact, it is rarely seen among experienced scuba divers. Most often the victims of air embolism are beginners who panic and hold their breath during emergency ascents. To prevent the occurrence of an air embolism, the scuba diver should always exhale continuously during his ascent. Furthermore, if he feels discomfort in his chest at any time, the diver should immediately exhale more forcefully to remove additional air from his lungs.

Resource Materials

Dacor Corporation
161 North Field Road
P.O. Box 157
Northfield, Illinois 60093

Professional Association of Diving Instructors (PADI)
P.O. Box 177
Costa Mesa, California 92627

National Association of Underwater Instructors (NAUI)
P.O. Box 630
Colton, California 92324

Scuba Pro, Inc.
3105 East Harcourt
Compton, California 90221

Underwater Explorers Club
Nassau, Bahama Islands

Activities

1. Invite a PADI or NAUI certified underwater instructor to speak to the class about the sports of skin and scuba diving.

2. Invite a diving equipment representative to speak to the class about the advantages and disadvantages of the various pieces of skin- and scuba-diving equipment.

3. Prepare a bulletin board display which demonstrates the various hazards presented by hostile marine life.

4. Conduct a survey of twenty-five adults to determine their attitudes toward scuba-diving safety. Summarize and discuss the results in a short paper.

5. Prepare a twenty-five question, true-false test dealing with the material in this chapter. Distribute a copy of the test to each member of the class.

Questions

1. Before attempting any skin diving, why should a person receive a complete physical examination and secure his physician's approval to participate in the sport?
2. When purchasing a mask, how can the person determine whether or not it fits properly?
3. What is the best way for the skin or scuba diver to enter the water?
4. When descending or swimming deeper, the skin diver will frequently experience discomfort in his ears and sinuses. How can he relieve this discomfort?
5. Why should the diver never enter a sunken naval vessel?
6. Why should the skin or scuba diver pause briefly about five feet below the surface of the water when ascending or rising to the surface?
7. What potentially hostile marine creature is often referred to as the "living fossil?"
8. What special precautions can the saltwater skin or scuba diver take to avoid attracting sharks?
9. Why is the underwater wristwatch an essential piece of equipment for the scuba diver?
10. What are three unique hazards of scuba diving?

Selected References

Carper, Jean. *Stay Alive!* Garden City, New York: Doubleday & Company, Inc., 1965.

Carrier, Rich and Barbara Carrier. *The Complete Book of Skin Diving.* New York: Wilfred Funk, Inc., 1963.

Ciampi, Elgin. *The Skin Diver—A Complete Guide to the Underwater World.* New York: The Ronald Press Company, 1960.

Conference for National Cooperation in Aquatics. 4th ed.; *The New Science of Skin and Scuba Diving.* New York: Association Press, 1974.

Duffner, Gerald J. "Scuba Diving Injuries," *The Journal of the American Medical Association,* February 4, 1961, 375-78.

Harper, Donald D. *Skin and Scuba Diving Fundamentals.* Columbus, Ohio: Charles E. Merrill Publishing Company, 1968.

Williams, Joy. "Tigers of the Sea," *Reader's Digest,* October, 1974, 156-60.

Hunting, Fishing, and Snowmobiling Accidents

19

Every year more than two thousand persons are killed in hunting, fishing, and snowmobiling accidents in the United States. Another forty-five thousand persons are seriously injured. Although most of the accidents involve persons between the ages of twenty and forty, more and more victims in recent years have been over sixty-five years of age. Moreover, many of the older victims are recent retirees. As a young woman, whose father was disabled in a fishing accident, sobbingly observed, "He worked hard all his life, and now, he'll have to spend his retirement in a wheelchair. It's not fair."

Hunting Accidents

Approximately nine hundred persons are killed annually in hunting accidents, and fifteen thousand persons are wounded. In nearly one-half of the accidents, young hunters, under twenty-one years of age, are judged to be at fault. Many of these young hunters are inexperienced, but contrary to popular belief, inexperienced hunters are not the most accident-involved segment of the hunting population. Actually, persons with three to five years of experience are most often involved in hunting accidents. Apparently because of their experience, the hunters often become over-confident and careless and, as a result, fail to handle their guns with the proper respect.

According to the nature of the mishap, hunting accidents may be classified as either intentional or unintentional discharge.

Intentional Discharge Accidents

Approximately sixty-five percent of all hunting accidents result from hunters' carelessly firing at game.

Choosing a Safe Companion

Most hunting injuries, both fatal and nonfatal, are not self-inflicted. Almost two-thirds of the injuries are inflicted by the victims' hunting companions. To lessen the possibility of being shot by a person in his own hunting party, the hunter should always choose companions who are responsible and careful. Whenever a hunting companion acts in a dangerous manner, the hunter should immediately reprimand him. If the companion continues to act dangerously, the hunter should stop his activity for the day and refuse to hunt with the individual again.

In addition, since beginners with double-gauges and autoloaders often become excited after a shot and carelessly fire again at the game, the hunter should always limit a beginning hunting companion to one shell in his gun. After the companion has proven that he is responsible and careful, usually after several trips, the hunter can then permit the beginner to carry additional shells in his gun.

Alerting Other Hunters

Because of the color of their clothing, hunters sometimes blend into the surrounding foliage. As a result, they are often mistakenly viewed as game by other hunters and then accidentally shot. From a safety viewpoint, camouflage-khaki is the worst type of hunting clothing. On the other hand, red clothing is undoubtedly more visible than grey or green outfits, but it is still not the safest hunting attire. In addition to appearing black at daybreak or dusk, red clothing is indistinguishable to the more than one-half million color-blind hunters who are in the fields and woods every year. Because fluorescent orange is exceptionally visible, even after sunset, and also can be easily seen by hunters with color-perception problems, this color is the safest for hunting attire. Thus, to alert other hunters that he is not game, the hunter should always wear a fluorescent-orange jacket, preferably in combination with a hat of the same color.

Preventing Stray Bullets

Occasionally, hunters are killed by stray bullets fired from the other side of hills, lakes, woods, or forests. Because some types of ammunition can travel several miles and still cause death, the hunter should always know the effective range of his ammunition. For example, rifle bullets and shotgun shells with slugs possess the greatest range, usually between three-fourths of a mile and three and one-half miles. On the other hand, shotgun shells loaded with shot possess the shortest range, usually between one hundred and fifty and three hundred yards, depending upon the gauge of the gun, the size of the shot, and the charge of the powder. For this reason, before firing at any game, the hunter should always remember that a missed shot may wound or kill another individual some distance away just as easily as a person nearby.

Unfortunately, missed shots are not the only type of stray missile which can kill. Hunters are sometimes killed by bullets or shot which had glanced off hard, flat surfaces. Referred to as ricochets, these stray shots can sometimes travel more than five hundred yards after striking hard surfaces, and can still often penetrate a board nine inches thick. Because of the danger of striking another hunter or himself with a ricochet shot, the hunter should always avoid shooting at trees, rocks, water, or other flat surfaces which could deflect a bullet or shot.

Keeping the Gun Free of Obstructions

An obstruction in the barrel is not a common cause of hunting accidents, but periodically, a few hunters lose their lives when their guns explode during discharge. Perhaps the most common, as well as the most dangerous obstruction, is the small shell which has been inadvertently inserted into a gun of a larger bore. (See Figure 18.1.) Since the smaller shell slides downward into the barrel of the larger gauge gun, the hunter may, after pulling the trigger, insert another shell, believing the gun has misfired. With this second shell of the correct size or gauge, the gun will explode in the hunter's face, thereby causing severe injury or death. To eliminate the possibility of inserting the wrong-size shell into his gun, the hunter should avoid carrying two gauges of shells. Furthermore, after returning from his hunting trip, he should immediately remove all of his shells from his jackets and vests, since a gun of another gauge may be used during his next trip.

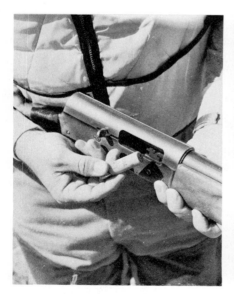 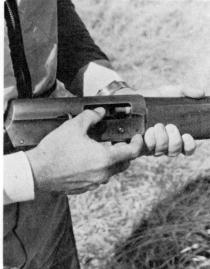

Figure 19.1   The insertion of a twenty-gauge shell into a twelve-gauge gun can easily produce an obstruction in the barrel.

While dirt, mud, sand, and similar substances rarely cause accidents, in sufficient amounts the materials can obstruct the barrel of a gun and cause an explosion. For this reason, after walking through thick underbrush or dropping or laying the weapon on the ground, the hunter should always unload his gun and check for foreign matter. If any material is present, he should immediately remove the obstruction. Obviously, because of the danger of an explosion, the hunter should never attempt to clear the barrel by firing the gun.

Identifying the Target

Not everything that moves in the field, woods, or forest is game. Yet, some hunters will automatically shoot in the direction of rustling sounds, shaking brush, and shadowy figures. Tragically, too often the intended game is another hunter! Seeing a "deer's horns" move, a Michigan hunter fired his gun; when he went to the location, he discovered a man, shot in the stomach. The only "horns" were the swaying branches of some balsam trees.

Because of such deceptions, the hunter should always know the identifying features of the game he intends to hunt, but, more important, before firing at any game he should always make certain of his target. Furthermore, if the hunter has a vision problem, he should wear either his contact lens or his glasses at all times.

Staying Out of the Line of Fire

Frequently hunters are killed when without any warning they suddenly move into other hunters' lines of fire. Often the hunters are unaware of the location of their companions, or they are too anxious to fire the first shot. Since most accidents of this type involve a hunter's "popping up" from cover to shoot as another hunter fires from behind, hunters in a group should always wait for game in a side-by-side formation, never in a pattern that places some individuals in front of others. Nevertheless, if the game appears suddenly at one end of the hunting formation, instead of in front or in back, only the hunter on that end should fire at the game.

Unintentional Discharge Accidents

Accidental discharges of guns account for approximately thirty-five percent of all hunting injuries.

Transporting the Gun

Although most unintentional discharges occur in the field, a few hunters are shot while getting into or out of automobiles with loaded guns. In many cases the discharges are the result of the hunters' accidentally bumping the guns against vehicles or dropping them on the ground. Other hunters are

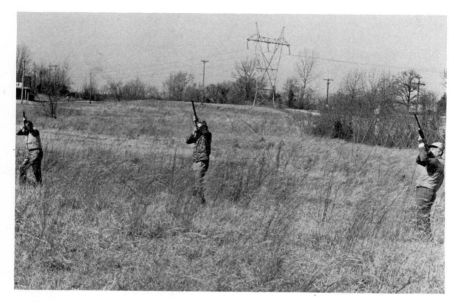

Figure 19.2   Hunters in a group should always walk and thus shoot in a side-by-side formation.

shot while riding in automobiles with loaded guns. In these cases the discharges are usually the result of hunting dogs' stepping on the guns or the vehicles' striking rough spots in the road and jolting the guns.

Before transporting any gun in a boat or an automobile, the hunter should always examine the weapon at the breach and remove all cartridges or shells. Furthermore, depending upon the particular weapon, the hunter should either break the gun down or leave its action open.

Carrying the Gun in the Field

Many hunters accidentally shoot their hunting companions or themselves when they brush their guns against bushes or branches, or when they stumble or fall over rocks, logs, clumps of dirt, tree roots, or other objects. To reduce the possibility of this type of accident, the hunter should always keep his gun on "safety" until just before he is ready to fire at the game. However, since the safety can be easily released during an accident, the hunter should also carry the gun so that its muzzle points away from himself and his hunting companions.

Ideally, hunters in a group should always walk in a side-by-side formation and point their muzzles downward and forward. However, if the hunters must walk in a formation that has some hunters in front of others, the lead hunter should point his muzzle downward and forward, and the other hunters should point their muzzles downward and to the side.

Crossing Field Obstacles

Often, while trying to cross fences, jump ditches, or climb trees, hunters will accidentally pull the triggers of their guns, thereby shooting themselves or their companions. Needless to say, all of the accidents occur because the hunters, either inadvertently or deliberately, fail to unload their guns before starting across the field obstacles.

Instead of crossing a fence or jumping a ditch with a loaded weapon, the hunter should always remove the shells from the gun, keep the action open, and pass the gun to the other side. After taking this precaution, he can then safely cross the fence or ditch. On the other hand, when the hunter is accompanied by a companion, each person should unload his gun and open its action. Then, while his companion holds both guns, the hunter can safely cross the obstacles. Once he is on the other side, the hunter should take the weapons from his companion, thus enabling him to also cross the fence or ditch safely.

While a tree may serve as an excellent hunting platform, the hunter should never attempt to climb the tree with his gun, either loaded or unloaded. Before climbing a tree to wait for game, the hunter should always unload the gun, keep its action open, and secure the end of a long rope around the stock of the gun. Securing the other end of the rope to his waist, he should climb the tree and firmly position himself in its branches. Once he is in place, the hunter can then safely pull the gun, stock first, upward into the tree.

Leaving the Gun Unattended

Occasionally, hunters are shot when they prop their weapons against bushes or trees and the guns fall to the ground and discharge. Since even a slight breeze may topple a gun from its resting place, the hunter should always unload the weapon before leaving it unattended. Furthermore, he should resist the temptation to rest a loaded gun on his foot. Although "foot resting" keeps the weapon out of the dirt, mud, or snow, this practice can easily lead to an accidental discharge. Accordingly, before resting the gun on his foot, the hunter should always unload the weapon.

Fishing Accidents

An ideal leisure pursuit for the entire family, fishing has long been one of the most popular water activities in this country. Today, more than thirty-five million individuals engage in this sport. Unfortunately, while it can be very enjoyable, fishing can also be extremely dangerous. Each year, besides producing over fifteen thousand injuries, most of them by barbed hooks, fishing accidents claim approximately one thousand lives.

Catching Fish Instead of People

Equipped with barbs to hold the fish and to keep the hook from backing out, fishhooks are notorious for causing injury. When they become firmly embedded in a person's body, fishhooks can easily tear the tissues, including muscles, tendons, nerves, and blood vessels.

Ideally, before they are transported, all hooks, flies, and plugs should be removed from the fishing lines and secured to the hook keeper within the tackle box. However, when this is impractical, the fisherman can still easily secure the hooks by pushing the barbs into a small cork, covering the cork with a folded handkerchief, and taping the handkerchief to the fishing rod.

After the fishing gear has been reassembled at the fisherman's destination, great caution must still be exercised if the person is to avoid hooking himself or someone else. Specifically, when he is casting his line, the fisherman should always check to make certain that no one is directly behind him or closer than several feet to either side of him. In addition, except when he is in the bow or the stern of a boat, the fisherman should use an overhead cast.

Fortunately, once the line has been cast and the hook is safely resting in the water, the greatest danger of the person's accidentally hooking himself, an onlooker, or another fisherman has passed. Nevertheless, upon hooking a fish and bringing it toward the shore or the boat, the fisherman should pull gently to prevent the hook from breaking loose and snapping toward him. Any sudden jerk can easily send the hook flying at a high rate of speed into the fisherman's body or, worse yet, someone else's body.

Staying in the Boat

Falling or being thrown overboard, sometimes in conjunction with the capsizing of the boat, is undoubtedly the most common type of boating accident involving fishermen. Each year such accidents account for almost five hundred deaths. Naturally, most of these drownings could be easily prevented if the individuals simply observed certain safe boating practices while fishing.

Since standing in a boat can easily result in a person's losing his balance, tipping the boat, and throwing his passengers into the water, the fisherman should always remain seated when casting his line or bringing in his catch. Contrary to what many people believe, most individuals can readily learn to cast their lines or reel in their fish as successfully from a sitting position as they can from a standing position.

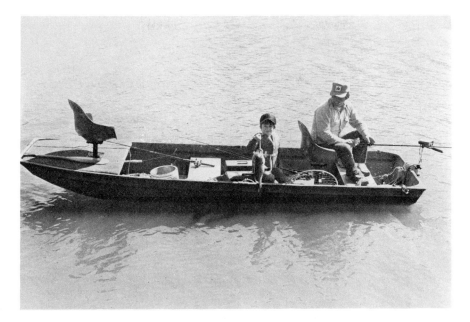

Figure 19.3   A poor-swimming fisherman should always wear a personal flotation device at all times while fishing from a boat.

In addition, upon getting ready to start back to shore, the fisherman should always remain seated when starting his motor. Far too often, forgetting that the motors are in gear, individuals will stand in their boats and pull the starting cords, acts which result in their being thrown into the water. In most cases, even if they are fortunate enough to avoid contact with the whirling propellers, the persons will usually drown, since they cannot climb back aboard the boats or use them for support until help arrives.

As a final note, any fisherman who is a poor swimmer or a nonswimmer should always wear some type of personal flotation device at all times. Although the device may not be particularly comfortable, it can save his life if he is unexpectedly thrown into the water. Furthermore, even if he is a good swimmer, the fisherman if he is not wearing a device should immediately don one whenever the weather or other circumstances cause the slightest concern for safety.

Escaping Wading Predicaments

While wading in ponds, lakes, and streams, fishermen are often drowned when they unexpectedly step into deep water. Most of these deaths can be

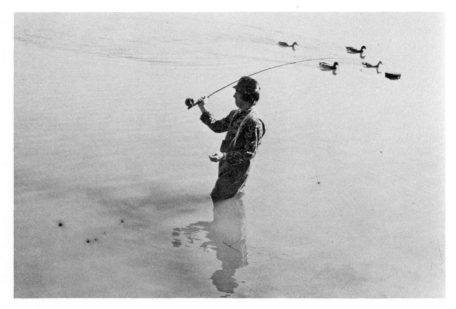

Figure 19.4 Waders, while they may complicate a water emergency, will not automatically pull the fisherman to the bottom if he suddenly steps into deep water.

prevented if the fishermen will simply test the bottom before taking each step. Yet, even when they are fully clothed and wearing water-filled hip boots or waders, most individuals can easily escape from a deep hole or a drop-off by remaining calm and taking appropriate action.

Fortunately, even with full outdoor gear the fisherman will not be pulled to the bottom. On the contrary, in most cases enough air will be trapped in his shirt or his jacket to bring him to the surface and help keep him afloat. Upon stepping into deep water and bobbing back to the surface, the fisherman should immediately turn in the direction from which he came and stroke forcefully with his arms. In most cases this procedure will bring him into contact with the ledge from which he stepped, but if it does not, the fisherman should then assume a floating position on his back and stroke with his arms until he can locate the ledge again and walk to the shore.

Fishing Safely on Ice

Although most fishing deaths occur in warm weather, a few persons are drowned during the winter season while fishing on frozen ponds, lakes, and rivers. Unfortunately, almost all of these deaths occur because the fishermen are ignorant of the various hazards associated with ice fishing.

Generally, spring and early winter are the most dangerous seasons for ice fishing. At these times, even ice which is thick and strong in the morning may melt and weaken in the afternoon heat and sun. For this reason, the ice fisherman should always restrict his activity to the mid-winter season when prolonged subfreezing temperatures cause the ice to freeze solidly. Yet, even then, before trying to fish on it, the person should make certain that the ice is at least three to four inches thick, a depth which will easily support the fisherman and several companions.

However, regardless of its thickness some ice is always too dangerous for fishing. A good example is ice formed over water which is constantly changing from one level to another. When the level of the water drops, an air space is left between the ice and the water. No matter how thick, the resulting "bridge of ice" is always weak. Equally unsafe is ice that has formed over swiftly flowing water, such as a stream or a river. Even though it may appear thick enough to support the fisherman's weight, the ice will usually have numerous weak spots where the current has worn away its undersurface. As a rule, small bodies of water, such as pools, ponds, slowly flowing streams, and small lakes, provide the safest surface for the ice fisherman, since they usually freeze more quickly than larger bodies of water and the ice remains firmer much longer.

Despite all his precautions, the ice fisherman may someday find himself in a drowning situation. In a typical instance, upon plunging through broken ice, the individual will suddenly panic and grab the edge of the ice in an effort to climb out of the cold water. However, instead of supporting the fisherman, the ice will only break again, forcing him back into the water. Instead of trying to climb out of the water after breaking through the ice, the person should stretch his hands and arms forward over the unbroken ice, kick his feet to the surface behind him, and try to wiggle chest-first onto the ice. If the ice breaks under his weight, he should simply maintain his position and wiggle forward again. Once he is on the ice, the fisherman should then wiggle or roll away from the broken area.

When trying to save a companion who has broken through the ice, the fisherman should resist the impulse to rush to the spot and to try to pull the person out by hand. Because of the weakened condition of the ice, the fisherman could easily find himself in the icy water along with the victim. Instead, he should lie on his stomach, crawl toward the victim, and extend a fishing rod, scarf, or other object to him. After the victim has grabbed the object, the fisherman should then pull him onto the ice and away from the hole. On the other hand, if several rescuers are present, they should lie on their stomachs, grasp each other's ankles, and crawl toward the victim, thus forming a human chain. After the lead person has seized the victim's wrists, they should then slowly and cautiously crawl back, pulling the victim along with them.

Nevertheless, despite repeated rescue efforts the victim may disappear below the surface of the water. When this happens the fisherman should never jump into the water and try to pull him out by hand. Although heroic in intent, such action is not only dangerous, but in most cases it is also futile. Even if the fisherman is fortunate enough to locate the victim, he may not be able to find the hole in the ice again. Thus, trapped beneath the ice, both the fisherman and the victim would drown.

Snowmobiling Accidents

A relatively new sport, snowmobiling has been steadily increasing in popularity over the past ten years. Today, wherever there is plenty of snow and open space, snowmobilers can usually be seen whizzing along on their machines. According to safety officials, slightly more than five million snowmobilers are active during the winter months in this country. Yet, while snowmobiles are fun to drive and have opened up areas which were previously inaccessible to hunters, fishermen, and adventurers, every year more than one hundred and fifty individuals are killed in snowmobiling accidents, and another eighteen thousand individuals are injured.

Wearing Protective Equipment

Of the various types of snowmobiling accidents, overturns and collisions are the most common. Realistically, because of the nature of his vehicle, the snowmobiler can never expect his machine to afford him much protection during an accident. However, he can considerably reduce the danger associated with his sport by wearing proper equipment.

To protect his eyes from flying objects and to prevent them from "tearing," the snowmobiler should wear either goggles or a face shield. More important, he should always wear a helmet, preferably one which is specially designed for snowmobiling. To assure adequate protection, the snowmobiler should immediately refurbish or replace the helmet if it sustains a severe "shock." However, even if the helmet has not received a shock, he should still refurbish or replace it at least once every four years, since dirt, sweat, and hair oil can destroy the helmet's lining and thus reduce its protective properties.

Although most snowmobile injuries result from accidents, each year a few snowmobilers suffer frostbite or cold exposure. Since his vehicle affords only minimal protection against the cold, the snowmobiler should always wear clothing that provides warmth and acts as a windbreak. For this purpose, instead of simply donning extra layers of clothing, he should wear garments which are specially designed for snowmobiling activities.

Necessary items include gloves or mittens, insulated boots, and a quilted windbreaking coverall which slips over the snowmobiler's regular clothing.

Maintaining a Safe Speed

Undoubtedly, excessive speed is the leading factor in most snowmobiling accidents. While many machines are capable of reaching speeds of more than sixty miles per hour, a reasonably safe speed is necessarily determined by the nature of the terrain. Thus a hole, rock, log, or other obstruction can easily lead to an accident when it is suddenly encountered by an unwary snowmobiler.

In rough, irregular, or unfamiliar areas or in unfavorable snow conditions, the snowmobiler should always restrict his speed to under fifteen miles per hour. Yet, even in open, flat areas which are well known to him, he should never drive faster than thirty miles per hour. In addition, since most machines can accelerate very quickly, the snowmobiler should control acceleration carefully to prevent being thrown off the vehicle.

Snowmobiling at Night

Although snowmobiling at night is extremely popular in certain areas of this country, it is undoubtedly more dangerous than snowmobiling in the daytime. In general, the snowmobiler should travel at night only when his snowmobile is equipped with headlights, taillights, and a brake light, and then only when absolutely necessary. As a further precaution, he should make certain that his machine is trimmed with retroreflective tape so that it will be more visible to other nighttime snowmobilers. In addition to these precautions, the snowmobiler should exercise extreme caution at all times, since at night any hazard may appear suddenly and unexpectedly.

Driving on Public Roads

Designed solely for use on trails and in open country, in most states snowmobiles are outlawed for travel on streets, roads, and highways. In spite of this, collisions with automobiles, trucks, and other motor vehicles are frequent occurrences.

Because snowmobiles provide a low profile and are small in size, they are difficult to spot on the road and often are not seen by motorists in time to avoid collisions. In addition, since the vehicles are exceptionally noisy, the snowmobiler usually has great difficulty hearing vehicles approaching from the rear. For these reasons, driving a snowmobile on a public road is always extremely dangerous. If the snowmobiler must travel on a road or highway to reach a trail outside of town and such travel is legally permitted in the area, he should always drive on the far right side of the road and continually check for traffic approaching him from the rear.

Resource Materials

American Snowmobile Association
13104 Crooked Lake Boulevard
Anoka, Minnesota 55303

International Snowmobile Industry Association
1755 South Jefferson Davis Highway
Arlington, Virginia 22202

Master Lock Company
2600 North 32nd Street
Milwaukee, Wisconsin 53210

National Rifle Association
1600 Rhode Island Avenue, N.W.
Washington, D.C. 20036

National Safety Council
444 North Michigan Avenue
Chicago, Illinois 60611

Sporting Arms and Ammunition Manufacturers' Institute
420 Lexington Avenue
New York City, New York 10017

Activities

1. Keep a scrapbook of newspaper articles which report hunting accidents in the local area. Determine what percentage of the mishaps involved intentional discharges and what percentage involved unintentional discharges.

2. Prepare a list of "safe hunting practices," and distribute the list to the class members.

3. Write a short paper on the incidence of fishing accidents among recent retirees.

4. Prepare a demonstration before the class on the proper way(s) to rescue a person who has broken through thin ice.

5. Conduct a survey of twenty-five adults to determine their attitudes toward the snowmobile and the snowmobile driver. Summarize and discuss the results in a short paper.

Questions

1. Why is fluorescent orange a safer color for hunting attire than green or red?
2. What is a ricochet?

3. What precautions can be taken to prevent the possibility of inserting the wrong-size shell into a gun?
4. Why is "foot resting" with a loaded gun extremely dangerous?
5. How should hooks, flies, and plugs be transported to the fishing site?
6. What is the most common type of boating accident involving fishermen?
7. When are the most dangerous times of the year for ice fishing?
8. What are the most common types of snowmobiling accidents?
9. What determines a reasonably safe speed for a snowmobile?
10. Why are snowmobiles dangerous to drive on public roads?

Selected References

The American National Red Cross. *Lifesaving and Water Safety*. Garden City, New York: Doubleday & Company, Inc., 1974.

Burgin, Bryan E. "Two-Thirds of Hunting Accidents Involve Hunters in the Same Party," *The Conservationist*. April-May, 1968, 16-17.

Carper, Jean. *Stay Alive!* Garden City, New York: Doubleday & Company, Inc., 1965.

Price, Franklin S. and Melvin A. Humphreys. *Safety Practices for Home and Leisure*. Dubuque, Iowa: Wm. C. Brown Book Company, 1966.

Seibel, Bill. "Guns: Is Your Youngster Ready?" *St. Louis Globe-Democrat*. Friday, December 20, 1974.

"Snowmobiles," *Consumer Reports*. January, 1973, 45-49.

"What You Should Know About Ice," *School Safety*. January-February, 1970, 20-22.

Disasters

20

"Galveston May Be Wiped Out by Storm" "Alaska Quake Measures 8.6 on Richter Scale" "Twisters Kill Hundreds in Midwest" "Buffalo Hit by Second Blizzard in Four Days" As these newspaper headlines suggest, disasters are always front-page news. However, as the National Safety Council emphasizes, the number of lives lost in disasters in the United States each year are relatively few in comparison to the day-to-day losses in ordinary accidents. (See Figure 20.1.) Still, disasters are noteworthy: annually, they kill several hundred individuals, injure thousands of persons, inflict widespread hardship and suffering, and damage millions of dollars worth of property.

In general, disasters are caused by either the forces of nature or by man himself. Yet, regardless of their cause, most disasters occur in an unpredictable manner, often without adequate warning. Consequently, advanced planning is essential for mitigating the effects of disasters. However, in reality, no one is ever really prepared for disasters, whether natural or man-made. The United States armed forces, with all of their emergency plans, antiaircraft installations, fighter planes, and the combined firepower of a major portion of the Pacific Fleet, were dealt a devastating surprise blow by the Japanese on December 7, 1941. Despite the hints of an impending war, few people really believed that the Japanese would have the audacity to attack the United States. To this day, Pearl Harbor is viewed as a classic example of "unprepared preparedness." Still, in any type of disaster, numerous lives can be saved and the severity of injuries can be reduced if people are reasonably prepared for the emergency and are familiar with the proper steps to take when it does occur.

Coping with Natural Disasters

Natural disasters may occur in a great variety of forms. Nevertheless, in this country thunderstorms, hurricanes, floods, earthquakes, and blizzards are the most common causes of disasters.

Largest U.S. Disasters by Category

	Type and Location	No. of Deaths	Date of Disaster
Floods:	Galveston tidal wave	6,000	Sept. 8, 1900
	Johnstown, Pa.	2,209	May 31, 1889
	Ohio and Indiana	732	Mar. 28, 1913
	St. Francis, Calif. dam burst	450	Mar. 13, 1928
	Ohio and Mississippi River valleys	380	Jan. 22, 1937
Hurricanes:	Florida	1,833	Sept. 16-17, 1928
	New England	657	Sept. 21, 1938
	Louisiana	500	Sept. 29, 1915
	Florida	409	Sept 1-2, 1935
	Louisiana and Texas	395	June 27-28, 1957
Tornadoes:	Illinois	606	Mar. 18, 1925
	Mississippi, Alabama, Georgia	402	Apr. 2-7, 1936
	Southern and Midwestern states	318	Apr. 3, 1974
	Ind., Ohio, Mich., Ill. and Wisc.	272	Apr. 11, 1965
	Ark., Tenn., Mo., Miss. and Ala.	229	Mar. 21-22, 1952
Earth-	San Francisco earthquake and fire	452	Apr. 18, 1906
quakes:	Alaskan earthquake-tsunami hit Hawaii, Calif.	173	Apr. 1, 1946
	Long Beach, Calif. earthquake	120	Mar. 10, 1933
	Alaskan earthquake and tsunami	117	Mar. 27, 1964
	San Fernando-Los Angeles, Calif. earthquake	65	Feb. 9, 1971
Marine:	"Sultana" exploded—Mississippi River	1,547	Apr. 27, 1865
	"Titanic" struck iceberg—Atlantic Ocean	1,517	Apr. 15, 1912
	"Empress of Ireland" ship collision—St. Lawrence River	1,024	May 29, 1914
	"General Slocum" burned—East River	1,021	June 15, 1904
	"Eastland" capsized—Chicago River	812	July 24, 1915
Aircraft:	Two-plane collision over New York City	134	Dec. 16, 1960
	Two-plane collision over Grand Canyon, Ariz.	128	June 30, 1956
	Scheduled jetliner crash in New York City	113	June 24, 1975
	Jetliner crash into mountainside near Juneau, Alaska	111	Sept. 4, 1971
	Scheduled plane crash near Miami, Fla.	101	Dec. 29, 1972
Railroad:	Two-train collision near Nashville, Tenn.	101	July 9, 1918
	Two-train collision, Eden, Colo.	96	Aug. 7, 1904
	Avalanche hit two trains near Wellington, Wash.	96	Mar. 1, 1910
	Bridge collapse under train, Ashtabula, Ohio	92	Dec. 29, 1876
	Rapid transit train derailment, Brooklyn, N.Y.	92	Nov. 1, 1918
Fires:	Peshtigo, Wisc. and surrounding area forest fire	1,152	Oct. 9, 1871
	Iroquois Theatre, Chicago	575	Dec. 30, 1903
	Cocoanut Grove nightclub, Boston	492	Nov. 28, 1942
	North German Lloyd Steamships, Hoboken, N.J.	326	June 30, 1900
	Ohio penitentiary, Columbus	320	Apr. 21, 1930
Explosions:	Texas City, Texas ship explosion	561	Apr. 16, 1947
	Port Chicago, Calif. ship explosion	322	July 18, 1944
	New London, Texas school explosion	294	Mar. 18, 1937
	Eddystone, Pa. munitions plant explosion	133	Apr. 10, 1917
	Cleveland, Ohio gas tank explosion	130	Oct. 20, 1944
Mines:	Monongha, West Va. coal mine explosion	361	Dec. 6, 1907
	Dawson, New Mexico coal mine fire	263	Oct. 22, 1913
	Cherry, Ill. coal mine fire	259	Nov. 13, 1909
	Jacobs Creek, Pa. coal mine explosion	239	Dec. 19, 1907
	Scofield, Utah coal mine explosion	200	May 1, 1900

Figure 20.1   Largest United States disasters by category. (Reproduced from *Accident Facts—1977 Edition,* p. 21, courtesy of the National Safety Council)

Although a particular disaster situation is often difficult or impossible to predict, the types which are most likely to affect a particular area of the country can be determined by historical analyses. For example, as indicated by the history of their area, persons along the Atlantic and Gulf coasts should expect to encounter hurricanes, individuals in the Northeast should expect to experience blizzards, and residents along the Pacific coast and in the Midwest should expect to encounter earthquakes. On the other hand, persons in some areas of the country such as the Northwest and the Midwest should be prepared to cope with a variety of disaster situations.

Thunderstorms

At any given moment, nearly two thousand thunderstorms are in progress over the earth's surface. Because of their frequency and potential for violence, thunderstorms are one of nature's greatest killers and destroyers.

Generated by temperature imbalances in the atmosphere, a thunderstorm is actually a cumulonimbus cloud. This cloud, which is shaped by winds into an anvil form, may appear as a lonely giant or as several smaller clouds moving abreast. Depending upon the particular storm system, the cloud may extend several miles along its base and tower over seven and one-half miles into the stratosphere. As a result, a thunderstorm may literally blot out the sun. Although a severe thunderstorm may develop from a shallow cloud formation, the most violent storms are usually the products of dense cloud systems. Thus, as a general rule, the darker the sky appears, the more likely the thunderstorm will be severe.

On the ground directly beneath the cloud, strong gusts of cold wind or heavy precipitation, either rain or hail, will normally accompany the storm. In addition, thunder and lightning are always present. These signs are nature's warnings that the thunderstorm is in its most violent stage. In some cases tornadoes may also be associated with the thunderstorm.

Strong Winds

Thunderstorm winds, which may reach velocities of nearly seventy-four miles per hour, are capable of unroofing houses, uprooting trees, and smashing mobile homes. During a recent storm in Tucson, Arizona, wind gusts of up to sixty-seven miles per hour severely damaged ten airplanes and unroofed several dozen houses. In Oklahoma City, Oklahoma, winds of over sixty-five miles per hour blew a man through a plate glass window of a department store and overturned several mobile homes, killing three small children. Because of their violent nature, the strong winds generated by a thunderstorm are often referred to as "killer winds."

In describing wind conditions, the United States Weather Bureau uses the Beaufort Scale. (See Figure 20.2.) Named for the British Admiral who first devised it, the Beaufort Scale is divided into thirteen categories of winds, ranging from calm, less than one mile per hour, to hurricane, above seventy-three miles per hour. In a thunderstorm the most dangerous and damaging winds are the gale and the whole gale winds.

During a period of increasing thunderstorm winds, the individual should quickly seek shelter inside a house or a large building. Mobile homes, especially when they are not tied down securely, are often inadequate protection against the strong winds. On the other hand, if the person is on the water in a boat when the winds first appear, he should immediately head for

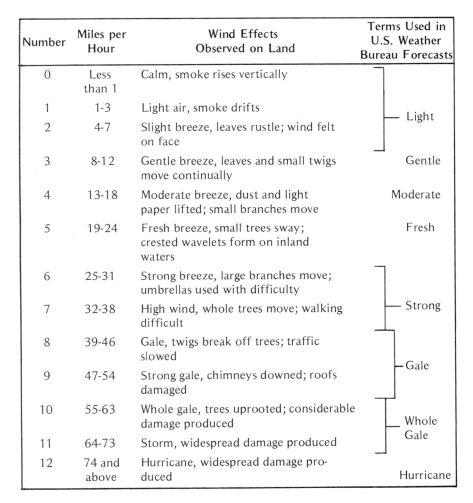

Number	Miles per Hour	Wind Effects Observed on Land	Terms Used in U.S. Weather Bureau Forecasts
0	Less than 1	Calm, smoke rises vertically	Light
1	1-3	Light air, smoke drifts	Light
2	4-7	Slight breeze, leaves rustle; wind felt on face	Light
3	8-12	Gentle breeze, leaves and small twigs move continually	Gentle
4	13-18	Moderate breeze, dust and light paper lifted; small branches move	Moderate
5	19-24	Fresh breeze, small trees sway; crested wavelets form on inland waters	Fresh
6	25-31	Strong breeze, large branches move; umbrellas used with difficulty	Strong
7	32-38	High wind, whole trees move; walking difficult	Strong
8	39-46	Gale, twigs break off trees; traffic slowed	Gale
9	47-54	Strong gale, chimneys downed; roofs damaged	Gale
10	55-63	Whole gale, trees uprooted; considerable damage produced	Whole Gale
11	64-73	Storm, widespread damage produced	Whole Gale
12	74 and above	Hurricane, widespread damage produced	Hurricane

Figure 20.2   Beaufort Scale of wind force.

shore, since high waves produced by the winds can easily capsize even the largest boat.

Heavy Rains

During a thunderstorm the water level in a small stream or river, especially near the headwater of a river basin, may rise dangerously high within a few hours. When this happens, the water can easily surge over the stream or river bank. Sometimes reaching heights of ten to twenty feet, the flash flood waves, moving at incredible speeds, can carve new channels, roll boulders,

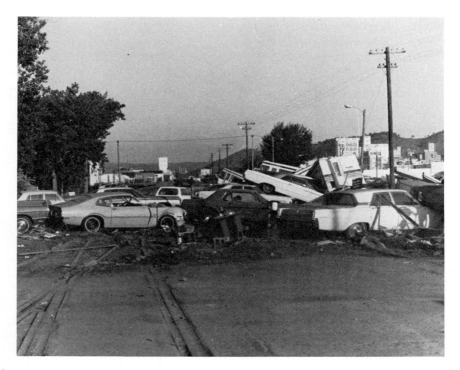

Figure 20.3   Flood waters in Rapid City, South Dakota, left cars and trailers piled in heaps. (Courtesy of the National Oceanic and Atmospheric Administration)

tear out trees, destroy bridges and buildings, and carry away cars and their occupants.

On June 9, 1972, stationary thunderstorms over the Black Hills resulted in flash floods that claimed the lives of more than two hundred and thirty persons in and near Rapid City, South Dakota. Trees, boulders, cars, and trailers were picked up, carried for great distances, and then deposited in huge piles. (See Figure 20.3.) Fortunately, however, most flash floods do not produce as large a death toll as the Rapid City floods. Typically, each year flash floods in this country take the lives of approximately one hundred persons.

Because of the potential danger presented by flash floods, the homeowner should familiarize himself with the elevation of his property in relation to nearby streams and rivers. If an area has been subjected to flash floods in the past, he should then prepare plans as to what steps to take and where to go in a flash-flood emergency. Similarly, the outdoorsman should investigate the flood history of the area in which he will be camping. Since water runs off the higher elevations very rapidly, thereby causing the natural drainage system to overflow with rushing floodwaters and deadly debris, the person should avoid camping on low ground at any time or hiking along natural streambeds, arroyos, and other drainage channels during and after a thunderstorm.

Unfortunately, certain communities are more susceptible to flash floods than others. Nevertheless, in many of these areas, the residents can obtain advance flash-flood information from the National Weather Service (NWS). If heavy rains are occurring in the area or if they are expected to occur, the NWS will issue a "flash-flood watch" to alert residents to the possibility of a flood emergency which would necessitate immediate action. When a flash-flood watch has been announced, the individual should listen to local radio and television stations for reports on flooding in progress and for a possible "flash-flood warning" from the NWS. The flash-flood warning means that flash floods are occurring or that they are imminent along certain streams or in designated areas, and that residents should immediately take certain precautions. When a flash-flood warning has been issued, the person should evacuate the area as quickly as possible. Often he may have only seconds to escape.

In moving out of the area, the individual should avoid locations that are already partially flooded. However, when this is impossible or impractical, certain precautions should always be taken. On foot, he should never attempt to cross a flowing stream where the water would rise above his knees, since the current could readily pull him under the water and carry him downstream to his death. Similarly, in a car the individual should never cross a dip without knowing the depth of the water, for the road may not be intact under the pool of water. If the vehicle stalls, he should immediately abandon the car and seek shelter on higher ground. Because the rapidly rising floodwaters may engulf the vehicle and persons in or near it, he should never attempt to move a stalled vehicle.

Once he is safely away from the flash-flood area, the person should listen to local radio and television stations for additional information about changing flood conditions. Even when the flash-flood warning has been cancelled by the National Weather Service, he should still listen for follow-up information. Although the flash floods may have ended, general flooding, which will be discussed later, may still occur along headwater streams and major rivers.

Hail

Instead of heavy rains, a thunderstorm may release precipitation in the form of lumps of ice, called hailstones. The size of the hailstones is an indication of the intensity of the thunderstorm. As a rule, hailstones may range in size from that of a pea to that of a grapefruit. Although occasionally they may be conical or irregular in shape with pointed projections, hailstones are usually round.

During a severe storm, hailstones can smash windows, shatter lighted signs, riddle trees, and batter cars and buildings. However, hail is most devastating to farm crops. A single heavy fall of hailstones may cover the ground so completely that every inch of the crop is mangled, battered, stripped, and destroyed. Contrary to popular belief, throughout this country greater property damage results from hail than from tornadoes.

Although these lumps of ice are some of nature's most powerful weapons, few deaths are attributed to hailstones. Apparently most persons know enough to seek shelter during a hailstorm. Yet, sometimes shelter is not readily available. Near Lubbock, Texas, a thirty-nine-year-old farmer was caught in open country during a hailstorm. He was pelted so furiously before he could reach shelter that he died within a few hours. According to safety experts, there is only one known defense against hail: the person must run fast and seek cover.

Thunder and Lightning

At any particular moment, almost one hundred strokes of lightning are occurring over the surface of the earth. In this country lightning associated with thunderstorms kills more persons annually than either tornadoes or hurricanes—approximately one hundred and twenty-five individuals. In addition, lightning injures more than five hundred persons each year and produces an annual property loss of hundreds of millions of dollars.

Of the various forces in nature, few are as instantly explosive as lightning. Flashing through the sky at over sixty thousand miles per second, a lightning bolt will last only a few thousandths of a second. Yet, during this minute period of time, the bolt may generate as much as 250,000 amperes of electric current and reach a temperature of 36,000 degrees Fahrenheit. Clearly, lightning is powerful enough and hot enough to move and to wither nearly everything in its path.

By description, lightning is a flashing rootlike system of light produced by electrification within a thunderstorm. (See Figure 20.4.) As the thunderstorm develops, the upper layers of the cloud develop a positive charge, and the lower layers develop a negative charge. Normally, the ground is negatively charged with respect to the atmosphere, but as the thunderstorm passes over the ground, the negatively charged base of the cloud induces a positive charge on the ground directly under and around the storm for a distance of several miles. Following the storm like an electrical shadow, the positive charge on the ground grows stronger as the negative charge on the base of the cloud increases. At the same time, the positive

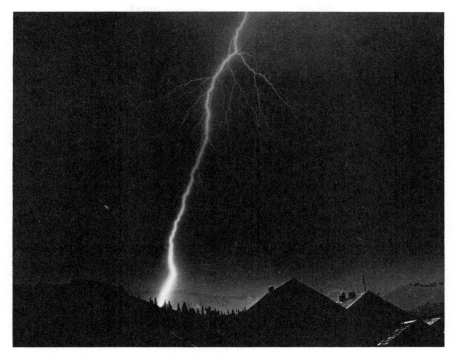

Figure 20.4   A bolt of lightning flashes across the sky. (Courtesy of the National Oceanic and Atmospheric Administration)

ground charge, in an attempt to establish a flow of current between the cloud and the ground, flows up trees, buildings, and other elevated objects. Eventually, when the differences between the ground and the cloud charges are large enough to overcome the insulating effect of the air, an electrical path is created between the ground and the cloud, and a discharge of lightning is produced. Similarly, since clouds are positively and negatively charged, lightning may also be discharged within the cloud or between the cloud and an adjacent cloud.

As lightning discharges during a storm, thunder, the explosive expansion of air which has been heated by the lightning bolt, is also produced. Even in the most favorable air currents, thunder cannot be heard more than twenty-five miles away. This accounts for the presence of "heat lightning" or distant lightning without thunder. Normally, however, thunder can be heard only ten miles away. When lightning is nearby, the thunder has a sound like a sharp crack. On the other hand, distant strokes of lightning will produce a growling and rumbling noise, as the sound is refracted and modified by the turbulent environment of the thunderstorm. In general, the more thunder that is heard and/or the more lightning that is observed, the more likely the thunderstorm will be severe.

Since the speed of light is approximately one million times the speed of sound, a lightning bolt can always be seen before the sound of the thunder can be heard. Thus the individual can easily estimate the distance in miles of an approaching thunderstorm by counting the number of seconds between the lightning and the thunder and then by dividing the number by five. For example, if five seconds have elapsed between the lightning and the thunder, the thunderstorm is approximately one mile away. To obtain the distance in feet, the person should simply multiply the elapsed time in seconds by one thousand.

When a thunderstorm and its accompanying lightning threaten, the person should immediately seek shelter inside a building. According to safety experts, the most reliable protection is afforded by a large steel or steel-framed building, followed by a lightning-rod protected building, a large unprotected building, and a small unprotected building. However, no building will offer complete protection. Lightning bolts can, and often do, enter buildings through chimneys, television antennae, telephone lines, and power lines, and even directly through roofs.

In Waterbury, Connecticut, a forty-year-old woman was preparing dinner during a thunderstorm when a bolt of lightning struck her home and raced through the electrical wiring to her stove. The lightning stroke knocked the woman unconscious and produced severe burns on her hands and forearms. Another woman in Tampa, Florida, was talking on the telephone during a thunderstorm when lightning flashed through the receiver and killed her. As these examples suggest, the person should always avoid taking a bath, talking on the telephone, or touching plumbing fixtures, appliances, electrical plugs, radiators, or other good conductors during a storm.

Paradoxically, when a building is not available for shelter, the individual can still obtain excellent protection by getting inside an all-metal car. In fact, according to some experts, the inside of an all-metal car, not a convertible, is the safest location for a person during a lightning storm. However, contrary to what many people believe, this is not because of the car's rubber tires. Actually, water is a good conductor of electricity, and in a thunderstorm wet rubber tires would offer very little protection against lightning current. As revealed by laboratory tests, when a car is struck by lightning, the electrical charge travels over the metal top and down along the springs, axles, and bearings to the wheels and then jumps past the rubber tires to the ground. Naturally, a person may suffer burns if he is in contact with any part of the metal; but lightning bolts strike cars so rarely that authorities have never verified a single injury case.

If he is caught outside and distant from any buildings or cars, the individual should immediately head for low ground, such as a ravine or a valley, or he should seek shelter in a cave or underneath a cliff. On the other hand, in a forest he should take refuge under a thick growth of small trees. Because lightning bolts are attracted by tall objects, the person should never stand under an isolated tree or next to a telephone pole.

In a level field or a prairie far from shelter, the individual should avoid being the tallest object in the area. Specifically, he should abandon any piece of metal farm equipment or any metal vehicle, such as a motorcycle, bicycle, or golf cart. If he is in a boat, the person should immediately head for shore and seek shelter. Many boaters have been electrocuted while they were on the water. Furthermore, since lightning can electrify water for several hundred feet, the person should never continue to fish, water ski, or swim when a thunderstorm threatens.

Whether on land or on water, the individual should always avoid holding any natural lightning rod, such as a golf club or a fishing rod, for the object will literally "draw in" the lightning bolts. Nevertheless, if he feels a tingling sensation or if his hair stands on end, the person should quickly drop to his knees, bend forward, and put his hands on his knees. Lightning may be ready to strike him. He should not lie flat on the ground. Fortunately, if a person is struck by lightning, he has a fifty percent chance of survival. On the other hand, if another person is available to administer artificial respiration or other needed first aid, he has at least a sixty to seventy-five percent chance of surviving the lightning stroke.

Tornadoes

Normally found in conjunction with severe thunderstorms, tornadoes are violently rotating columns of air, usually moving in a counterclockwise direction, which have descended from storm cloud systems. Because of their rotating appearance, tornadoes are often referred to as "twisters." "Of all the winds that sweep this planet's surface, tornadoes are the most violent."[1] Every year in this country tornadoes claim approximately one hundred lives and produce hundreds of millions of dollars in property damage.

In order to form, a tornado requires layers of air with contrasting properties of temperature, moisture, density, and wind flow. Complicated energy transformations, which are not yet fully understood by scientists, produce the vortex of the tornado, a whirlpool formation of winds rotating about a hollow cavity in which a partial vacuum has been produced by centrifugal forces. Although many theories have been proposed to explain the type of energy transformation which is necessary to produce a tornado, none has received general acceptance. However, the two most frequently encountered

---

1. U.S. Department of Commerce/National Oceanic and Atmospheric Administration, *Tornado* (Washington, D.C.: U.S. Government Printing Office, Rev. 1976), p. 1.

theories suggest that either the effect of the thermally induced rotary circulations or the mechanical effect of the converging rotary winds is responsible for the generation of a tornado. Currently, most scientists seem to believe that the combined effects of both thermal and mechanical forces are probably responsible for tornado formation.

As a tornado develops, condensation occurs around the vortex, and a pale cloud appears in the characteristic form of a funnel. (See Figure 20.5.) In addition, as the storm moves along the ground, the rotating winds which surround the funnel become dark with dust and debris. If the funnel remains in contact with the ground for a long enough period of time, the entire tornado will eventually appear dark. On the other hand, if the storm moves along water, the funnel will appear as a cloud of spray instead of dust and debris found over land. A funnel cloud which forms over a lake or other body of water and then touches the water is referred to as a "waterspout."

Although most twisters are recognized by their appearance, a tornado at night or a tornado hidden by low-hanging clouds, heavy rain, or buildings

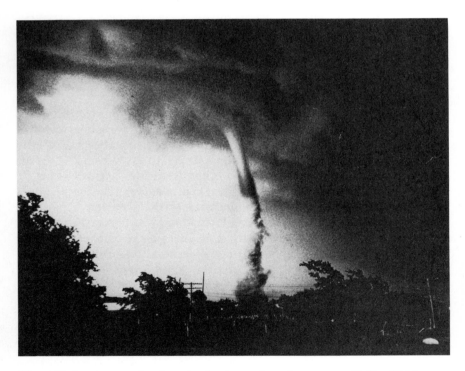

Figure 20.5   A tornado funnel cloud touches down near Enid, Oklahoma. (Courtesy of the National Oceanic and Atmospheric Administration)

can still be detected. It has a distinctive roar which can be heard for several miles. Some people have described the sound as a jet airliner; others have described it as several trains. According to scientists, the tornado's "roar of wind" is actually a continual noise generated by the discharge of a lacework of lightning.

On the average, tornado paths are only about a quarter of a mile wide and seldom more than sixteen miles long. However, in spectacular cases tornadoes have caused heavy destruction along paths of over a mile wide and nearly three hundred miles long. On May 26, 1917, a tornado traveled two hundred and ninety-three miles across Illinois and Indiana, and lasted for seven hours and twenty minutes. Its forward movement was forty miles per hour, an average speed for tornadoes.

Although tornadoes occur in many parts of the world, no area is more favorable to their formation than the United States. Each year approximately seven hundred tornadoes are formed in this country. In the last thirty years tornadoes have occurred in every state in the Union. As a rule, the fewest number of tornadoes occur during December and January; the greatest number, approximately one-half of the yearly total, occur during April, May, and June. In February, when tornado activity begins to increase, the center of maximum frequency rests over the central Gulf states. During March the center shifts eastward to the southeast Atlantic states, where tornado frequency peaks in April. Then during May the center of maximum frequency moves to the southern plain states, and during June it moves northward to the northern plains states and Great Lakes area, and sometimes as far eastward as western New York State. The reason for these shifts is the increasing penetration of warm, moist air from the south into the continental land mass, while contrasting cool, dry air still rushes in from the north and the northwest. Where these air masses collide, tornadoes are generated with the greatest frequency.

Although they may occur at any hour of the day or night, tornadoes form most readily, because of the meteorological combinations which produce them, during the warmest hours of the day. The greatest number of tornadoes, over eighty percent, occurs between noon and midnight, but the greatest single concentration, almost twenty-five percent, occurs between the hours of 4:00 and 6:00 P.M.

Basically, tornadoes perform their destructive tasks through the combined action of their strong rotary winds and the partial vacuum created in the center of the funnels. As a tornado passes over a home, the winds, estimated at between two hundred and three hundred miles per hour, twist and rip at the outside of the building. At the same time the partial vacuum effects a reduction in pressure around the house, and this, in conjunction with the greater relative pressure inside the building, causes the structure to literally explode. The debris of the explosion, assisted by the strong winds, is propelled through the air in a deadly barrage.

As most people realize, anything can happen in a tornado. According to verified reports, tornadoes have driven wheat straws more than an inch into a tree trunk; stripped chickens of all of their feathers; pulled a wheel off a car; carried a bedroom dresser one hundred yards without breaking the mirror; and blown a home away so cleanly that not even a splinter remained. They have also pulled up fence posts and stacked them neatly; ripped the bedding and the mattress from underneath a sleeping boy; carried a pair of trousers thirty-nine miles; picked up a farm worker, plastered him with mud, and set him down over one hundred feet away; and lifted an eighty-three-ton railroad coach and its one hundred and seventeen passengers, carried them through the air for eighty feet, and dropped them into a ditch.

Naturally, however, not all tornado damage is freakish. On March 18, 1925, a tornado moved through Missouri, Illinois, and Indiana, finally dissipating after two hundred and nineteen miles and more than three hours of destruction. Along its mile-wide path more than six hundred persons were killed, nearly two thousand were injured, and approximately seventeen million dollars in property was destroyed. The tornado was the most deadly twister in the history of the United States.

Unfortunately, meteorologists still cannot predict exactly when a tornado will form or precisely where a mature tornado will touch ground. However, they can follow the movements of a thunderstorm and establish when and where the probabilities of tornadoes are expected to be dangerously high. When tornadoes are expected to develop, the National Weather Service (NWS) will issue a "tornado watch" to alert the residents in a particular area to the possibility of tornado development during a specified period of time. Except to listen for additional weather information on the radio or television or to watch the sky for tornadoes, especially to the south and the southwest, the person should not interrupt his normal routine during a tornado watch. On the other hand, when a tornado has actually been sighted or indicated on radar, the NWS will issue a "tornado warning" to alert residents in an area to the presence of the tornado. The warning will specify the location of the tornado at the time of its detection, the area through which it is expected to move, and the time period during which it will move through the area. When a tornado warning has been issued, the individual should immediately seek suitable shelter.

According to safety experts, the best protection against a tornado is provided by a special storm cellar. Commonly built by persons in the Midwest states and other areas where tornadoes are comparatively frequent, these storm cellars are underground concrete-reinforced excavations with heavy doors. Significantly, no person has ever been killed by a tornado while he was inside a storm cellar. To obtain instructions at a reasonable cost for building a storm cellar, the homeowner should write to the U.S. Government Printing Office in Washington, D.C. (See Resource Materials at the end of this chapter.)

Surprisingly, when a storm cellar is not available, the person can still obtain excellent protection by seeking shelter under a workbench, table, or other piece of sturdy furniture in the basement of his home. In a home without a basement, the individual should take cover on the ground floor in the center of the house under sturdy furniture or in a closet, bathroom, or other small room. To help lessen damage to his house, he should also leave the windows and doors open on the sides away from the tornado. However, because of the possibility of encountering flying debris, he should stay away from the openings. Since mobile homes are especially vulnerable to overturning during strong winds, the person should never remain in a trailer home during a tornado.

Unfortunately, not all tornadoes occur when a person is at home and can easily take shelter. Nevertheless, in towns and cities, adequate protection is almost always available somewhere. In shopping centers the person should move quickly to a designated shelter area, not to a parked car. A rolling, pitching, twisting automobile would automatically become a death trap for the person. In a school, office building, or factory, he should seek protection in an interior hallway on the lowest floor, or preferably, if it is available, in a basement. Since structures with wide free-span roofs are subject to collapse during a tornado, the person should always avoid gymnasiums, auditoriums, and similar areas.

Ideally, when a tornado approaches, the individual should seek shelter in a steel-framed or reinforced concrete building of substantial construction. However, if he is caught outside on foot and cannot find suitable shelter in time, he should lie flat in the nearest depression, such as a ditch, culvert, excavation, or ravine. On the other hand, if he is inside a moving car, the individual should drive away from a tornado at a right angle to its path. Since a tornado travels at an average speed of only forty miles per hour, he can usually escape with relative ease. However, if the tornado is moving at a faster speed and he cannot outdistance it, the person should stop the car immediately and seek shelter in the nearest depression.

Storm Warning Service

Thunderstorms, with their accompanying winds, rains, hail, lightning, and tornadoes, are short-lived and difficult to forecast precisely. Nevertheless, the National Severe Storms Forecast Center, which is operated by the National Weather Service, in Kansas City, Missouri, can predict general areas where severe thunderstorms, as well as flash floods and tornadoes, are most likely to develop.

Basically, meteorologists at the Center in Kansas City use radar summaries, satellite photographs, meteorological upper-air profiles, reports from pilots, and surface data from hundreds of points to monitor conditions in the North American atmosphere. From these thousands of pieces of information, the meteorologists can determine the area where the probability of severe thunderstorm and/or tornado development is greatest. They will then issue information concerning this area to National Weather Service Offices and to the general public in the form of a "watch bulletin."

Normally, a severe thunderstorm or tornado watch bulletin will identify an area about one hundred and forty miles wide by two hundred miles long and specify the length of time that the area should expect the storm to threaten. Yet, the bulletin does not mean that the storm will not occur outside the watch area or beyond the projected time span. Since a watch bulletin is only an indication of where and when the probabilities are greatest, persons within at least seventy-five miles of the watch area should also be alert to threatening weather conditions. Except to listen to the radio or the television for further severe weather information and to watch for threatening weather, individuals in and near the watch area should continue their normal routines.

When a severe thunderstorm or tornado has actually been sighted in the area or indicated on radar, the National Weather Service will then issue a severe thunderstorm or tornado "warning bulletin." The warning will describe the downstream area that may be affected. Generally, this area is determined from the location, direction, and speed of the storm. When a warning has been issued, persons near the storm should seek shelter immediately, especially in the case of a tornado warning. Furthermore, individuals who are not in the direct path of the storm should be prepared to seek shelter if threatening conditions are sighted. However, since tornadoes are not always sighted by severe storm spotters or indicated by radar, a tornado warning may not always be issued. For this reason, during a severe thunderstorm persons should always be alert to the possibility of tornadoes.

To keep the public advised of current information, especially when a watch or a warning bulletin is in effect, the National Weather Service will prepare "severe weather statements." These are issued at least once every hour in normal storm situations and more frequently in rapidly-changing storm situations.

Whenever the threat of severe thunderstorms or tornadoes has ended in the area previously designated by the warning bulletin, the National Weather Service will issue an "all-clear bulletin." However, when a warning has been cancelled but a watch is still in effect for the area or an adjacent area or when a warning has been cancelled but a warning is still in effect for an adjacent area, the Service will issue a "Severe Weather Bulletin." This bulletin, which is a qualified weather message, will also be issued when the watch is cancelled for a portion, but not all, of the watch area. Through the use of Severe Weather Bulletins, the National Weather Service can provide a continuous alert in the path of the storm.

Hurricanes

Bringing destruction to islands and coastlines in their paths, hurricanes are tropical storms in which the winds reach speeds of at least seventy-four miles per hour and move in a large counterclockwise spiral (Northern Hemisphere) around the "eye," a relatively calm center. Tropical storms of the same type are referred to as cyclones in the Indian Ocean, typhoons in the North Pacific, and baguios in the Philippines. Each year in this country hurricanes kill more than one hundred persons and produce almost two hundred million dollars worth of property damage.

While the exact processes in hurricane formation are unknown, the storm apparently begins as a relatively small tropical cyclone, technically referring to any rotating storm, which becomes embedded in the westward-blowing tradewinds of the tropics and drifts gradually to the west-northwest in the Northern Hemisphere. Under certain conditions the small cyclone increases

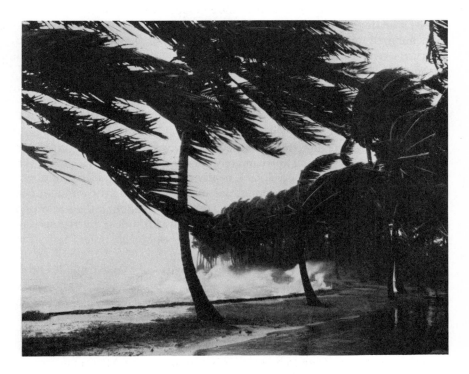

Figure 20.6   Hurricane winds and waves batter the Gulf coast. (Courtesy of the National Oceanic and Atmospheric Administration)

in size, speed, and intensity until it becomes a full-fledged hurricane. Driven by the heat released through condensing water vapor and by external mechanical forces, the hurricane moves forward very slowly in the tropics, usually at fifteen miles per hour or less, and sometimes hovers for short periods of time. Then, as it moves farther from the equator, the hurricane increases its forward speed until at middle latitudes and in extreme cases it may exceed sixty miles per hour. However, once it moves over the land, the hurricane soon begins to dissipate because of the lack of water and heat energy and also because of the friction generated by contact with the landscape. As a rule, an August storm will continue the longest time, approximately twelve days, while a July or November storm will last the shortest, approximately eight days. On the average, a hurricane will last about nine days.

Stated very simply, a hurricane is a giant whirlwind in which the air moves in a large, tightening spiral around a center of extreme low pressure. With a one-hundred-mile core of thunderclouds and torrential rain, a hurricane is analogous to a squashed doughnut which spreads outward as far as four hundred miles from its hole in the center. In the center or "eye" of the hurricane, which has an average diameter of about fourteen miles, the wind moves very slowly, approximately fifteen miles per hour or less. Because of the relative calmness of the winds, the "eye," which is unique to hurricanes, is especially deceptive to the unwary person. Unfortunately, many individuals have been injured or killed when the calm "eye" lured them out of their shelters, thus causing them to become trapped by the winds, which move in the opposite direction because of the cyclonic circulation, at the far side of the "eye." Within approximately twenty-five miles of the center, the winds move at their greatest velocity, nearly one hundred and fifty miles per hour. By comparison, at the outer rim of the hurricane the winds move rather slowly, approximately thirty miles per hour. Although the size of the storm and the intensity of the winds decrease with altitude, a hurricane may nevertheless tower more than seven and one-half miles into the stratosphere.

Despite their formation along the west coast of Mexico and Central America, hurricanes seldom produce destructive effects as far north as California. On the contrary, virtually all of the hurricanes that strike the United States are formed in the subtropical North Atlantic Ocean, the Caribbean Sea, and the Gulf of Mexico. Although most hurricanes threaten the Atlantic and Gulf coasts in August, September, and October, the six-month period from June to November is considered the Atlantic hurricane season. As a rule, early in the season, May and June, most hurricanes originate in the western Caribbean and the Gulf of Mexico. In July and August, the origin of the storms shifts eastward, and by September, most hurricanes form in the area from the Bahamas southeastward to the Lesser

Antilles and eastward to the Cape Verde Islands off the west coast of Africa. After mid-September, the origin shifts back, and once again most hurricanes originate in the western Caribbean and the Gulf of Mexico. On the average, six Atlantic hurricanes occur every year.

Once it has formed, a hurricane is undoubtedly the most powerful force in nature. In 1945, the atomic bomb dropped over Nagasaki, Japan, exploded with a blast equivalent to twenty-two thousand tons of TNT. By comparison, the average hurricane that sweeps across the Atlantic Ocean has a blast equivalent to eleven billion tons of TNT or nearly five hundred thousand times the explosive power of the Nagasaki bomb. Fortunately, a hurricane is spread over an area of approximately 126,000 square miles and may travel for one or two thousand miles before it strikes land. Naturally, if the power of a hurricane were unleashed along the relatively limited path of a tornado, the impact of the storm would completely destroy towns, cities, states, and even countries.

For persons in its path, a hurricane presents a triple threat in the form of strong winds, high tides, and heavy rains. Although wind speeds are somewhat reduced when the storm crosses an island or strikes a section of the mainland, the maximum wind velocities of an average hurricane may still reach one hundred and twenty-five miles per hour. In most cases the storm will continue to deliver these hurricane-force winds to the area for almost twelve hours. Yet, for persons living on or near the coast or in coastal or inland lowlands, high tides and heavy rain are usually a greater threat than the strong winds. As the storm approaches and travels across the coastline, it brings huge waves which raise tides fifteen or more feet above normal. In many cases the elevated tides approach so rapidly that flash floods are produced in coastal lowlands; in other cases the tides strike as giant waves (often mistakenly referred to as "tidal waves") which pound and demolish seawalls, docks, and buildings. In still other cases the elevated tides produce strong currents that erode beaches and seawalls, undermine building structures, and wash away highway and railroad beds. As the storm moves inland and its winds diminish, the torrential rains continue and produce extensive flooding. In most instances the hurricane will release between six to twelve inches of rainfall over the area, often in a few hours.

On September 8, 1900, a hurricane struck Galveston, Texas, and produced a storm tide that crested at fifteen feet above normal. When the water receded, six thousand persons were dead, and thirty million dollars worth of property was destroyed. According to Hoehling,

> Everywhere amid the debris was a thick slime, as a dazed, half-naked, bruised populace picked its way in search of loved ones. Death rested upon the whole sandbar, singly, in groups, in long windrows: corpses of horses, cows, pigs, and mules interspersed with those of men, women, and children. Some protruded from the broken timber of buildings; others lay stark and cold under the unkind

glare of daylight. Still others were found on beaches as distant as fifty miles up and down the coast.[2]

Tragically, the Galveston hurricane was the worst disaster in American history.

Today, through the efforts of the National Weather Service, the possibility of another "Galveston disaster" is very remote. During summer and autumn, meteorologists at the National Hurricane Center in Miami and at Weather Service Hurricane Warning Offices in Boston, New Orleans, San Juan, Washington, Honolulu, and San Francisco maintain a continuous watch for tropical disturbances which could develop into destructive hurricanes. By analyzing hemispheric summaries, cloud photographs and other satellite data, ship and aircraft reports, weather station measurements, aircraft reconnaissance information, tidal records, and radar trackings, meteorologists can determine whether or not a particular disturbance will intensify, remain unchanged, or dissipate. If an intensification is indicated, they can then predict the general path, speed, and direction of the storm. The meteorologists will then issue information to the general public in the areas threatened by the storm.

When a hurricane moves within a few hundred miles of the coast, the National Weather Service (NWS) will issue an "advisory" to warn small-craft operators to take precautions. During a small-craft warning, the boater should not venture into the open ocean. Even at a great distance from the storm, the waves may reach gigantic proportions. When winds of 38-55 miles per hour (33-48 knots) are expected, the NWS will add a "gale warning" to the advisory message. On the other hand, when winds of 55-74 miles per hour (48-64 knots) are expected, a "storm warning" will be added to the advisory. Gale and storm warnings specify the coastal region to be affected by the warning, the length of time that the warning will apply, and the expected intensity of the disturbance.

If the hurricane continues to advance and threatens coastal and inland regions, the National Weather Service will issue a "hurricane watch" in conjunction with the advisory message. The hurricane watch, which covers a specified area and time period, means that storm conditions may threaten within twenty-four hours; it does not mean that hurricane conditions are imminent. Except to listen to the radio or the television for additional NWS advisories, the person should continue his normal activities.

When hurricane conditions are actually expected within twenty-four hours, the National Weather Service will issue a "hurricane warning" in addition to the advisory. The hurricane warning will identify the coastal regions where winds of at least seventy-four miles per hour are expected to

2. A. A. Hoehling, *Disaster: Major American Catastrophes* (New York: Hawthorn Books, Inc., Publishers, 1973), p. 26.

occur. Also, the warning may specify coastal areas where dangerously high water or exceptionally high waves are expected, even though the winds may not be of hurricane force. As a rule, hurricane warnings are seldom issued more than twenty-four hours beforehand. In fact, if the path of the hurricane is unusual or erratic, the warnings may be issued only a few hours before the start of the hurricane conditions.

When a hurricane warning has been issued, the individual should plan his time before the storm hits and avoid any last-minute hurry which could leave him unprepared or marooned. If he lives in a mobile trailer or in a low-lying area that may be swept by high tides or storm waves, he should evacuate his home and seek shelter on high ground away from the ocean. On the other hand, if he lives on high ground and in a sturdy building, the person should stay at home during the storm.

Regardless of whether he stays at home, goes to a building on high ground, or moves to a designated shelter, the individual should first, if time safely permits, secure his home. Specifically, he should board up windows or protect them with tape or storm shutters. While large windows may be broken by the pressure of the winds, small windows are usually broken by wind-driven debris. Next, the person should bring outside possessions inside

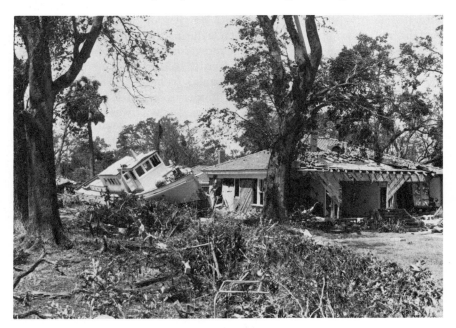

Figure 20.7   A private residence was destroyed, and a fishing boat was driven ashore in Biloxi, Mississippi, by a hurricane. (Courtesy of the National Oceanic and Atmospheric Administration)

the house or tie them down securely. In hurricane-force winds, trash cans, garden tools, lawn furniture, awnings, bricks, lumber, signs, toys, and other objects may become destructive, deadly missiles. Then he should store as much drinking water as possible in cooking utensils, bottles, jugs, and even clean bathtubs. After the storm has passed, the town's water supply may be contaminated by flooding or damaged by hurricane floods. Next the person should carefully check his battery-powered equipment. After the passage of the hurricane, a radio may be his only link with the outside world. Furthermore, if utilities are interrupted, flashlights, portable lights, and emergency cooking facilities will be essential. Finally, if he owns a boat the individual should store it in a garage, if it is small, or moor it in a narrow creek or canal, if it is larger.

During a hurricane the person should remain indoors. Since winds and tides will be whipping through the area, travel is extremely dangerous and often impossible. In some cases a sudden lull will occur in the winds, but this lull is simply an indication that the "eye" of the storm is directly overhead. At the other side of this calm storm center, the winds are whirling at hurricane force in the opposite direction. Depending upon the size of the "eye" and the forward speed of the storm, the lull will last from a few minutes to more than one-half hour. Unless emergency repairs are absolutely necessary, the individual should not permit himself or any of the members of his family to be lured outside during this stage of the hurricane.

After the passage of the storm, the individual should listen to local radio and television stations for complete disaster information. As a rule, unless he is qualified to help he should stay away from any disaster sites where rescue personnel are present. Besides hindering organized operations, the person may encounter numerous hazards, such as.weakened buildings, downed power lines, and leaking gas mains. However, if he must travel at a disaster site, the person should drive carefully along the debris-filled streets and avoid areas that are partially flooded.

River Floods

Floods are natural and inevitable occurrences along rivers. Each year nearly seventy-five thousand Americans are forced to evacuate their homes because of river floods. In addition, almost one hundred persons are killed, and over $250 million worth of property is damaged or destroyed.

Most often floods begin when soil and vegetation cannot absorb falling rain or melting snow and when water drains from the land in such quantities that it cannot be carried in normal river channels or retained in ponds and reservoirs. As the water level rises, the river whirls, churns, roars, and plunges until finally it surges over its banks and natural levees and flows onto the nearby floodplains. Persons who are caught in the path of the water,

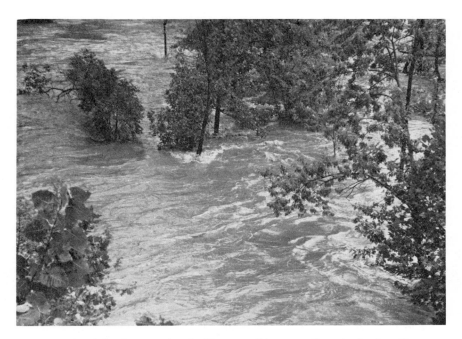

Figure 20.8   After heavy rains the Potomac River overflows its banks. (Courtesy of the National Oceanic and Atmospheric Administration)

as well as pets and livestock, may be drowned or severely injured by the current-borne debris. In addition, bridges, buildings, and farmlands may be damaged; personal possessions may be lost or destroyed; and water, power, and communication facilities may be disrupted.

Unfortunately, the transformation of a peaceful river into a raging, destructive flood occurs hundreds of times every year. No area in the country is completely free from the threat of floods. However, some areas are more susceptible than others. For example, certain regions of the country, such as the Pacific Northwest, the Rocky Mountains and Great Basin areas, and Southern California, are subjected to seasonal floods. Other sections, such as the Southeast and Gulf states, may experience periodic floods without any seasonal pattern. Still other regions, such as the Northeast and Mississippi River areas, may be subjected to floods at any time but are most likely to experience floods during a fairly well-defined period of the year.

Because of the threat of floods the National Weather Service (NWS) maintains a special river and rainfall reporting network and continually analyzes river and rainfall data. When rain falls in sufficient quantities to cause rivers to overflow their banks or when melting snow combines with rain to produce similar effects, the NWS will issue "flood forecasts and warnings."

The flood warnings are communicated to the general public by radio and television and through local emergency agencies. Each warning message specifies the expected degree of flooding (minor, moderate, or severe), the affected river, and when and where flooding will begin. On major tributaries, flood warnings can be issued hours to days in advance of the flood peak. However, main river flood forecasts can be issued as far in advance as several days or even weeks.

When a flood warning has been issued by the National Weather Service, the individual should always determine how many feet his property is below or above the predicted flood levels. If he lives in a low-lying area, he should secure his home and then evacuate the area before the flood begins. If time safely permits, the person should carry furniture and other movable objects to the upper floor of his house. However, if he cannot move the objects or if the house does not have an upper floor, he should disconnect electrical appliances and equipment and place any small, valuable possessions on tables, counters, and kitchen appliances. Finally, the person should lock the windows and the doors of his home and seek shelter on high ground.

Since flood waters may disrupt the town's services and utilities during and after the flooding, the individual in a high-lying area who remains at home still should prepare for the emergency. Generally, he should store as much drinking water as possible in cooking utensils, bottles, jugs, and clean bathtubs. When service is restored, he should boil the tap water until city officials announce that the water is unpolluted by the flood and safe to drink. Next the individual should check his supply of food and secure items that require little cooking and no refrigeration. After a flood, electrical services may be disrupted for several days. Then he should check his portable radio, emergency cooking equipment, flashlights, and portable lights to make certain they are in perfect working order. If utilities are interrupted, these items will be essential for a relatively normal routine. Finally, the individual should refuel his automobile and park the vehicle in a high, but readily accessible, location. In rare instances he may, in spite of these preparations, be forced to evacuate his home.

During an evacuation, the person should avoid areas that are already partially underwater. However, when this is impossible, certain measures should always be taken by the person. In a car he should never cross a dip without knowing the depth of the water. Often the water will hide a bridge or a part of the road that has been washed out. However, if the vehicle stalls, the individual should immediately leave the car and seek shelter on higher ground. On the other hand, if he is on foot, the person should never attempt to cross a flowing stream where the water would rise above his knees, since the current could pull him underwater and carry him downstream.

Once he has evacuated the area, the individual should listen to local radio and television stations for additional information on changing flood conditions and on emergency assistance projects in the community. Furthermore, unless he is a member of a rescue team or a cleanup group, he should avoid returning to the disaster area immediately after the flooding has ended. Besides hampering organized rescue and other emergency operations, the person may encounter numerous hazards, such as downed power lines, leaking gas mains, debris-filled streets, or washed-out bridges and roads.

Earthquakes

One of nature's most catastrophic phenomena, earthquakes are shakings or tremblings of the earth's crust. According to seismologists, every hour at least five quakes are occurring throughout the world. They range in size from minor tremors which are barely perceptible to devastating shocks. In the history of the world, the February 2, 1556 earthquake in China, which devastated three large provinces and killed 830,000 persons, is unequaled in terms of property and human destruction. By comparison, the worst earthquake in this country occurred in San Francisco, California, on April 18, 1906, and killed approximately four hundred and fifty persons.

Reconciling the evidence produced by geology, seismicity, gravity, and geomagnetics, scientists have developed the "plates theory" to explain the causative mechanisms of earthquakes. According to this theory, the earth is acted upon by the periodic forces of the solar system. In addition, in geologic time the earth is shifting on its axis. As a result, the molten and relatively plastic material from the upper mantle, which lies directly under the earth's crust, pushes upward along the mid-Atlantic ridge and causes movement of large plates or blocks of the earth's crust. Apparently, these plates interact by overlapping, rubbing together, or spreading where new crust is formed. As the plates move in relationship to each other, stresses develop and accumulate until a fracture or abrupt slippage occurs. These shaking and trembling movements, which are referred to as an earthquake, tend to relieve the stresses and thereby reestablish equilibrium.

The point at which the stresses are relieved by the movements is the focus of the earthquake. Although it may be located over four hundred miles beneath the surface of the earth, the focus is usually situated within a depth of forty miles. From the focus a succession of seismic waves radiate in all directions. When they reach the earth's surface, the waves spread outward and travel along the ground for many miles. Consequently, the damage caused by the earthquake, while normally insignificant at the point of origin, may be extensive at a great distance from the focus.

In describing the strength or magnitude of the quake at its origin or focus, not the damage caused by the shock itself, scientists use the Richter Scale. The smallest earthquakes identifiable by instruments have magnitudes of just above zero; the smallest earthquakes felt by man have magnitudes of above three; and the largest earthquakes have, theoretically, no upper limit. In the history of the world, however, no earthquake has reached a magnitude of greater than 8.9. In this country the San Francisco (1906) and the Alaska (1964) shocks had the greatest magnitude. According to seismologists, the San Francisco quake had a Richter reading of 8.3, and the Alaska quake had a reading of 8.6.

In 1945, the nuclear bomb dropped over Hiroshima, Japan, exploded with a blast equivalent to twenty thousand tons of TNT. By comparison, an earthquake with a magnitude of 8.5 on the Richter Scale is equivalent to an energy release of 240 million tons of TNT or nearly twelve thousand times the destructive power of the Hiroshima bomb. Naturally, however, the intensity or extent of damage caused by an earthquake is not always dependent upon the magnitude of the shock. For a quake to be intense, it must occur near an area of human habitation. Fortunately, most earthquakes originate beneath the oceans, where they cause little concern unless tsunamis, giant waves, are generated.

As a rule, the onset of a major earthquake is indicated by a deep rumbling sound or by a rushing sound of disturbed air. These sounds are quickly followed by a series of violent shakings and tremblings of the ground. Inside a building, the person will usually hear creaking, squeaking, and groaning sounds as the building strains with the movement of the ground. As the ground movements continue, buildings, bridges, dams, tunnels, water tanks, cliffs, and other rigid structures are set in motion in a vibrational pattern. If the motions are violent enough, the structures will then crack, spall, and even collapse. Depending upon the particular structures which are destroyed, the disaster site may then be subjected to fires, floods, and landslides. In addition, during an earthquake the ground may violently fissure or split, thereby leaving cracks and horizontal or vertical displacements in the earth.

While they may occur anywhere in the world, earthquakes are especially abundant along well-defined tracts called seismic belts. The greatest belt, the Circum-Pacific Belt, borders the Pacific Ocean from the Tonga and Fiji Islands through the Philippine and Ryukyu Islands, Japan, the Aleutian Islands, southern Alaska, and the Pacific coast of the United States, Central America, and South America. Of the three major belts and the numerous minor belts throughout the world, the Circum-Pacific Seismic Belt presents the greatest threat to the United States. However, while Alaska and the Pacific coastal states are most vulnerable to shocks, earthquakes may, and occasionally do, occur in other regions, such as Missouri, New England, and South Carolina.

Although much information has been gathered in recent years, scientists still cannot predict exactly when and where an earthquake will occur. For

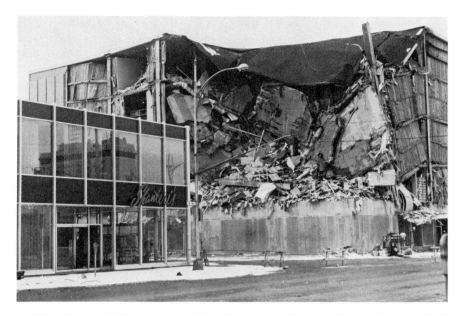

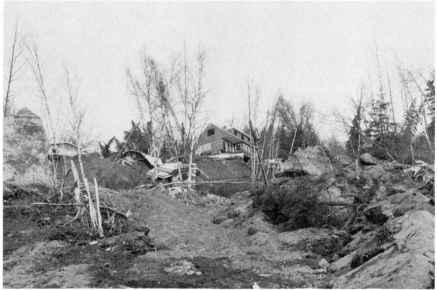

Figure 20.9   The Alaska earthquake on March 27, 1964, claimed one hundred and seventeen lives and produced $300 million in property damage. The city of Anchorage, as shown in these photographs, sustained the most damage. (Courtesy of the National Oceanic and Atmospheric Administration)

this reason, if he lives in a high-risk area, the person should always be prepared for an earthquake. In the construction of a new home, the individual should follow local building codes and other sound practices which are designed to reduce earthquake hazards. In addition, he should bolt down water heaters and other gas appliances, brace or anchor tall or top-heavy furniture, wire or anchor overhead fixtures, and store large or heavy objects on lower shelves in closets and other storage areas.

During an earthquake the person should remain as calm as possible and seek appropriate shelter. If he is indoors, he should sit or stand against an inside wall in the basement. However, if his home does not have a basement, he should take cover under a desk, table, or bench, preferably against an inside wall or in an inside doorway. When he is outdoors and on foot, the person should stay away from overhead electric wires, telephone poles, cornices of tall buildings, and other objects which might shake loose and fall to the ground. On the other hand, if he is outdoors and in a moving car, he should pull off the road and stop as soon as possible. However, until the quake subsides, he should remain within the hard, protective shell of the vehicle.

After an earthquake the individual should thoroughly survey his home, particularly foundations and chimneys, for any structural damage. In addition, he should check for fallen or damaged electrical wires, leaking gas pipes, and damaged sewer lines. If damage is detected, he should immediately implement all applicable emergency procedures given by local officials and then report any hazardous situations to the proper authorities. While he is entering or working in buildings after an earthquake, the individual should always use extreme caution, since a damaged or weakened structure may collapse suddenly without any warning and thereby trap or kill him.

Blizzards

By their simplest description, blizzards are winter storms in which strong winds whip huge amounts of snow into a horizontal fury. At times the snow, which is usually in the form of fine powderylike particles, may reduce visibility to only a few yards. Of all winter storms, blizzards are the most dramatic and dangerous. Each year in this country blizzards claim nearly one hundred lives and produce millions of dollars in property damage.

The storms are generated, as are many summer thunderstorms, by contact between cold polar and warm tropical air masses. Along the boundary between them, the air masses, with their different temperatures and densities, wage a perpetual struggle between instability and equilibrium. If the resulting disturbance becomes an intense low-pressure system, the cold front may churn over tens of thousands of miles in a great counterclockwise sweep.

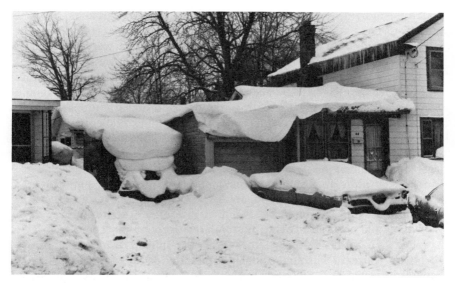

Figure 20.10 After repeated blizzards near Syracuse, New York, cars and homes were covered by five to seven feet of snow. (Courtesy of the National Oceanic and Atmospheric Administration)

In the Pacific area, disturbances form along the polar fronts off the east coast of Asia and travel northeastward toward Alaska and sometimes southeastward toward California. In some cases the disturbances cross the Rocky Mountains in this country and Canada, redevelop to the east, and then converge over the Great Lakes, thus affecting the Midwest states. In addition, disturbances form over the Great Lakes and move southward, while other disturbances drift northward to the midwest from the southern plains and the Gulf of Mexico. On the Atlantic coast, disturbances form along the polar front near the coast of Virginia and the Carolinas and in the area east of the southern Appalachian Mountains, and then travel northward along the coast.

In some regions of this country, blizzards are a threat from mid-September to mid-May. During any one of the colder months from November to March, several different blizzards may affect an area at the same time or they may affect it on succeeding days. When blizzards strike a region, they completely immobilize large areas, isolating and killing persons and livestock in their paths. In the northern parts of the United States, the severity of the storms makes them a seasonal threat.

As winter approaches, the meteorologists of the National Weather Service (NWS) monitor atmospheric conditions to detect disturbances which could develop into severe winter storms. When a storm has formed and is approaching the area, the NWS will issue a "blizzard watch." During a watch the individual should begin to take precautionary measures. Since he may be isolated at home for one or two weeks, especially in rural areas, the person should stock an emergency supply of food and water, as well as emergency cooking equipment. Because of a possible power failure, some of the food should be of the type that does not require refrigeration. Since regular fuel supplies may be curtailed by the blizzard, the person should keep an adequate supply of heating fuel on hand and use it sparingly. If necessary, he should conserve fuel by keeping the house cooler than usual or by "closing off" some rooms temporarily. In addition, he should stock some kind of emergency heating equipment and fuel so that he can keep at least one room of his house warm enough to sustain normal activities. Finally, the individual should check his battery-powered equipment and secure a plentiful supply of extra batteries. During and after a blizzard he may need a radio to obtain weather and disaster information, as well as flashlights and portable lights to maintain relatively normal routines.

When a blizzard is imminent, the NWS will issue a warning in one of two forms. A "blizzard warning" indicates that considerable falling or blowing snow is expected in conjunction with winds at speeds of at least thirty-five miles per hour. Under these conditions, visibilities are dangerously limited, thus making it very easy to become lost or stranded. On the other hand, a "severe blizzard warning" means that a great density of falling or blowing snow, winds with speeds of at least forty-five miles per hour, and a temperature of ten degrees Fahrenheit or lower are expected. When either warning has been issued, the individual should remain in his home until the passage of the blizzard. However, if he becomes trapped in his car by the storm, he should stay in the vehicle. Moving on foot in open country during a blizzard is almost certain death. In addition, he is more likely to be found if he remains in his car. To make the vehicle more visible to work crews, the person should activate the emergency flashers, turn on the dome light, and hang a dark-colored piece of cloth from the radio antenna or the car window. Then, while waiting to be rescued he should periodically change sitting positions and exercise occasionally by clapping his hands and moving his arms and legs vigorously. If he needs more warmth, the person can run the engine and heater sparingly. However, to protect himself against carbon monoxide gas, he should open the downwind window for ventilation.

After the passage of a blizzard, the individual should avoid overexertion in the cold. Many unnecessary deaths occur because persons suddenly engage in more strenuous physical activity than they are accustomed. Although cold weather by itself places an extra strain on the body, physical exertion in the cold, such as shovelling snow or pushing an automobile, may tax the circulatory system to the utmost. Consequently, even for persons in apparently good physical condition, the cold-exertion combination may result in a stroke, heart attack, or other bodily damage.

Planning for Man-made Disasters

Of the various types of man-made disasters, public fires and nuclear attack present the greatest threats to the general population. Each year fires in public places kill almost as many people as all of the natural disasters combined. On the other hand, nuclear attack has the potential to produce more deaths and widespread devastation than all of the disasters, both natural and man-made, in the history of this country.

Public Fires

Any escape from a fire is difficult. However, in a public fire most persons feel utterly helpless to escape. Typically, in competition with each other, individuals run, push, shove, and even fight others in their desperation. Tragically, each year in this country, approximately six hundred persons are killed by fires in public places.

In addition to the basic fire information which was presented in Chapter 8, the individual should remember one basic rule during a public fire: do not attempt to escape through the main entrance. In their panic most persons try to escape by the same route through which they entered, thereby crushing each other in the process. After the Iroquois Theater fire in Chicago, Illinois, on December 30, 1903, firemen found bodies piled four feet high at the main entrance. The balcony doors through which the occupants could have escaped had not even been opened. Altogether, five hundred and seventy-five persons were killed in the fire. As a general rule, when entering a public place, the person should always look for the nearest exits and then plan to use one of them during an escape emergency.

Nuclear Attack

Possessing only 6 percent of the world's population, the United States uses nearly one-third of the world's total energy production. At present this energy production is based predominantly on fossil fuels, such as coal, oil, and natural gas. However, the fossil fuels are not inexhaustible. Consequently, scientists have turned to a new source of power: the atom. By 1985, nuclear power plants are expected to produce 40 to 50 percent of the energy in this country.

Despite the unlimited number of peaceful uses for nuclear energy, one fact still remains: nuclear energy was originally developed for a single purpose, the production of death and destruction. This was clearly demonstrated at Hiroshima and Nagasaki during the closing days of World War II. In explosions that cast lights "brighter than a thousand suns," more than 100,000 persons were killed immediately, and thousands of buildings were leveled. In recent years, with the development of nuclear weapons throughout the world, a nuclear attack on the United States has become a definite threat.

In a nuclear attack the main effects are flash (intense light), heat, blast, and radiation. However, the intensity of the effects is dependent upon the size and type of weapon, the distance from the explosion, the height of the explosion, the nature of the terrain, and the weather conditions.

As a rule, persons close to the explosion will be killed or seriously injured by the heat or the blast. On the other hand, those who are a few miles away in the "fringe area" of the explosion will be endangered by the heat and the blast and by the fires started by the explosion. However, most of the persons will survive the hazards.

Outside the fringe area, individuals are not affected by the heat, blast, or fires, but they are threatened by the radioactive fallout. According to studies by the Department of Defense, in any nuclear attack on this country, tens of millions of persons will be outside the fringe areas.[3]

When a nuclear weapon explodes close to the ground, thousands of tons of pulverized earth and debris are sucked upward into a mushroom-shaped cloud, which may reach an altitude of sixteen miles or more before leveling off. Within the cloud, radioactive gases produced by the explosion condense in and upon the dirt and debris, thereby producing radioactive particles. After a short time the particles, referred to as "fallout," then fall back to the earth. On their way down and after they reach the ground, these particles give off invisible streams of radiation that can injure or kill persons.

In simple terms, nuclear radiation damages the body by causing physical and chemical changes in the cells. The extent of the damage depends upon the amount of radiation that the person has received and the period of time that he was exposed. Typically, a person suffering from radiation sickness will exhibit a lack of appetite, nausea, vomiting, fatigue, drowsiness, weakness, headache, sore mouth, loss of hair, bleeding gums, diarrhea, and bleeding under the skin. In cases of extreme exposure, he may die within hours or days. However, if he survives, the person may suffer from fever and mouth ulcers for a period of seven to eight weeks.

Depending upon wind currents, weather conditions, and other factors, radioactive particles in a nuclear cloud may be carried for miles and then disseminated in all directions. Consequently, no one can predict how soon, or to what extent, the particles will fall back toward the earth or even where they will land. However, as a rule, areas close to a nuclear explosion will receive fallout within fifteen to thirty minutes. On the other hand, areas between one hundred and two hundred miles away may not receive any fallout

---

3. Department of Defense/Office of Civil Defense, *In Time of Emergency* (Washington, D.C.: U.S. Government Printing Office, 1968), p. 11.

for five to ten hours. According to defense officials, after a nuclear attack no area in the United States can be sure of not getting fallout, and most areas can be reasonably certain of receiving at least some fallout.

Generally, after the fallout begins to settle, the first twenty-four hours is the most dangerous period. The heavier particles which fall first are still highly radioactive and thus give off strong rays. However, the lighter particles which remain airborne longer will lose much of their radiation high in the atmosphere and therefore will emit weaker rays.

In all cases of radioactive fallout, three kinds of radiation are emitted: alpha, beta, and gamma. The penetrating power of these particles and rays varies greatly. Alpha particles will penetrate very thin metal foils, but they are stopped by a piece of paper; beta particles will penetrate thin sheets of metals, but they are stopped by ordinary clothing; and gamma rays will penetrate several inches of metal, but they are stopped by a foot of lead. Thus, because of their greater penetrating power, gamma rays present the greatest threat to human life.

In all probability a nuclear attack on the United States by a foreign power would be preceded by a period of international tension or crisis. This crisis period should help to alert Americans to the possibility of attack. However, if an attack actually occurs, this country's network of warning systems would almost certainly detect the incoming missiles in time for citizens to seek shelter. In some locations the warning time may be as little as five to fifteen minutes; in other locations it may be as much as one hour or longer.

Depending upon where he happens to be at the time, the person may hear the attack warning on a radio or television broadcast, or from another person by word-of-mouth. Furthermore, in some cities, towns, and villages, he may receive the alert from an outdoor warning system. In this case the signal will be a three to five-minute wavering sound on sirens, or a series of short blasts on whistles, horns, or bells. Regardless of the method by which he receives the warning, the person, unless the local government has instructed otherwise, should immediately seek protection in a public fallout shelter. Once he is safely inside the shelter, he should turn on his portable radio and listen to a local station for official disaster information. Until he receives other instructions, the individual should remain inside the shelter and follow all recommended attack procedures. After a nuclear war the individual, as well as others in the community, may be forced to stay in the shelter for several days or weeks.

Resource Materials

National Safety Council
444 North Michigan Avenue
Chicago, Illinois 60611

Superintendent of Documents
U.S. Government Printing Office
Washington, D.C. 20402

Activities

1. Select one of the disaster "case histories" given in this chapter, research the incident thoroughly, and write a short report on your findings.

2. Prepare a twenty-five-question true or false test over the material on "thunderstorms," and administer the test to fifty adults. Discuss the test questions and the test results with the class.

3. Invite a local meteorologist to speak to the class about the National Weather Service and its many functions.

4. Conduct a survey of ten adults to determine their preparedness for a nuclear attack on the United States by a foreign power. Summarize the results, and discuss with the class the adults' plans for survival in a nuclear war.

5. Prepare a scrapbook of newspaper articles which report disasters. When at least twenty articles have been collected, write a two-page, statistical summary of the disasters.

Questions

1. What are the five dangers associated with thunderstorms?
2. What is the Beaufort Scale?
3. If ten seconds have elapsed between the lightning and the thunder, how far away is the thunderstorm?
4. What is another name for a tornado?
5. What type of shelter offers the best protection against a tornado?
6. What does a "thunderstorm watch" mean?
7. What is the "eye" of a hurricane, and why can it lead an unwary person to his death?
8. What is the Richter Scale?
9. What precautionary measures should be taken during a blizzard watch?
10. What is the most dangerous period after a nuclear attack?

Selected References

Carper, Jean. *Stay Alive!* Garden City, New York: Doubleday & Company, Inc., 1965.

Dunn, Gordon E. and Banner I. Miller. *Atlantic Hurricanes.* n.c.: Louisiana State University Press, 1964.

Hoehling, A. A. *Disaster: Major American Catastrophes.* New York: Hawthorn Books, Inc. Publishers, 1973.

"How Do Precipitation and Temperatures Affect the Occurrence of Floods?," *Science Digest,* March, 1973, 56.

U.S. Department of Commerce/National Oceanic and Atmospheric Administration. *Tornado.* Washington, D.C.: U.S.Government Printing Office, (Rev) 1976.

———. *Floods, Flash Floods and Warnings.* Washington, D.C.: U.S. Government Printing Office, (Rev) 1973.

———. *Severel Local Storm Warning Service and Tornado Statistics, 1953-1973.* Washington, D.C.: U.S. Government Printing Office, (Rev) 1974.

———. *Thunderstorms.* Washington, D.C.: U.S. Government Printing Office, 1976.

———. *Winter Storms.* Washington, D.C.: U.S. Government Printing Office, (Rev) 1975.

———. *Hurricane Information and Atlantic Tracking Chart.* Washington, D.C.: U.S. Government Printing Office, 1974.

U.S. Department of Defense/Office of Civil Defense. *In Time of Emergency.* Washington, D.C.: U.S. Government Printing Office, March, 1968.

Appendix

Contents

Basic Review Guide for General First Aid

1. First Aid Guidelines

"*First aid* is the immediate care given to a person who has been injured or has been suddenly taken ill."[1] Besides reassuring the victim with verbal encouragement, competent handling, and a willingness to help, the first-aider should enlist the aid of bystanders to:

1. telephone for medical assistance,
2. telephone the appropriate authorities (police department or highway patrol), and
3. protect the accident scene (direct traffic, position safety flares, or keep onlookers at a distance).

While help is being summoned, the first-aider should attend to the following:

1. maintain breathing by opening the airway and, if necessary, by performing mouth-to-mouth or mouth-to-nose artificial respiration,
2. control severe bleeding,
3. give first aid for poisoning, or
4. control for shock.

The first-aider should also:

1. refrain from any unnecessary manipulation of the victim,
2. examine the victim for clues to the nature of his injury or illness (color of skin, nailbeds, or mucous membranes on the inside of the mouth; presence or absence of carotid pulse at the side of the neck; size of pupils of victim's eyes; and observable injuries), and
3. perform any additional first aid measures which appear to be necessary.

2. Traumatic Shock

Injury-related shock, commonly called traumatic shock, is a depression of numerous vital body functions. It usually accompanies injuries or emotional upsets and may cause death even though the victim's original condition would not otherwise be fatal.

---

1. The American National Red Cross, *Standard First Aid and Personal Safety* (Garden City, New York: Doubleday & Company, Inc., 1973), p. 11.

Signs and Symptoms

1. Skin, nailbeds, and mucous membranes on the inside of the mouth or under the eyelids are pale in color.
2. Skin is cold.
3. Skin may be moist and clammy from perspiration.
4. Pulse is usually rapid but weak.
5. Breathing is usually increased but may be shallow, deep, or irregular.
6. Pupils of the eyes are often widely dilated.
7. Nausea or vomiting may be apparent.

First Aid Measures

1. Keep the victim lying flat on his back with his feet or the foot of the stretcher elevated eight to twelve inches. However, if the victim experiences additional pain or increased breathing difficulty, lower the feet again. In special cases one of the following shock positions may be used:
   a. Flat on his back with his head and shoulders elevated eight to twelve inches—red face or breathing difficulty.
   b. On his side—nausea, vomiting, or severe wounds of the lower part of the face and jaw (especially if the victim is unconscious).
   c. Flat on his back—head injury, suspected spinal fracture, or doubt about the proper position.
2. Place a sheet, a blanket, or several articles of clothing over and under the victim to keep him warm. However, the victim should not be made to perspire.
3. Give fluids (water, tea, coffee, etc.) by mouth only under the following conditions:
   a. Medical help will *not* be available for one hour or more.
   b. The victim is *not* unconscious, nauseated, vomiting, convulsing, or suffering from a head injury or abdominal injury. In addition, do *not* give fluids if the victim is likely to require emergency surgery or a general anesthetic.

The following fluid mixture may be used if the ingredients are available: 1 teaspoon salt, 1/2 teaspoon baking soda, and 1 quart water (neither hot or cold). Give an adult victim four ounces (1/2 glass) every fifteen minutes. Approximately two ounces (1/4 glass) should be given to children between the ages of one and twelve, and one ounce (1/8 glass) should be given to infants under the age of one.

3. Wounds

Wounds may be classified as either open or closed. In an open wound the skin or the mucous membrane is broken. Open wounds include abrasions, incisions, lacerations, punctures, and avulsions. In a closed wound, referred to as a bruise or a contusion, the tissues underlying the area of contact are injured, but the skin or the mucous membrane is not broken.

Heavily Bleeding Open Wounds

Damage to a vein or an artery usually results in a rapid loss of blood. Such a loss can easily lead to shock, unconsciousness, and death within a matter of minutes.

First Aid Measures

1. Place a clean handkerchief, cloth, or pad directly over the wound and press firmly with the palm of your hand (direct pressure). Then, unless a fracture is evident, raise the injured part (elevation) until the wound is above the level of the victim's heart. If blood saturates the pad, do not remove it; instead, place additional pads over the original pad and continue direct pressure.
2. Firmly bandage the pads in place and secure the bandage with a knot directly over the pads (pressure bandage).
3. If the bleeding does not stop after the use of direct pressure, elevation, and a pressure bandage, apply pressure over the artery supplying the injured part (pressure point). The most frequently used pressure points are shown in Figure A.1. When applying a pressure point, continue to use both direct pressure and elevation of the injured part.
4. After the bleeding has been stopped, perform the necessary measures to control shock.
5. Summon medical help as soon as possible.

WARNING

A tourniquet is rarely required to control bleeding. It should be used only when an arm or a leg has been amputated, mangled, or crushed or when bleeding from an arm or a leg threatens life and cannot be controlled by other means. According to the American National Red Cross, "The decision to apply a tourniquet is in reality a decision to risk sacrifice of a limb in order to save life."[2]

---

2. The American National Red Cross, p. 28.

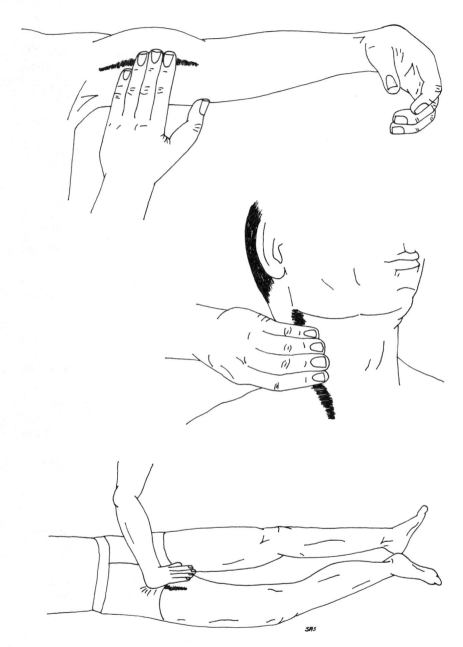

Figure A.1   Pressure points—(top) brachial artery, (middle) carotid artery, and (bottom) femoral artery.

To apply a tourniquet, use a strong, wide (at least two inches) piece of cloth. Never use wire, twine, rope, or similar material. Wrap the tourniquet band around the limb just above the wound. However, if the wound is at a joint or just below the joint, place the tourniquet band immediately above the joint. Tie a half-knot; place a short, strong stick, or similar object on the half-knot; tie a full-knot over the stick; twist the stick to tighten the tourniquet just enough to stop the bleeding; and secure the stick in place with the loose ends of the tourniquet or another strip of cloth. Mark the letters "TK" and the time of application on the victim's forehead. Do not cover the tourniquet or loosen it except on the advice of a physician.

Internal Bleeding

Whenever a violent force has been exerted on the body, the first-aider should expect a closed wound with the possibility of internal bleeding.

Signs and Symptoms

1. Skin, nailbeds, and mucous membranes on the inside of the mouth or under the eyelids are pale in color.
2. Skin is cold.
3. Skin may be moist and clammy from perspiration.
4. Pulse is usually rapid but weak.
5. Breathing is usually increased but may be shallow, deep, or irregular.
6. Pupils of the eyes are often widely dilated.
7. Victim may exhibit uncontrolled restlessness and excessive thirst.
8. Blood may be vomited or coughed up, or it may be apparent in the urine or feces.
9. Victim may complain of pain and tenderness in the area where the injury is suspected.
10. Swelling, discoloration, or a deformity in the injured area may be visible.

First Aid Measures

1. Keep the victim lying flat on his back. However, if he vomits or coughs up blood, turn his head to the side to permit the substance to drain out the side of his mouth. Always maintain an open airway in the victim.
2. Place a sheet, a blanket, or several articles of clothing over and under the victim to keep him warm. However, the victim should not be made to perspire.

3. Even though he complains of extreme thirst, do *not* give the victim any fluid by mouth.
4. Summon medical help for the victim as soon as possible.

Impaled Object

Often a penetrating foreign object, such as a stick, metal rod, gearshift lever, or section of glass, will remain fixed in the victim's body. This impaled object should be removed only by a physician.

First Aid Measures

1. Place the victim in a flat, lying-down position. If the object will not permit this action, leave the item in place but cut it off at a distance from the skin.
2. Place massive pads around the object to hold it firmly in place.
3. Cover the victim wherever possible with a sheet, a blanket, or several articles of clothing. Do *not* cause the victim to perspire, and do *not* cover the object with the sheet, blanket, or clothing.
4. Summon medical help as soon as possible.

Head (Brain) Injury

Whenever the victim has sustained a blow to the head, the first-aider should expect possible, direct or indirect, damage to the brain.

Signs and Symptoms

1. Victim may experience semiconsciousness or unconsciousness.
2. Clear or blood-tinged fluid may drain from the nose or ears.
3. Bleeding from the nose, ears, or mouth may be apparent.
4. Pupils of the eyes may be of unequal size.
5. Partial or complete paralysis of a body part may exist.
6. Victim may exhibit dizziness, slurred speech, convulsions, vomiting, or a loss of bowel and bladder control.

First Aid Measures

1. Keep the victim lying flat on his back and gently turn his head to the side to allow vomit, blood, or other secretions to flow out the side of the mouth. Always maintain an open airway for the victim.
2. Cover the victim with a sheet, a blanket, or clothing to keep him warm. However, the victim should not be made to perspire.
3. Control severe bleeding, but do *not* place direct pressure over a suspected skull fracture.

4. Even though the victim desires water, do *not* give any fluids by mouth.
5. Seek medical aid immediately.

Abdominal (Stomach) Wounds

Because of the possibility of damage to internal organs, abdominal wounds are especially dangerous.

First Aid Measures

1. Place the victim on his back with a pillow, rolled blanket, or other object under his knees.
2. If the intestines or abdominal organs protrude from the wound, cover them with a sterile dressing, a clean towel, a sheet of plastic, or a piece of metal foil. If medical help will be delayed, moisten the material with cool, boiled water.
3. If breathing difficulty is apparent, elevate the victim's head and shoulders about eight to twelve inches.
4. Cover the victim wherever possible with a sheet, a blanket, or several articles of clothing. Do *not* give the victim enough covering to cause him to perspire.
5. Since surgery will be necessary, do *not* give the victim any fluids by mouth.
6. As rapidly as possible, obtain medical help.

Sucking Wound of the Chest

A deep, open wound of the chest wall through which air can flow in and out during the breathing process is referred to as a sucking wound of the chest. Unless air is prevented from entering the chest cavity, the victim's lung on the injured side will collapse.

Signs and Symptoms

1. A characteristic sucking sound can be heard when the victim breathes.
2. If the lung has also been punctured, the victim may cough up bright-red, frothy (bubbly) blood.
3. Victim will exhibit or complain of breathing difficulty.

First Aid Measures

1. After the victim has breathed out, place a large sterile gauze pad, a clean cloth, a sheet of plastic, or a piece of metal foil over the

wound. Secure the pad, which should form an airtight seal, with tape, a belt, or a bandage.

2. To ease the victim's breathing, place him on his injured side, or, if the victim desires, place him flat on his back with his head and shoulders elevated eight to twelve inches.

3. Place a sheet, a blanket, or several articles of clothing over and under the victim to keep him warm. Do *not*, however, cause the victim to perspire.

4. Seek medical assistance as soon as possible.

4. Respiratory Emergencies

A respiratory emergency occurs when normal breathing stops or when breathing is so reduced that the resulting oxygen intake is not sufficient to maintain life. If the brain is deprived of oxygen for four or more minutes, the result is either irreversible brain damage or, more likely, death. Typical causes of respiratory emergencies include:

1. heart attack,
2. water submersion,
3. electric shock,
4. gas poisoning (particularly carbon monoxide gas),
5. depressant-drug overdose,
6. choking on food, objects, or fluids,
7. tongue's dropping back and obstructing the throat,
8. hanging,
9. heavy object's pressing on the chest, and
10. swelling of the throat from a blow or burns.

Signs and Symptoms

1. Breathing movements have stopped.
2. Victim is unconscious.
3. Victim's tongue, lips, and fingernail beds are blue.
4. Pupils of the eyes are widely dilated and in extreme emergencies will not constrict when light strikes them.

First Aid Measures

1. Whenever necessary, such as in electric shock or carbon monoxide poisoning, remove the victim to safety.
2. If the victim is choking on food or a foreign object, stand behind the victim, wrap your arms around his waist, and clasp your hands

together against his stomach. Then, apply pressure quickly and forcefully just below the victim's rib cage. The object should "pop" out of the mouth.

3. Quickly tilt the victim's head backward so his chin is pointing upward.
4. If breathing remains stopped, pinch the victim's nostrils shut with your thumb and index finger. Then, with your mouth sealed tightly around the victim's mouth, blow into the victim until his chest rises. Remove your mouth and permit the victim to breathe out. Continue this procedure once every five seconds for an adult or once every three seconds for a child. (Note: Although the mouth-to-mouth method was described in this step, the first-aider may be required in special cases to use either the mouth-to-nose, the mouth-to-mouth and nose (child), the mouth-to-stoma (laryngectomee), or a manual method of artificial respiration. However, regardless of the method, the first-aider should still complete one cycle every five seconds for an adult or one cycle every three seconds for a child.)
5. Continue artificial respiration until the victim is able to breathe by himself or until he is pronounced dead by a physician.
6. After the victim begins to breathe for himself, cover him with a sheet, a blanket, or several articles of clothing to control shock.
7. Obtain medical assistance as rapidly as possible.

5.   Cardiac Arrest

In cardiac arrest, circulation is either absent or inadequate to sustain life. Typical causes of cardiac arrest include:

1. cardiovascular collapse (shock, various drugs, or severe bleeding),
2. ventricular fibrillation (heart attack, electric shock, or fresh-water submersion), and
3. cardiac standstill (carbon monoxide poisoning or suffocation).

Signs and Symptoms

1. Breathing movements have stopped.
2. Victim is unconscious.
3. Victim's tongue, lips, and fingernail beds are blue.
4. Pupils of the eyes are widely dilated and will not constrict when they are exposed to light.
5. Carotid pulse in the neck will not be present.

First Aid Measures

A. Witnessed cardiac arrest (Arrest is seen, and cardiopulmonary resuscitation is started within one minute.)
1. Quickly tilt the victim's head backward so his chin is pointing upward, or if the head tilt alone is unsuccessful in opening the airway, perform the jaw thrust maneuver by lifting the lower jaw upward, tilting the head backward, and drawing the lower lip downward to open the mouth.
2. Feel for the carotid pulse in the neck.
3. If the pulse is absent, place your clenched fist eight to twelve inches above the victim's chest and deliver a quick, firm blow over the middle of the sternum with the fleshy part of your fist (precordial thump maneuver).
4. Check for signs of a breathing stoppage. If breathing is absent, give four quick, full lung inflations.
5. If the pulse and breathing are not immediately restored, quickly begin cardiopulmonary resuscitation (CPR).
   a. One-rescuer method on adult victim: compress the lower one-half of the sternum at a rate of eighty times per minute and quickly give two full lung inflations after every fifteen compressions.
   b. Two-rescuer method on adult victim: compress the lower one-half of the sternum at a rate of sixty times per minute while your fellow rescuer quickly gives a full lung inflation after every five compressions.
   c. Method on child: compress the midsternum at a rate of eighty to one hundred times per minute while providing one quick lung inflation after every five compressions.
6. Periodically check the carotid pulse and pupils of the eye to determine the effectiveness of the CPR or the return of a spontaneous heartbeat.
7. As rapidly as possible, secure medical help.
B. Unwitnessed cardiac arrest (Arrest is unseen or CPR is not started within one minute.)
1. Quickly tilt the victim's head backward so his chin is pointing upward, or when the head tilt does not sufficiently open the airway, perform the jaw thrust maneuver by lifting the lower jaw upward, tilting the head backward, and drawing the lower lip downward to open the mouth.
2. Check for signs of a breathing stoppage. If breathing has stopped, give four quick, full lung inflations.

3. Feel for the carotid pulse in the neck.
4. If the pulse is absent, quickly begin CPR.
    a. One-rescuer method on adult: compress the lower one-half of the sternum at a rate of eighty times per minute and quickly give two full lung inflations after every fifteen compressions.
    b. Two-rescuer method on adult: compress the lower one-half of the sternum at a rate of sixty times per minute while your assistant quickly gives a full lung inflation after every five compressions.
    c. Method on child: compress the midsternum at a rate of eighty to one hundred times per minute while providing one quick lung inflation after every five compressions.
5. To determine the effectiveness of the CPR or the return of a spontaneous heartbeat, periodically check the carotid pulse and the pupils of the eye.
6. As soon as possible, obtain medical assistance.

WARNING

CPR should be performed only by persons who have been specially trained in the recognition of cardiac arrest and have practiced extensively on manikins. A fractured sternum, separations of the rib cartilages, lung contusions, and lacerations of the liver are all complications that may result even with properly performed CPR. Obviously, the danger of serious injury is much greater when the rescuer is inexperienced or lax in performing proper CPR.

---

6. Poisoning

Poisons may enter the body in any one of four ways:

1. by mouth (orally),
2. by injection,
3. by inhalation, or
4. by absorption.

Each mode of entry requires strikingly different first aid measures.

Oral Poisoning

The most common means by which poisons enter the body is by mouth or orally.

Signs and Symptoms

The signs and symptoms of poisoning vary greatly according to the type of poison that has been swallowed.

A. Noncorrosives (Examples include aspirin, barbiturate drugs, opium derivatives, tranquilizers, ant paste, vitamins, and plants.)
    1. Victim may experience restlessness or dizziness.
    2. Pulse is slow, and breathing is shallow.
    3. Victim will usually appear drowsy.
B. Corrosives (Examples include acids, such as hydrochloric, sulfuric, and nitric, and alkalies, such as drain cleaner, lye, washing soda, ammonia, and bleach.)
    1. Burns will be apparent around the lips or mouth.
    2. Victim will complain of extreme pain.
C. Petroleum products (Examples include gasoline, kerosine, fuel oil, lighter fluid, and furniture polish.)
    1. Victim will have a strong "petroleum-like" odor on his breath.
    2. Victim may choke, gasp, and cough.
    3. Victim may experience abdominal pain, dizziness, drowsiness, and shallow breathing.

First Aid Measures

A. Noncorrosives
    1. Give the victim one or two glasses (three or four for an adult) of milk or water to dilute the poison.
    2. Induce vomiting by giving "syrup of ipecac" in the dosage recommended on the label. If ipecac is not available, insert your finger or the blunt end of a spoon into the back of the victim's mouth. Do *not* give mustard water, soapy water, or salt water as a means of inducing vomiting.
    3. When vomiting occurs, place or hold the victim face down to prevent vomitus from entering the lungs.
    4. To absorb any poison remaining in the stomach *after* vomiting, give the victim one glass of a mixture of water and activated medicinal charcoal. To mix the fluid, slowly add water to the charcoal until the mixture has a "soupy" appearance.
    5. If the victim is conscious and has taken aspirin, tranquilizers, barbiturates, paregoric, opium-containing drugs, or drinking alcohol, give stimulant drinks, such as coffee or strong tea.
B. Corrosives
    1. Give the victim two or three glasses (three or four for an adult) of milk or water to dilute the poison. Do *not* induce vomiting; do *not* give a neutralizing fluid; and do *not* administer a demulcent, such as olive oil or egg whites.

C. Petroleum products
   1. Give the victim one or two glasses (two or three for an adult) of milk or water to dilute the poison. Do *not* induce vomiting.
   2. If vomiting does occur, place or hold the victim face down to prevent vomitus from entering the lungs.
   3. To absorb the poison, give the victim a mixture of activated charcoal and water in a dosage of not less than five times the estimated amount of poison ingested, if the stomach is empty of food, or not less than ten times the estimated amount of poison ingested, if the stomach is filled with food. As a general rule, this dosage should never be less than one glass. To mix the fluid, slowly add water to the medicinal charcoal until the mixture has a "soupy" appearance.

General Poisoning Guidelines

1. Regardless of the type of poison, immediately give a conscious victim milk or water to dilute the substance.
2. If a specific antidote is printed on the product's label, perform the listed first aid measures.
3. When no antidote is listed, classify the poison, and carry out the steps suggested for that particular class of products. However, if you are unsure about the poison's proper classification, immediately seek advice from the local poison control center, a physician, or hospital personnel.
4. After performing any first aid measures, transport the victim to the hospital as rapidly as possible. Always bring along the poison's container for identification of the substance and, if the victim has vomited, a sample of the vomited material.

Poisonous Injections by Insects, Spiders, and Scorpions

Stings by bees, wasps, yellow jackets, hornets, and ants occasionally result in death. In most cases these deaths are caused by extreme allergic reactions, rather than by the venom itself. Bites by black widow and brown recluse spiders and stings by scorpions, on the other hand, result in severe localized or generalized reactions from the venom. While nearly all the victims recover, an occasional death may result.

Signs and Symptoms

A. Insect stings
   1. Redness, swelling, and an itchy feeling are apparent at the site of the sting.
   2. Victim may appear flushed shortly after the sting, but later he will appear pale.

3. Swelling of the hands, feet, and throat may occur.
4. Victim may experience extreme difficulty in breathing.
B. Spider bites
   1. Black widow spider
      a. Victim will develop only a slight localized reaction, but he will usually experience severe pain.
      b. Victim may exhibit profuse sweating and difficulty in breathing and speaking.
      c. Victim may experience nausea, vomiting, and extremely painful abdominal cramps.
   2. Brown recluse spider
      a. A generalized rash may develop within 24 to 48 hours.
      b. Victim may experience chills, fever, joint pains, nausea, and vomiting.
      c. A severe local reaction, which results in an open ulcer within one or two weeks, will be apparent at the bite site.
C. Scorpion stings
   1. Victim may experience extreme pain at the site of the sting, as well as abdominal pain.
   2. Victim may exhibit vomiting, convulsions, and shock.

First Aid Measures

1. If the sting or bite is on the victim's arm or leg, apply a constricting band above the injection site. If the device is applied correctly, you should be able to slip your index finger under the band. Do *not* leave the band in place longer than thirty minutes.
2. Keep the injection site below the level of the victim's heart.
3. To reduce swelling, relieve pain, and slow the spread of the venom, apply cold cloths or ice wrapped in a towel or plastic bag over the sting or bite.
4. As quickly as possible, transport the victim to a hospital.

Injections by Poisonous Snakes

Four kinds of poisonous snakes are found in the United States:

1. rattlesnakes,
2. copperheads,
3. cottonmouths, and
4. coral snakes.

Because they possess a heat-sensitive pit between the eye and the nostril on each side of the head, the first three snakes are called pit vipers.

Signs and Symptoms

A. Pit vipers
    1. One or more puncture marks produced by the fangs may be visible at the bite site.
    2. Victim usually experiences extreme pain and rapid swelling at the bite area.
    3. Bite site will usually appear markedly discolored.
    4. In extreme cases the victim may experience weakness, nausea, vomiting, shortness of breath, and shock.

B. Coral snakes
    1. Victim experiences only slight pain and mild swelling at the bite area.
    2. Since corals inject their venom by chewing on the victim, the area of the bite often appears abraded.
    3. In extreme cases the victim may experience drooping eyelids, blurred vision, slurred speech, increased salivation, profuse sweating, drowsiness, nausea, vomiting, difficulty breathing, paralysis of various body parts, convulsions, shock, and possibly coma.

First Aid Measures

A. Pit vipers
    1. Instruct the victim to remain quiet and inactive.
    2. If the bite is on an arm or a leg, immobilize the part in a position that keeps the bite site below the level of the victim's heart.
    3. If the bite is on an arm or a leg, apply a constricting band two to four inches above the bite. After the band has been applied, you should still be able to slip your index finger under the band.
    4. Using a blade from a snakebite kit or a knife which has been sterilized with a flame, make a single incision, parallel to the body part, at each fang mark and over the suspected point of the venom deposit. The incisions should only extend through the skin, never deeper, and measure less than one-half inch long.
    5. Apply suction for approximately thirty minutes with a suction cup from a snakebite kit or your mouth. Although pit viper venom is not a stomach poison, do *not* swallow it. Always rinse the venom from your mouth whenever water is readily available.
    6. To relieve pain, apply cold cloths or ice wrapped in a towel or plastic bag over the bite site.
    7. Transport the victim to the hospital for the administration of antivenin. Since the victim may be extremely sensitive to antivenin, do *not* administer the drug yourself.

B. Coral snakes
1. Instruct the victim to remain quiet and inactive.
2. If the bite is on an arm or a leg, apply a constricting band above the bite. You should be able to slip your index finger under the band.
3. As soon as possible transport the victim to the hospital for an antivenin injection.

Poisonous Injections by Jellyfish

Jellyfish and the Portuguese man-of-war possess stinging cells (nematocysts) on their tentacles and inject venom whenever they come into contact with swimmers, waders, or sunbathers. Such stings, however, are rarely serious and usually produce only localized reactions.

Signs and Symptoms

1. Victim usually complains of a burning pain in the area of the sting.
2. Small, rashlike eruptions develop on the skin at the sting site.
3. In extreme cases the victim may experience nausea, vomiting, muscle cramps, breathing difficulty, and shock.

First Aid Measures

1. Wipe the affected area with a dry towel to remove any tentacles remaining on the skin.
2. Thoroughly wash the sting area with diluted ammonia or rubbing alcohol.
3. Give the victim aspirin for pain relief.
4. If symptoms are severe, seek medical help as soon as possible.

Poisonous Injections by Stingrays

Besides injecting poison into their victims, stingrays produce severe wounds. Most stings involve waders who accidentally step on the stingrays.

Signs and Symptoms

1. A puncture or laceration, often with fragments of the stingray's spine embedded in it, will be present at the sting site.
2. Victim may experience nausea, vomiting, diarrhea, muscular paralysis, and shock.

First Aid Measures

1. Soak the sting area in hot water.
2. Apply a dressing over the wound.

3. If fragments of the spine remain in the wound, obtain medical help as soon as possible.

Poisoning by Inhalation

Poisonous gases, such as carbon monoxide, ammonia, sulfur dioxide, chlorine, and carbon tetrachloride, will readily cause a breathing stoppage when they are inhaled for a prolonged period of time. Regardless of the type of gas, all cases of inhalative poisoning should be handled as a respiratory emergency (see page 334).

Poisoning by Absorption

Some of the most common and most severe cases of absorptive poisoning result from contact with poison ivy, poison oak, and poison sumac.

Signs and Symptoms

1. A severe rash, characterized by redness, blisters, swelling, itching, and intense burning, will develop in the contact area.
2. Victim may develop a high fever and remain acutely ill for several days.

First Aid Measures

1. Remove all contaminated clothing and wash the affected area thoroughly with soap and water. Then, apply rubbing alcohol to the skin.
2. If the rash is mild, apply a soothing skin lotion over the area.
3. If severe signs and symptoms appear, seek medical assistance.

7. Heat Injury and Illness

A burn is an injury that results from direct contact with heat, chemicals, electricity, or radiation; heat stroke, heat exhaustion, and heat cramps are illnesses that result from prolonged, indirect exposure to high temperatures.

Burns

Burns are classified in two ways: (1) according to the depth or degree and (2) according to the extent of the total body area involved.

Signs and Symptoms

A. Depth of burn
   1. First-degree
      a. Skin will appear red or discolored.

      b.   Mild swelling may be apparent in the burned area.

      c.   Victim will usually complain of pain.

  2. Second-degree

      a.   Skin will appear red or mottled, and blisters will develop over the burned area.

      b.   Considerable swelling will develop over a period of several days.

      c.   Due to the loss of plasma through the damaged skin, the burned area will appear wet.

  3. Third-degree

      a.   Burned area will appear white or charred.

      b.   Tissues underlying the skin, such as nerves, muscles, and bones, may be visible.

B.   Extent of body area involved—Surface area can be easily and quickly calculated by the "Rule of Nines." This is shown in Figure A.2. Generally, hospitalization will be required for an adult with burns over fifteen percent of his body. Similarly, a child with burns over ten percent of his body, will usually need hospitalization.

First Aid Measures

A.   Small first or second-degree burns

  1. Immediately submerge the burned part in cold water (not ice water). However, if submersion is difficult, immerse clean towels or cloths in ice water, wring out the water, and apply the material to the burned part. In either method continue cold application until the victim can remove the burned part from the cold without feeling pain.

  2. Apply dry, sterile gauze or clean cloth to protect the burn. Do *not* break any blisters, and do *not* apply any home remedy to the burn.

  3. If a limb is affected, elevate the body part.

B.   Third-degree burns or extensive burns

  1. Do *not* remove particles of clothing that adhere to the burn, and do *not* immerse the burn in cold water or apply cold applications to the burned part.

  2. Cover the burns with thick, sterile dressings, a clean sheet, or an unused plastic dry-cleaning bag.

  3. If the arms, the legs, or the head has been burned, keep the victim in a flat lying-down position and elevate the affected body part.

  4. As quickly as possible, call for an ambulance. If medical help will *not* arrive within one hour and the victim is conscious, *not* nauseated, and *not* vomiting, give portions of the following fluid

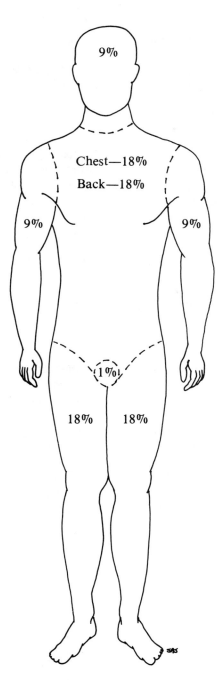

Figure A.2   Body-area percentages for the adult burn victim.

mixture: 1 teaspoon salt, 1/2 teaspoon baking soda, and 1 quart water (neither hot or cold). Give an adult victim four ounces (1/2 glass) every fifteen minutes. Two ounces (1/4 glass) should be given to children between the ages of one and twelve, and one ounce (1/8 glass) should be given to infants under the age of one.

Heat Stroke

Caused by a disturbance of the body's sweating mechanism, heat stroke is an illness in which the body temperature has become extremely high. Because of this abnormally high temperature, the victim may easily die or, if he recovers, may suffer permanent damage to many of his vital organs.

Signs and Symptoms

1. Body temperature may be 105 ° F or higher.
2. Skin is red, hot, and dry.
3. Pulse is rapid and very strong.
4. Victim may be semiconscious or unconscious.

First Aid Measures

1. Remove as much clothing from the victim as modesty allows and repeatedly sponge the bare skin with cool water or apply cold packs continuously. If this fails to cool the victim sufficiently, pour water over his entire body, thus saturating any remaining clothes, or place him in a tub of cold water.
2. If fans or air conditioners are available, use these to further cool the victim.
3. After the victim's temperature drops below 102° F, discontinue the cooling measures. However, carefully monitor the victim, and if his temperature begins to rise again, repeat the cooling steps.
4. Obtain medical assistance for the victim.

Heat Exhaustion

Heat exhaustion is an illness which results from an excessive loss of fluids through sweating.

Signs and Symptoms

1. Body temperature is nearly normal.
2. Skin, nailbeds, and mucous membranes on the inside of the mouth or under the eyelids are pale in color.
3. Skin is clammy, and perspiration is profuse.

4 Victim may complain of headache, fatigue, weakness, dizziness, or nausea.
5. Victim may faint or vomit.

First Aid Measures

1. Place the victim flat on his back and elevate his feet from eight to twelve inches.
2. Loosen the victim's clothing and apply cool, wet cloths on the bare skin.
3. If fans or air conditioners can be obtained, use these to further cool the victim.
4. If the victim is conscious and *not* vomiting, give portions of the following fluid mixture: 1 teaspoon of salt in 1 glass (8 ounces) of water. Over a period of about one hour, give an adult victim four ounces (1/2 glass) every fifteen minutes. Two ounces (1/4 glass) should be given to children between the ages of one and twelve, and one ounce (1/8 glass) should be given to infants under the age of one.
5. If the victim vomits, do *not* give any more fluid. Instead, transport the victim to a hospital.

Heat Cramps

Heat cramps are muscular pains or spasms which result primarily from the loss of salt through sweating. Frequently, heat cramps occur in conjunction with heat exhaustion.

Signs and Symptoms

1. Victim complains of extreme pain in the affected area.
2. Generally, the muscles of the legs and the stomach are affected first.

First Aid Measures

1. With your hands exert firm pressure over the cramped muscles or gently massage the area.
2. Over a period of one hour, give the victim portions of the following fluid mixture: 1 teaspoon salt in 1 glass (8 ounces) of water. An adult should receive four ounces (1/2 glass) every fifteen minutes, a child between the ages of one and twelve should receive two ounces (1/4 glass) every fifteen minutes, and an infant under the age of one should receive one ounce (1/8 glass) every fifteen minutes.

8. Cold Injury and Illness

Whenever the body is exposed to abnormally low temperatures, frostbite and/or cold exposure (hypothermia) may result. Generally, the effect of both conditions is accelerated by water and wind.

Frostbite

Frostbite is an injury caused by freezing. The most commonly affected parts are the nose, cheeks, ears, fingers, and toes.

Signs and Symptoms

1. Before frostbite develops the skin is pink in color.
2. As frostbite develops the skin changes to a white or grayish-yellow color.
3. Initially the victim experiences pain, but it quickly subsides.
4. Victim feels cold and numb and is usually unaware of his condition.

First Aid Measures

1. Until the victim can be brought indoors, cover the frostbitten part with extra clothing or a warm hand. If the hand or fingers are affected, encourage the victim to hold the part in his armpit, next to his body.
2. Once indoors, remove all wet or frozen clothing and cover the victim with a blanket.
3. Rewarm the frostbitten part in warm water that has a temperature between 102° and 105° F. However, if warm water is not available or is impractical to use, gently wrap the frostbitten part in a sheet and warm blankets. Do *not* rub the affected part or expose it to direct heat, such as a hot water bottle, an electrical heating pad, a heat lamp, or an open fire.
4. During the rewarming process, give the victim a warm, nonalcoholic drink.
5. When the part has been rewarmed, encourage the victim to exercise the fingers and the toes. Do *not,* however, permit the victim to place any pressure on the part.
6. Raise the frostbitten part and protect it from direct contact with a blanket or other bedclothes. In addition, if the fingers or toes are involved, separate them with dry, sterile gauze pads.
7. Secure medical assistance as soon as possible.

Cold Exposure

Cold exposure or hypothermia is an illness in which the body temperature has dropped abnormally low. Unless the victim is warmed, he may easily die from his weakened condition.

Signs and Symptoms

1. Victim usually exhibits violent shivering, mental confusion, and slurred speech.
2. Victim will often complain of numbness and drowsiness.
3. The body temperature will be markedly below 98.6 ° F.

First Aid Measures

1. Bring the victim indoors as quickly as possible and remove all wet or frozen clothing.
2. Cover the victim with a blanket or place him in a tub of warm (102 °-105 ° F.) water.
3. If the victim is conscious, give him a warm nonalcoholic drink.
4. Seek medical help whenever possible.

9. Bone, Joint, and Muscle Injuries

Common injuries to the skeletal system and/or the adjacent soft tissues include:

1. fractures,
2. dislocations,
3. sprains, and
4. strains.

Fractures

A fracture is a crack or a break in a bone. Depending upon whether or not the break is related to an open wound, fractures may be classified as either closed or open. In closed fractures the break is not directly associated with an open wound, although a laceration or similar wound may exist over the fracture site. In open fractures, on the other hand, the break is directly related to an open wound, since the broken bone ends tore through the skin in making the wound or an object penetrated the skin, thus making the wound, while enroute to breaking the bone. Since the fracture area is contaminated and may become infected, open fractures are always more serious than closed fractures.

Signs and Symptoms

1. Victim may report that he felt or heard a bone break.
2. Victim may complain of tenderness or pain over the fracture site, difficulty in moving the injured part, or, if the part is moved, a grating sensation (crepitus) as the broken bone ends rub together.
3. Affected part may appear swollen, discolored, deformed, or irregular in shape or length.

First Aid Measures

1. Cut away the victim's clothing over the suspected fracture site.
2. If an open wound exists, control bleeding. Then, cover the entire wound with a large, sterile pad or a sanitary napkin. Do *not* attempt to replace any bone fragments which protrude from the wound.
3. Without causing discomfort to the victim, place the body part in as natural of a position as possible. Then, apply padded splints which extend well beyond the joints above and below the fracture site. Splints for the various body areas are shown in Figures A.3-A.7.
4. Cover the victim with a sheet, a blanket, or clothing to keep him warm, but do *not* make the victim perspire. Periodically, check the victim to make sure the splints are not restricting circulation in the fractured part.
5. As soon as possible call for medical help.

Dislocations

The displacement of a bone end from its joint is referred to as a dislocation.

Signs and Symptoms

1. Dislocated part may be swollen, discolored, and extremely painful.
2. A noticeable bulge or deformity will usually be apparent at the involved joint.

First Aid Measures

In general, dislocations should always be handled in the same manner as closed fractures.

Sprains

Sprains are injuries to the ligaments and other soft tissue which surround the skeletal joints.

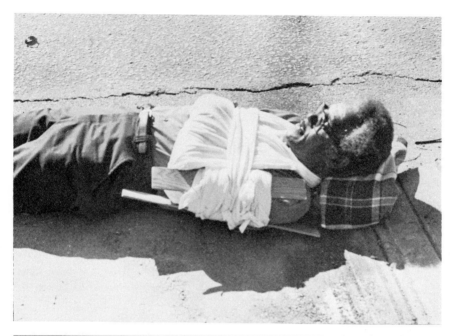

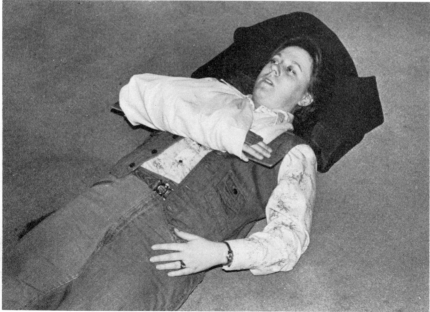

Figure A.3   (Top) Splint for arm. (Bottom) Splint for forearm.

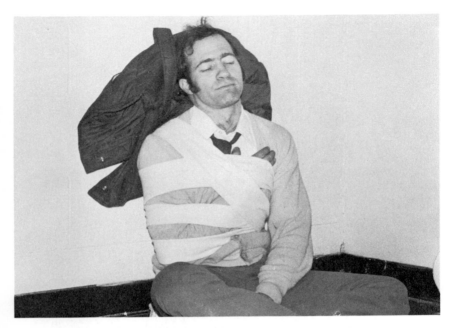

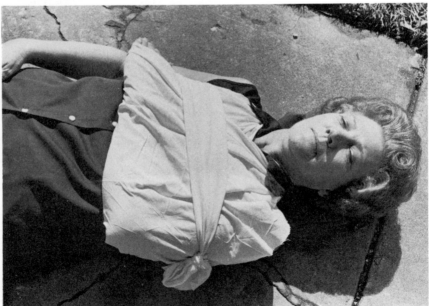

Figure A.4   (Top) Immobilization of ribs. (Bottom) Immobilization of collarbone.

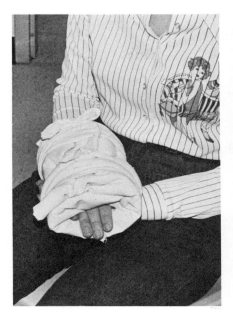
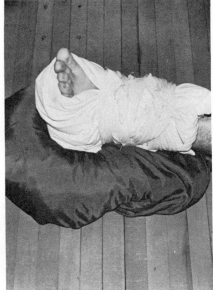
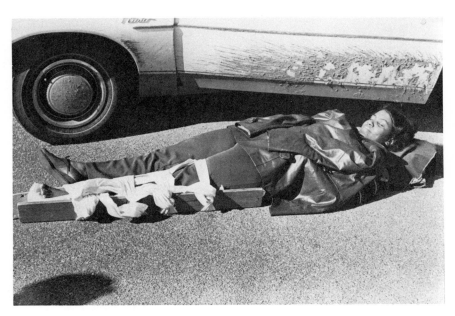

Figure A.5 (Top left) Immobilization of hand. (Top right) Immobilization of foot. (Bottom) Splint for lower leg.

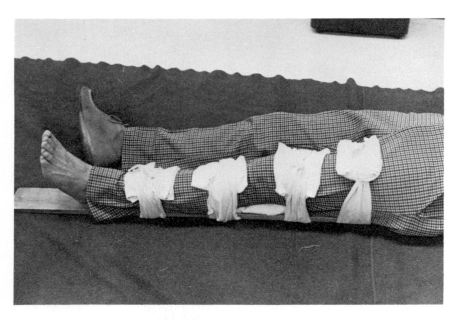

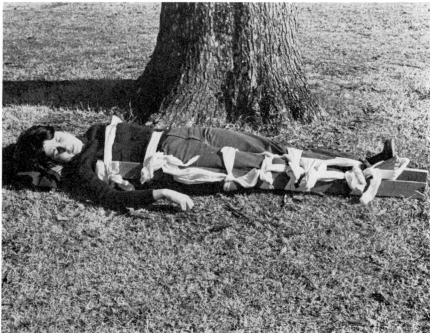

Figure A.6   (Top) Splint for kneecap. (Bottom) Splint for thigh.

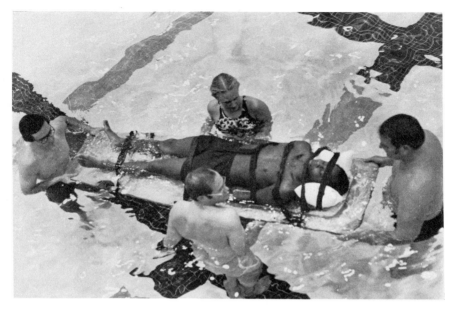

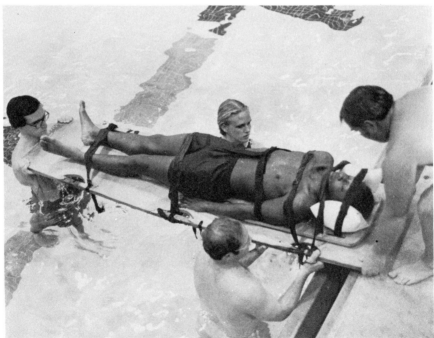

Figure A.7   Shallow-water rescue—splint for neck and back.

Signs and Symptoms

1. Swelling, as well as discoloration in many cases, appears shortly after the injury.
2. Tenderness is usually present in the sprained area.
3. Victim may report a dull, aching pain while resting the affected part or a sharp pain while trying to move it.
4. Because of the pain, the victim may be reluctant to move the injured part.

First Aid Measures

Since a great amount of swelling usually accompanies a sprain, it is often difficult to determine whether or not a fracture has occurred in association with a sprain. In such cases the injury should always be handled as if it were a fracture. However, when the injury appears to be a simple sprain, the following measures should be taken.

1. Elevate the sprained part to reduce blood flow to the area. In mild sprains, keep the injured part elevated for at least twenty-four hours, and if the ankle or knee is affected, do *not* permit the victim to walk.
2. To relieve pain and reduce internal bleeding, place over the area a cold, wet pack or a small bag of crushed ice which has been wrapped inside a towel. Continue this form of cold application for several hours.
3. If the swelling and the pain persist for several days, seek medical assistance.

Strains

Strains are injuries to the muscles.

Signs and Symptoms

1. Victim may report that he felt a sharp pain at the time of the injury.
2. When moving the affected part, the victim will experience tenderness and pain.
3. Discoloration and swelling may be apparent at the strain site.

First Aid Measures

1. Apply dry heat or warm, wet applications to the strained area. However, if the victim experiences greater pain with the application of heat, suspect a major strain and immediately apply cold, wet packs or bags of crushed ice wrapped in a towel over the area.

2. Instruct the victim to rest the affected part. If the back has been strained, place a board under the mattress of a bed for firmer support.
3. If the pain persists for several days, obtain medical help.

10. Common Emergencies

Some emergency problems, while largely unrelated, share a common factor: they all appear suddenly and they all demand immediate action. The emergency problems which are most often encountered by the first-aider include:

1. heart attack,
2. angina,
3. stroke,
4. appendicitis, and
5. convulsions.

Heart Attack

Often called coronary, coronary thrombosis, coronary occlusion, or myocardial infarction, heart attack refers to the blockage of one of the coronary arteries which supply the heart with blood. Most often, this blockage is the result of a blood clot in the vessel.

Signs and Symptoms

1. Victim will experience persistent chest pain, usually under the breastbone but sometimes along the left shoulder and arm.
2. Victim may complain of weakness, coldness, or nausea, or he may actually vomit.
3. Skin, lips, and fingernail beds may be bluish in color.
4. Victim may exhibit gasping and a shortness of breath.

First Aid Measures

1. If breathing is absent, quickly begin artificial respiration. (If the pulse is absent and you are trained in external cardiac compression, immediately begin cardiopulmonary resuscitation.)
2. As soon as possible, instruct someone to call for an ambulance equipped with oxygen.
3. If the victim is conscious and has been under medical care for a heart condition, assist him in administering any prescribed medicine.

4. To ease breathing, place the victim in a half-sitting position and loosen any tight clothing.
5. To control shock, cover the victim with a light blanket or an article of clothing. Do *not* cause the victim to perspire.

Angina

Angina or angina pectoris refers to a severe pain in the chest caused by an insufficient supply of blood to some portion of the heart. In general, the signs and symptoms of angina are quite similar to those of a heart attack. However, unlike in heart attack, chest pain in angina persists for only a few minutes (or even seconds).

First Aid Measures

1. If the victim is conscious and has been under medical care for angina, assist him in administering his prescribed medicine, either nitroglycerine or amyl nitrite.
2. If he desires, place the victim in a half-sitting position to ease his breathing.
3. If the chest pain and the shortness of breath does not subside within a few minutes, call for an ambulance with an oxygen supply.
4. If breathing stops, immediately begin artificial respiration. (When you are trained in external cardiac compression and the victim's pulse is absent, quickly begin cardiopulmonary resuscitation.)

Stroke

Sometimes referred to as apoplexy or cerebrovascular accident, a stroke usually involves a sudden rupture of a blood vessel in the brain or the presence of a blood clot in the vessel which disrupts the blood supply to the brain.

Signs and Symptoms

1. Victim may be semiconscious or unconscious.
2. If conscious, the victim may complain of a headache and nausea, or he may vomit. Often, however, the victim is unable to speak, or if he can speak, his sentences are slurred.
3. Pupils of the eyes may be of an unequal size.
4. Victim may experience a loss of bladder and bowel control, breathing difficulty, and numbness, weakness, or paralysis on one side of the body.

First Aid Measures

1. Place the victim on his back and elevate his head and shoulders; if vomiting occurs, roll the victim onto his side to permit the vomitus to flow out the side of his mouth.
2. Cover the victim with a light blanket or an article of clothing if shock is apparent. However, do *not* cause the victim to sweat.
3. As soon as possible, summon medical help.

Appendicitis

Appendicitis is an inflammation of the appendix. Since the victim may suffer intense discomfort and pain or may die if the appendix ruptures, the first-aider should always seek medical help immediately.

Signs and Symptoms

1. At the onset the victim will usually report feeling severe pain in the naval area; after several hours he will often complain of severe pain in the lower right side of the abdomen.
2. Victim may experience weakness, loss of appetite, nausea, vomiting, and abnormal bowel movements (constipation, most often, or diarrhea).
3. Slight fever may be apparent.

First Aid Measures

1. Place the victim on his back in a semireclining position and keep his knees bent.
2. To further relieve pain, apply an ice bag, wrapped inside of a towel, to the abdominal area.
3. Immediately transport the victim to a hospital.

Convulsions

Common causes of convulsions include fever, head injury, and epilepsy.

Signs and Symptoms

1. Victim will suddenly become unconscious and quite rigid.
2. After a short period of time, the victim will exhibit jerking movements, foaming or drooling at the mouth, and a bluish color of the lips and face. In addition, he may bite his tongue or lose control of his bladder and bowel.

3. After the attack the victim will usually appear drowsy and disoriented for a short time.

First Aid Measures

1. Protect the victim by removing any nearby objects. Do *not* place a blunt object between the victim's teeth.
2. After the attack move the victim to a quiet place, turn him on his side, cover him with a light cover, and permit him to rest.
3. If repeated convulsions occur, summon medical help at once.

11. Emergency Childbirth

Although the onset of labor is usually gradual, thereby providing sufficient time for transportation to a hospital, certain situations may require the first-aider to assist in emergency childbirth. Miscalulation about the anticipated date of delivery, premature onset of labor after an accident or extreme emotional trauma, and delay in transportation are factors which may cause a pregnant woman's labor to begin unexpectedly.

Signs and Symptoms

1. Labor contractions are approximately two minutes apart.
2. Woman may be straining or pushing down with the contractions, crying out constantly, or warning of the baby's coming.

Delivery Measures

1. Remove any underclothing from the woman and place her on her back with her knees bent, feet flat, and thighs widely separated. If you are in a public place, instruct onlookers to stand around the woman with their backs toward her to shield the scene from others.
2. If newspapers, a clean sheet, or clothing are available, place the material under the woman's buttocks. Then, if water is readily available, wash your hands.
3. As the baby's head emerges, guide and support it with your hands to keep it away from blood, mucus, and fecal matter. Do *not* place your hands or fingers into the birth canal at any time, and do *not* try to hold back the baby's head.
4. As soon as possible, wipe out the baby's mouth with gauze, clean cloth, or facial tissues. If the bag of water failed to break with the emergence of the head, tear the bag with your fingers to permit the fluid to escape. In addition, if the umbilical cord is wrapped

around the baby's neck, gently but quickly insert your index finger between the cord and the baby's neck and slip the cord over the baby's head. However, if the cord cannot be slipped over the head, immediately cut the cord to prevent strangulation and squeeze the cut ends together with your fingers until ties can be applied.

5. As the baby's shoulders emerge, lift them slightly with one hand while supporting the baby's head and neck with your other hand.

6. After being expelled from the mother, the baby will usually begin breathing and crying within one or two minutes. To assist him, firmly grasp his ankles (preferably over a clean cloth to prevent slipping) with one hand and support his chest and head with your other hand. Then, with a milking motion, stroke the baby's neck from his chest toward his mouth. If the baby does not begin to cry and breathe, rub his back or flick the bottoms of his feet with your fingers. If this fails, begin artificial respiration.

7. When the baby is breathing well, cover him with a clean cloth, position him on his back, and place a pad under his shoulders, thereby tilting the head back and maintaining an open airway. However, if the mother can help, she may wish to hold the baby on her abdomen.

8. Shortly after the baby's birth, the mother will resume contractions in preparation for the expulsion of the placenta or afterbirth. Allow the expulsion to proceed without interference. After the placenta emerges, place your hand over the mother's lower abdomen and gently but firmly massage the area for several minutes. Since the massaging stimulates contraction of the uterus and helps control bleeding, repeat the massage every five minutes until medical help arrives. Place the placenta in a plastic bag and take it to the hospital for examination.

9. For convenience and sanitary reasons, do *not* cut the umbilical cord. Medical personnel will perform this procedure at the hospital. However, if the cord must be cut to prevent strangulation when the baby's head emerges, ties should be applied. Using new white shoelaces or narrow strips of clean white cloth which have been boiled in water for twenty minutes, tie a square knot four to six inches (never closer) from the baby and a second square knot approximately eight inches from the baby (thus, two to four inches between knots). Then, using a new razor blade or scissors which have been boiled in water or soaked in rubbing alcohol for twenty minutes, cut the cord between the two knots.

10. Gently clean the mother's vaginal opening, from above toward the rectum, with a clean moist towel and rinse the area with warm

water. Cover the vaginal opening with a sanitary napkin or other clean cotton material.

11. Cover the mother to keep her warm and give her hot, nonalcoholic drinks.

12. Transportation

Transportation of the victim should always be limited to situations in which an immediate danger to the life of the victim exists or to situations in which professional ambulance or rescue personnel are not available. Under these circumstances, the first-aider should observe the following guidelines:

1. Unless his life would be in further danger, never move the victim until his breathing has become adequate, his bleeding has been controlled, and his fractures or dislocations have been splinted. If, for his immediate safety, the victim must be moved before such measures can be taken, always protect and support the injured parts during the move.
2. If there is no immediate danger, employ a practice "victim" and direct the helpers to rehearse the lifting-and-carrying procedure. (Inexperienced individuals usually find it difficult properly to lift and carry a victim.)
3. Whenever possible, bring the transportation device (litter or vehicle) to the victim rather than carrying him to it.
4. When lifting and carrying the victim, gently support the head, neck, back, and extremities, keeping the body aligned at all times.
5. When transporting an injury-victim, never force him to travel in a sitting position; instead, always place the victim in a reclining or semireclining position, the necessary space being best afforded by a station wagon, van, or truck.
6. Since the few minutes saved by a high-speed ride is almost always unimportant for the victim's recovery, drive within the posted speed limits and reduce speed whenever necessary, especially on curves and turns. (Often, a high-speed ride will only worsen the victim's condition and cause him further anxiety.)

Index

elements in, 189
epidemiological accident prevention/mitigation model and, 191
evaluation of, 194-195
faculty and, 190
instructional (behavioral) objectives in, 192
junior and senior high, 196-197
organization of, 189-195
policy of, 189-190
program objectives for, 191-192
safety coordinator in, 190-191, 194-196
safety council and, 194
superintendent and, 189
teaching methods in, 193
Scuba
  divers
    equipment for, 270-271
    unique hazards for, 271-273
  -diving
    accidents, 269-273
    equipment
      depth gauge, 270
      exposure suit, 271
      self-contained underwater breathing apparatus, 270
      underwater compass, 270-271
      underwater wristwatch, 270
Seat belts, see "Safety belts"
Second Interval Concept, 47, 63
Secondary escape route, 107
Seismic belts, 314
Seismologists, 313, 314
Severity rate, 207
Sharks
  behavior of, 268-269
  hatred and fear of, 268
  reason for attack by, 269
  skin diver and, 269
  spearfisherman and, 269
Shoot-out, 149
Shops and laboratories (school)
  dangerous work habits in, 171
  good housekeeping in, 170-171
  safety and teachers of, 170
Sidewalks
  and falls, 95-96
  surfaces of, 95-96
Skateboarding, as cultural fad in accident causation, 15
Skills, in accident causation, 13
Skin
  divers
    and partners, 265
    barracudas and, 267-268
    discomfort in ears of, 266

equipment for, 262-265
moray eels and, 267
physical
  abilities of, 262
  condition of, 262
  examination and, 262
sharks and, 268-269
spearfishing and, 266
sunken ships and, 266
diving
  abilities necessary for learning, 262
  aspects of, 261
  choosing sport of, 261-262
  equipment for, 262-265
  hostile marine life and, 267
  physical condition and, 262
  popularity of, 261
  skills in, 262
  spearguns and, 266
  strenuous nature of, 261
  sunken ships and, 266
  survival in, 265-267
-diving
  accidents, 261-269
  equipment
    diver's flag, 265
    fins, 263-264
    float, 264-265
    inflatable vest, 264
    knife, 264
    mask, 262
    snorkel, 262
Skull and crossbones, 125
Sleet, in accident causation, 15
Slow-moving vehicle emblem
  description of, 227
  development of, 227
  federal law and, 227-228
  function of, 227-228
  position of, 228
  replacement of, 228
Smoke
  and dangerous locations in home, 101
  and escape from fire, 108
  and relatively gas-free layer, 101
  as real killer in fire, 99, 108
  color of, 101
  detectors
    and bedroom doors, 104
    factors in selection of, 102-103
    installation of, 104
    ionization, 102
    photoelectric, 102
  gases in, 100
  keeping out of room, 107
  physics of, 101